CURRENT ADVANCES IN AMYOTROPHIC LATERAL SCLEROSIS

Edited by **Alvaro G. Estévez**

Current Advances in Amyotrophic Lateral Sclerosis
http://dx.doi.org/10.5772/56966
Edited by Alvaro G. Estévez

Contributors

Cédric Raoul, Melissa Bowerman, Thierry Vincent, Frédérique Scamps, William Camu, Laura Ferraiuolo, Kathrin Meyer, Brian Kaspar, Alvaro G. Estévez, Fabian Rossi, Maria Clara Franco, Jin Hee Shin, Jae Keun Lee, Arun Aggarwal, Cassandra Dennys, Luca Diamanti, Stella Gagliardi, Cristina Cereda, Mauro Ceroni, Kiyohiko Abe, Tommaso Bocci, Elisa Giorli, Lucia Briscese, Silvia Tognazzi, Fabio Giannini, Ferdinando Sartucci

Published by InTech

Janeza Trdine 9, 51000 Rijeka, Croatia

Publishing Process Manager Sandra Bakic
Technical Editor InTech DTP team
Cover InTech Design team

Additional hard copies can be obtained from orders@intechopen.com

Current Advances in Amyotrophic Lateral Sclerosis, Edited by Alvaro G. Estévez
p. cm.
ISBN 978-953-51-1195-5

For EU product safety concerns:
IN TECH d.o.o., Prolaz Marije Krucifikse Kozulić 3, 51000 Rijeka, Croatia,
info@intechopen.com or visit our website at intechopen.com.

Meet the editor

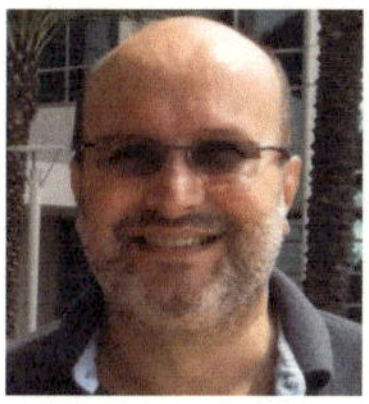

Alvaro G. Estevez, Ph.D. is an Associate Professor of Medicine at the Burnett School of Biomedical Sciences, College of Medicine, University of Central Florida. Dr. Estevez performed his graduate studies at the University of Buenos Aires and was a post-doctoral fellow with Dr. Joseph S. Beckman at the University of Alabama at Birmingham, where he become Assistant Professor in the Department of Physiology and Biophysics. Dr. Estevez was also a faculty member at the Weill Cornell Medical College, the Burke Medical Research Institute and Oregon State University. Dr. Estevez research focalizes on oxidative mechanisms of motor neurons death in ALS. He published over 60 papers and reviews and his work is founded by the NIH/NINDS.

Contents

Preface

The research in amyotrophic lateral sclerosis (ALS) has dramatically increased in the last 20 years, greatly improving our understanding of the pathological mechanisms involved in the disease. The number of hypothesis on the pathogenic causes of ALS and the mechanisms of motor neuron death keeps growing. Twenty years ago there was a general agreement that ALS was a motor neuron disease. All other symptoms were secondary to the primary cause that was the death of upper and lower motor neurons. Today there are several hypotheses suggesting that dysfunction in other cell types, such as astrocytes, is the primary cause of the disease that leads to motor neuron death. Twenty years ago there were not animal models for ALS, now there are multiple rodent and non-mammalian models of the disease.

The more accepted hypotheses for the causes of ALS are reviewed in the first chapter by Rossi and coauthors. This chapter reviews the potential pathogenic mechanism involved in the etiology of ALS providing short description of each mechanism.

The chapter by Shin and Lee reviews the cellular mechanisms found to potentially participate in the degeneration of motor neurons in ALS. This chapter provides a cellular approach to the proposed mechanisms of motor neuron death in ALS, supporting the hypothesis that multiple molecular pathways could be involve in motor neuron death in different patients.

Diamanti and collaborators provide further support for the hypothesis of multiple molecular mechanisms in ALS by reviewing correlations between genotype and disease presentation. Using studies of Italian ALS patients, the authors provide evidence showing the correlation between different phenotypic presentations of ALS with known genetic causes of the disease.

The chapter by Bowerman and collaborators reviews up to day evidence of the role of neuroinflammation in the pathology of ALS. The role of astrocytes and other inflammatory cells is reviewed in detail. The authors also discuss in depth the possible inflammatory mediators and molecular mechanism involved in the induction of motor neuron death.

Franco and collaborators review the highly controversial participation of oxidative stress in the pathology of ALS. The chapter focuses on the oxidative mechanisms proposed to explain the gain-of-function of ALS-linked mutant SOD.

Ferraiuolo and coauthors provide a new interpretations of the ALS literature based on the recent discovery that a plethora of new genetic mutations affecting a variety of genes are linked to ALS. The review provides an unique perspective on the strengths and weaknesses of classic and new animal models of the disease based on performance and similarities to the human disease.

The chapter by Aggarwal describes studies in at risk presymtomatic individuals carrying mutant SOD. The research uses MUNE to determine motor neurons status and the therapeutic benefits of riluzole. The methods described in this chapter could provide and early diagnosis in patients carrying mutations linked to ALS allowing presymtomatic treatments.

Bocci and collaborators found by Macro-EMG, that there is a possible compensatory overbranching in ALS motor neurons, which provides a possible explanation for the adult onset of the disease.

Abe and collaborators provided a review of the last advances of eye-gaze systems, which allows ALS patient to communicate after almost other voluntary mobility is lost. The technology reported here is relatively inexpensive and for those patients unable to communicate by other means could represent a significant improvement on quality of life.

Alvaro G. Estévez, Ph.D.
Burnett School of Biomedical Sciences,
College of Medicine,
University of Central Florida,
USA

Chapter 1

Pathophysiology of Amyotrophic Lateral Sclerosis

Fabian H. Rossi, Maria Clara Franco and
Alvaro G. Estevez

Additional information is available at the end of the chapter

http://dx.doi.org/10.5772/56562

1. Introduction

Amyotrophic lateral sclerosis (ALS) is a progressive neurodegenerative disorder characterized by death of pyramidal neurons in the motor cortex (upper motor neurons) and motor neurons in the brain stem and central spinal cord (lower motor neurons). This results in muscle weakness, progressive motor disability, and finally death by respiratory failure or an associated infection (Shook and Pioro, 2009). There are two types of ALS familiar (fALS) and sporadic ALS (sALS). They are both clinically undistiguishale one from the other; fALS accounts for 10% of all cases being the rest of the cases sALS (Pasinelli and Brown, 2006). In the last few years, there had been an explosion of genetic studies associating ALS with several genetic mutations in genes codifying for different proteins: Cu/Zn superoxide dismutase, (SOD1), transactive response binding protein 43 (TARDBP), fused in sarcoma (FUS), and valosin containing protein (VCP). Most recently, a genetic defect was identified with an expansion of the noncoding GGGGCC hexanucleotide repeat in the chromosome 9, open reading frame 72 (C9ORF72), associated with ALS with and without frontotemporal dementia (Boeve et al., 2012).

Despite of all these discoveries the etiology of ALS remains elusive. A number of potential pathogenic mechanisms have been associated with ALS including excitotoxicity, mitochondrial dysfunction, apoptosis, glial activation, RNA-processing, growth factor abnormalities, etc. These potential pathogenic processes are reviewed in this chapter.

2. Pathology

ALS is characterized by upper motor neuron (corticospinal motor neurons) and lower motor neuron (bulbospinal motor neurons) degeneration and death as well as reactive gliosis replacing death neurons (Leigh and Garafolo, 1995). As corticospinal motor neuron degenerate the cells suffer from a retrograde axonal loss with secondary myelin pallor and gliosis. These changes are most severed at the brainstem and upper spinal cord, but are extended throughout the spinal cord (Brownell et al., 1970). ALS motor cortex shows astrocytic gliosis, especially in the deeper layers at the gray matter and underlying the subcortical white matter. Irregular immunoreactivity to GFAP is identified in the motor strip (Kamo, et al. 1987; Ince, 2000). The lysosomal marker CD68 also revealed that most of the glial response at the cortical and spinal tracts corresponds to microglia activation and active macrophages (Cagnin et al., 2001; Sitte et al., 2001). ALS affects spinal motor neurons of the ventral horn and brainstem motor neurons. The autopsy of ALS patients shows loss of motor neurons and atrophic motor neurons with basophilic appearance suggesting a programmed cell mechanism (Martin, 1999). The ventral roots become thin with loss of large myelinated fibers in motor nerves leading to denervation atrophy with evidence of reinnervation in affected muscles. Frontal temporal dementia ALS (FTD-ALS) is a neurodegenerative disorder associated with ALS that presents typical pathological findings of the disease in addition to neuronal loss of the frontal or temporal cortex, hippocampus and amygdale, and spongiform changes of the neocortex with (Leigh PN and Garofolo, 1995). Non-motor findings encountered in ALS pathology are posterior columns demyelination and reduced density of myelinated sensory fibers (Ince, 2007)

2.1. Inclusion bodies

The hallmark finding of lower motor neuron (LMN) pathology in ALS is the presence of intracellular inclusion bodies in neuronal soma and proximal dendrites as well as glia (Barbeito et al., 2004).

2.1.1. Ubiquitylated Inclusions (UBI)

UBI are the most common and specific inclusion in ALS, found at LMN of the spinal cord and brainstem (Matsumoto et al., 1993) and also at the corticospinal tract upper motor neurons (UMN) (Sasaki and Maruyama, 1994). UBI morphological spectrum goes from thread-like ubiquitylated profiles, through skeins of different compactness to more spherical bodies (Ince et al, 1998). The compacted lesions may be eosinophilic, basophilic and "Lewy-like" in appearance. The composition of UBI remains unknown but several proteins were identified in UBI such as ubiquitin (Leigh et al., 1991), peripherin (He and Hays, 2004), Cu/Zn SOD1 (Shibata 1996) and dorfin (Niwa et al., 2002). UBI are present in near 100% of sALS (Ince et al., 2003). However, UBI are found in FTD with ubiquitin positive/tau negative inclusions. In both fALS and sporadic types of ALS-FTD, UBI are found in cortical frontal and temporal lobe neurons.

2.1.1.1. TAR DNA binding Protein 43 (TDP-43)

TDP-43 is a major component of ubiquinated inclusions in sALS, FTD with ubiquitin-positive but tau-negative inclusions (non-tau FTD), FTD-ALS, and non-SOD1 fALS. TDP-43 inclusions are practically not present in mSOD1-related fALS.

2.1.1.2. Fused in Sarcoma protein (FUS)

Recently, mutations in the gene codifying for the fused in sarcoma protein (FUS) have been linked to fALS. Indeed, spinal cord LMNs in fALS and sALS but not in mSOD1-fALS are immunoreactive for FUS inclusions. These inclusions also present immunoreactivity for TDP-43 and ubiquitin (Chaudhuri et al., 1995).

2.1.2. Bunina bodies

Bunina bodies are eosinophilic paracrystalline bodies present in the LMNs of many cases of ALS (Piao et al., 2003). They are immunoreactive for a cysteine protease inhibitor called cystatin C (Okamoto et al., 1993).

2.1.3. Hyaline Conglomerate Inclusions (HCI)

HCI consist of intracellular accumulation of intermediate filament proteins, especially hyperphosphorylated neurofilament subunits and peripherin (Corbo and Hays, 2002), and are found in the motor cortex neurons (Troost et al., 1992). HCI are much less frequently encountered in spinal motor neurons than UBI and they are mainly associated with some types of mSOD1 fALS. They form a larger conglomeration than UBI and are positive for silver staining, contrary of UBI. (Ince PG and Wharton S, 2007).

3. Oxidative stress

Mutations in the gene of copper/zinc superoxide dismutase type 1 (SOD1) are the most common cause of fALS (Rothstein, 2009; Boillee and Cleveland, 2008; Robberecht and Phillips, 2013). Recent reports indicate that SOD1 mutations may also be the cause of between 0.7 - 4% cases of sporadic ALS (sALS) (Robberecht and Phillips, 2013). SOD1 is primarily an antioxidant metalloenzyme that catalyzes the conversion of superoxide radical ($O_2^{\cdot-}$) to oxygen (O_2) and hydrogen peroxide (H_2O_2). However, SOD1-linked fALS is most likely not caused by loss of the normal SOD1 activity, but rather by a gain of a toxic function. One of the hypotheses for mutant SOD-linked fALS toxicity proposes that an aberrant SOD1 chemistry is responsible for the toxic gain-of-function, which allows small molecules such us peroxynitrite or hydrogen peroxide to produce damaging free radicals. Other hypotheses for mutant SOD1 neurotoxicity include inhibition of the proteasome activity, mitochondrial damage, and formation of intracellular aggregates. SOD1 aggregation is an early event in ALS and could mediate motor neuron degeneration via sequestration of cellular components, decreasing chaperone activity and the ubiquitin proteasome pathway. Also, SOD1 mutations seem to disrupt RNA processing in the cells.

Defining the role of oxidative stress, and particularly nitrative stress in neurodegeneration has been extremely difficult because of the multiplicity of potential targets that can be damaged by oxidation and nitration. Certain proteins are particularly susceptible to tyrosine nitration by the oxidant peroxynitrite ($ONOO^-$). Tyrosine nitration is a well-established, early biomarker in ALS and it has been proposed that in fALS mutant SOD1 produces motor neuron death by allowing peroxynitrite formation and catalyzing tyrosine nitration, which in turn inhibits trophic signals (Estevez et al., 1999; Beckman et al., 1993; Crow et al., 1997; Ischiropoulos et al., 1992; Franco and Estevez, 2011). Motor neurons are highly dependent on a continuous supply of trophic factors to survive both *in vivo* and *in vitro*. Deprivation of trophic support *in vivo* by ventral root avulsion in adult animals and axotomy in newborns, but not in adults, triggers apoptosis (Li et al, 1994; Oppenheim, 1997; Gould and Oppenheim, 2011). Induction of apoptosis in these conditions is preceded by induction of neuronal nitric oxide synthase (nNOS) and nitric oxide production. Motor neuron death induced by trophic factor deprivation requires protein synthesis and caspase activation both *in vivo* and *in vitro* (Milligan et al., 1994; Li et al, 1998; Yaginuma et al, 2001). Cultured motor neurons deprived of trophic factors induce nNOS expression, production of nitric oxide and peroxynitrite formation that is followed by tyrosine nitration, which precedes motor neuron death (Estevez et al., 1998). Inhibition of nitric oxide production and peroxynitrite formation prevents rather than delays motor neuron death, suggesting that peroxynitrite is acting at decision-making points in the apoptotic cascade. Deprivation of trophic factors activates the Fas pathway in motor neurons, and inhibition of the Fas pathway prevents motor neuron death. Fas activation in motor neurons triggers two parallel pathways: the classical extrinsic pathway recruiting FADD and Caspase 8; and a seemingly motor neuron specific pathway, that activates DAXX/ASK1/p38 and the induction of neuronal NOS, increasing production of nitric oxide, peroxynitrite formation and tyrosine nitration (Raoul et al, 2002).

4. Excitotoxicity

4.1. Glutamate

A dominant hypothesis of ALS pathogenesis is glutamate excitotoxicity. Glutamate is the major excitatory neurotransmitter found in mammalian central nervous system (CNS) however, in high concentrations is toxic to motor neurons. Some of the evidence supporting glutamate excitotoxicity was based on the observation that exposure of neuronal cell cultures to excess glutamate leads to cell death (Choi et al 1988). A similar observation was made in anterior horn cells in tissue cultures of rat spinal cord where incubation with high concentrations of glutamate is associated with cell loss (Silani et al 2000). In addition, defects in glutamate transport leading to elevated glutamate levels have been reported in mSOD1 mice and significant number of patients with sALS (Dunlop et al., Lin et al., Rothstein et al.,). Elevated glutamate levels were found in serum and spinal fluid of patients with sALS (Al-Chalabi, et al 2000; Rothstein et al., 1990; Shaw, et al, 1995). Another study showed that 40% of about 400 patients with sALS have an elevation in glutamate levels that correlates with the severity of the disease (Spreux-Varoquax et al., 2002)

The mechanism of glutamate neurotoxicity remains elusive. Excessive glutamate levels lead to activation of glutamate ionotropic AMPA receptors in neurons and glial cells. AMPA receptor activation triggers mitochondrial changes such as reduction in ATP synthesis, decreased cellular oxygen consumption, oxydative phosphorylation uncoupling, and increase in mitochondrial reactive oxygen species (ROS) production, causing a loss in the mitochondrial calcium buffer properties and apoptosis (Heath and Shaw 2002) (Fig. 1). Rapid clearance of glutamate at the synapsis cleft is an essential step in the prevention of motor neuron excitotoxicity. This step accomplished by the astrocyte glutamate transporter excitatory amino acid-2 (EAAT2) (Rothstein et,al 1996). In transgenic mice, depletion of EAAT2 has been implicated with neuronal death (Rothstein et,al 1996). Abnormalities in EAAT2 expression were identified in two rodent models of fALS. In the SOD1^{G85R} transgenic mice a ~ 50% decrease in EAAT2 expression was observed in the spinal cord at the end of the disease (Bruijin et al., 1997), while in the spinal cord ventral horn of transgenic SOD1^{G93A} rats EAAT2 expression was decreased before the symptomatic stage of the disease and was almost undetectable at the end of the disease (Howland et al., 2002). Reduction in the expression of EAAT2 was found in motor neuron disease (Fray et al 1998) and decreased glutamate transport was identified in motor cortex and spinal cord in ALS (Rothstein et al., 1992) (Fig. 1).

4.2. Glutamate receptor

An alteration in the expression of the glutamate receptor was found in motor neurons expressing mutant SOD1, suggesting that excitotoxicity is not only induced by increased glutamate levels but also by alterations in the glutamate signaling pathway (Spalloni et al., 2004). In oocytes co-expressing A4V or I113T-SOD1 with EAAT2, the mutants but not the wild type SOD1 selectively inactivated the glial glutamate transporter in the presence of hydrogen peroxide. This suggests that EAAT2 may be a target for mutant SOD1 toxicity (Trotti et al., 1999). On the other hand, overexpression of EAAT2 in mutant SOD1 expressing mice delayed the onset of motor neuron disease and decreased caspase 3 activation, the final step of the apoptotic pathway (Guo et al 2003). In motor cortex and spinal cord extracts from ALS patients, 25% of the patients showed almost complete loss of EAAT2 protein, and 80% of the patients showed some sort of protein abnormality (Rothstein et al., 1995) (Fig.1).

Glutamate receptor dysfunction is other possible route of excitotoxicity. Glutamate toxicity in motor neurons is primarily mediated via alpha-amino-3-hydroxy-5-methyl-4 isoxazole propionic acid (AMPA) receptors (Van Den Bosch et al., 2000). In patients with ALS, a deficiency in the AMPA receptor mRNA expression was found in spinal motor neurons (Kawahara, et al., 2004). This defect results in an increase in calcium influx through the receptor leading to cell damaged. The increased entry in calcium in addition to the reduction in the calcium buffer capacity due to abnormal mitochondria result in an increase in free intracellular calcium levels, leading to motor neuron death (Bogaert et al., 2010) (Fig.1). Additionally, the expression of the glutamate receptor subunits is reduced in ALS motor neurons (Williams et al 1997). Another pathway leading to excitotoxicity is via deficiency in glutamate dehydrogenase activity (Pioro et al., 1999).

The modest protection conferred by the antigluaminergic drug riluzole in ALS patients as well as in mutant SOD1 mice seems to support the effect of glutamate toxicity in the pathogenesis of ALS (Lacomblez et al., 1996; Gurney et al., 1996). However, whether riluzole protects by a mechanism related to its antiglutaminergic properties needs to be established.

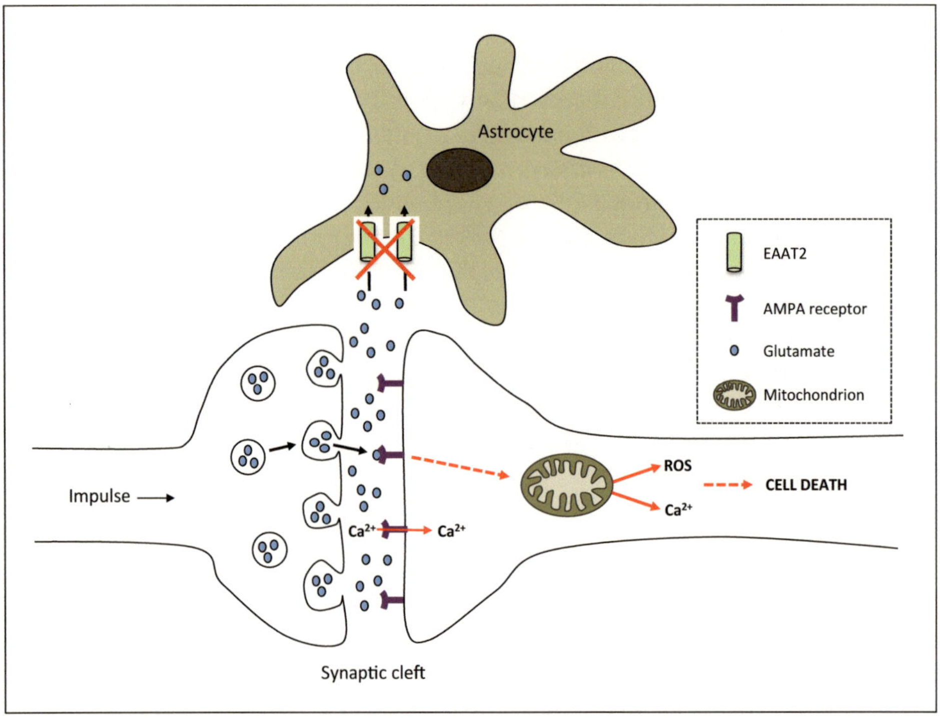

Figure 1. Induction of motor neuron death by glutamate excitotoxicity. Red arrows/lines indicate the pathways that are affected or induced in ALS.

5. Mitochondrial abnormalities

The mitochondrion is a vital organelle with multiple functions within cells. Mitochondria are the main source of ATP, maintain calcium homeostasis and participate in calcium signaling, and play a key role in the intrinsic apoptotic pathway. Mitochondrial malfunction turns motor neuron more vulnerable to damage, especially in aging and stress neurons. Mitochondrial malfunction is an important hypothesis in ALS pathogenesis (Bruijn et al., 2004; Manfredi et al., 2005).

5.1. Mitochondrial morphology

Indeed, mitochondria morphological and ultrastructural changes as well as bioenergetic malfunction have been reported in ALS. SOD1 is localized mainly in the cytoplasm, but has been found also in the mitochondria and other organelles (Okado et al., 2001; Sturtz et al., 2001). Mutant SOD1 protein is present in the mitochondrial intermembrane space, matrix and outer membrane of mitochondria (Higgins, et al, 2002; Vijayvergiya et al., 2005; Vande Velde et al., 2008; Kawamata et al., 2008). This abnormal SOD1 protein may fail to fold properly

http://dx.doi.org/10.5772/56562

resulting in mitochondrial protein retention and mitochondrial dysfunction with damaged of the mitochondrial membrane and loss of mitochondrial membrane potential and swelling (Wong et al., 1995; Kong et al., 1998). Severe mitochondrial morphological changes were found in NSC34 cells overexpressing mutant SOD1 (Raimondi et al., 2006; Menzies et al., 2002). In addition, mitochondrial swelling and vacuolization in motor neuron axons and dendrites were reported in mSOD1 mice even before disease onset (Wong et al., 1995; Kong et al., 1998; Borthwick et al., 1999). The presence of abnormal mitochondrial clusters was also described in mutant SOD1 rat motor axons (Sotelo-Silveira et al., 2009) as well as in lumbar spinal cord motor neurons and proximal axons of sALS patients (Sasaki et al., 1996; Hirano et al., 1984).

5.2. Electron transport chain

Abnormal respiratory complex activities, disrupted redox homeostasis and decreased ATP production were described in ALS (Borthwick et al., 1999; Jung et al., 2002; Bowling et al., 1993; Ferri et al., 2006). Biochemical studies showed several abnormalities in mitochondrial electron transport chain. The enzymatic activity of the electron transport chain complexes I, II, IV was reduced in mSOD1 mice and cell cultures from patients with fALS (Jung et al., 2002; Mattiazzi et al., 2002). The interaction between cytochrome c and the inner mitochondrial membrane in addition to the activity of complex IV were reduced in the $SOD1^{G93A}$ transgenic mice (Kirkinezos et al., 2005). Decreased oxygen consumption, lack of ADP-dependent respiratory control, and decreased membrane potential were also reported in mutant SOD1 rat spinal astrocytes (Cassina et al., 2008) (Fig. 2).

5.3. Calcium homeostasis

Mitochondria play an important role in the intracellular calcium homeostasis as a calcium buffer, accumulating or releasing calcium depending on the cytosolic levels. Abnormalities in mitochondrial calcium homeostasis were reported in ALS patients and in mutant SOD1 animals (Kruman et al., 1999; Carri et al., 1997; Reiner et al, 1995; Jaiswal et al., 2009). The release of calcium from the mitochondria leads to excessive intracellular calcium levels. This abnormal calcium homeostasis induces motor neuron death through several mechanisms including: 1) toxic generation of reactive oxygen species (ROS), as reported in $SOD1^{G93A}$ transgenic mice (Kruman et al., 1999); 2) release of cytochrome c from the mitochondria (Martin et al., 2009); 3) glutamate excitotoxicity (Nicholls et al., 2003), and others. All these mechanisms may have a special role in motor neurons because these cells contain less mitochondrial density per volume compared to non-neuronal cells, thus making neurons more deficient in mitochondrial calcium buffering properties (Grosskreutz et al., 2007) (Fig. 2). In addition, ALS patients show a deficiency in calcium binding proteins calbidin and paralbumin in cortical motor and spinal motor neurons. These two proteins regulate intracellular calcium levels and their deficiency may result in neuronal loss. On the contrary, oculomotor neurons or neuron from the Onuff's nuclei contains normal levels of calbidin and paralbumin levels and they are preserved despite ALS progression (Alexianu, et al. 1994; Celio, 1990; Ince et al., 1993, Palecek et al., 1999).

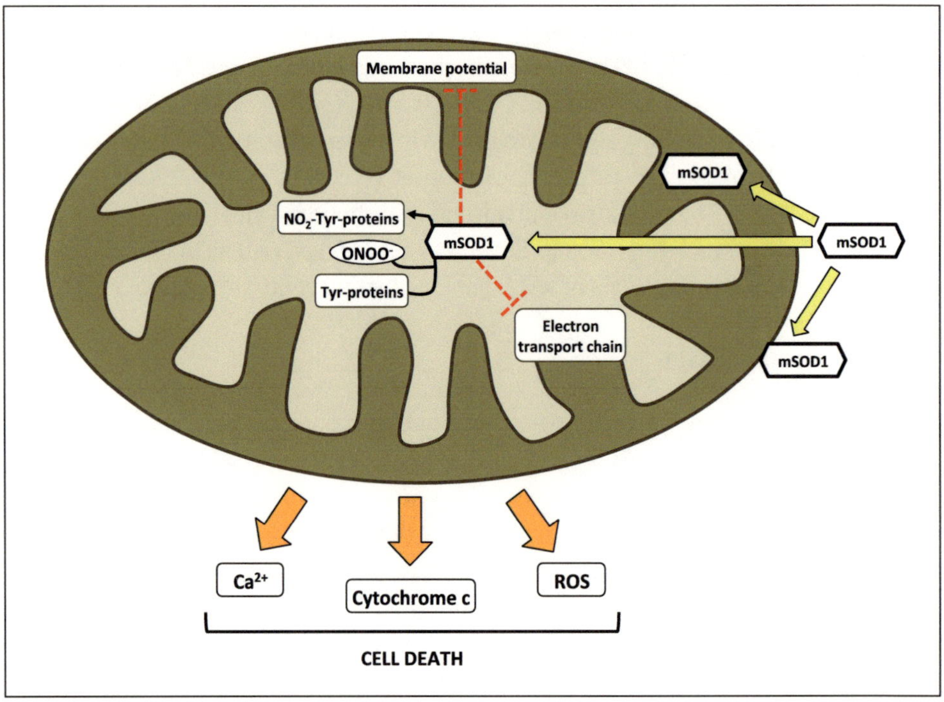

Figure 2. Mitochondrial abnormalities associated with mutant SOD1 (mSOD1). Mutant SOD1 translocates to mitochondrial intermembrane space and matrix, and is associated with the mitochondrial outer membrane. The expression of mutant SOD1 is linked to decrease of mitochondrial membrane potential and electron transport chain activity. The release of calcium and cytochrome c to the cytosol, and the production of ROS lead to cell death in ALS.

6. Axonal transport abnormalities

Transport of proteins, vesicles, and organelles between cell body and terminal axons is a vital process in neuronal development, function and survival. Cytoskeletal proteins such as neurofilament (NFs) confer structure and shape to motor neurons, and are involved in axonal anterograde and retrograde transport between soma and motor axons. NFs are intermediate filaments made from the assembly of light, medium, and heavy subunits (Maragakis and Galvez-Jimenez, 2012). Disorganization of NFs affects axonal transport resulting in axonal strangulation and accumulation of axonal cargo (Collard et al., 1995). A hallmark of ALS pathology is the abnormal accumulation of NFs in the neuronal cell bodies and proximal axons. Animal models and patients with ALS show that axonal transport is a critical component in ALS pathogenesis (Morrison et al., 1998; Lin et al., 2006). Transgenic models of fALS and sALS are associated with mutations of the heavy NF subunits (Figlewicz et al., 1994; Al-Chalabi et al., 1999). In addition, reduction in light subunit mRNA levels was found in motor neurons from the spinal cord of patients with ALS (Wong et al., 2000). Abnormal axonal transport, vacuolization and degeneration of axons and motor neurons have been reported in transgenic mice overexpressing or with reduced expression of NF subunits (Collard et al., 1995; Cote et al., 1993). In neurons, mitochondria are frequently found in axon terminals due to the high demand of ATP and calcium handling at the synapses (Shepherd et al., 1998; Rowland et al., 2000). Mitochondria are transported in both anterograde and retrograde directions via kinesin and dynein motor complexes (Nangaku et al., 1994; Zhang, et al 2004; Varadi et al., 2004). The disruption of the mitochondrial axonal transport has been implicated in neurodegenerative diseases including ALS (Hollenbeck et al., 2005; De Vos et al., 2007; Magrane et al. 2009). Mitochondria display saltatory movement along microtubules. In SOD1^{G93A} transgenic mice and cortical neurons transfected with G93A-SOD1, mitochondrial transport was selectively reduced in the anterograde direction (De Vos et al., 2007). In addition, in NSC34 cells overexpressing mutant SOD1 mitochondrial transport was altered in both anterograde and retrograde directions (Magrane et al., 2009). Abnormalities in axonal transport cause abnormal renewal of mitochondria and autophagosomes at distal motor axons resulting in mitochondrial accumulation, deficit in energy production, accumulation of ROS, and released of pro-apoptotic agents leading to neuronal death. Slow axonal transport impairment has been described as one of the earliest pathological events in mSOD1 mice (Williamson et al., 1999; Zhang et al. 1997). Fast axonal transport is mediated by kinesin while dynein motor complexes mediate the transport of membrane-bound organelles necessary for axonal and synaptic functions. In patients and transgenic rodent models of ALS there are impairments in the kinesin-mediated anterograde transport and dynein-mediated retrograde axonal transport (Williamson et al., 1999; Breuer et al 1987; Breuer et al., 1988; Collard et al., 1995; Sasaki et al., 1996; Ligon et al., 2005; Parkhouse et al., 2008). Disruption of kinesin heavy chain KIF5B causes perinuclear clustering of mitochondria in mice neurons, indicating that KIF5B is essential for mitochondrial dispersion (Tanaka et al., 1998). Abnormalities in the transport of other proteins such as dynactin, myosin and actine were also identified in transgenic mutant SOD1 models (LaMonte et al., 2002). Dynactin mutations have been associated with autosomal familiar motor neuron disease (Puls et al 2003; Puls et al 2005). Peripherin, another intermediate transport filament was found in neuronal inclusions of sALS (Corbo et al., 1992). Overexpression of peripherin in transgenic mice is associated with axonal degeneration. Inflammatory cytokines increased peripherin levels, suggesting an association between inflammation and axonal transport disorders (Sterneck, et al 1996).

7. Growth factors

Several growth factors (GFs) has been investigated and potentially implicated in the pathogensis of ALS. One of the most studied GFs is the vascular endothelial growth factor (VEGF), a protein involved in vasculogenesis and angiogenesis, and in restoration of oxygen supply upon limited blood circulation. Animal data suggest that VEGF may be neuroprotector. Overexpression of VEGF delayed onset and progression motor neuron disease, as shown in a double transgenic mice generated by crossing mice expressing human mutant SOD1 with mice overexpressing neuronal VEGF (mSOD1/VEGF). The mSOD1/VEGF transgenic mice showed a delayed in motor neuron loss, motor impairment, and a prolonged survival compared with mutant SOD1 transgenic mice (Wang et al., 2007). Intracerebroventricular administration of VEGF in a $SOD1^{G93A}$ rat model of ALS delayed motor neuron degeneration and onset of paralysis, improved motor performance, preserved neuromuscular junction, and extended survival (Storkebaum et al., 2005). This study also showed that in $SOD1^{G93A}$ mice, neurons expressing a transgenic VEGF receptor prolonged mice survival. Also supporting the VEGF neuroprotective role, a single injection of a VEGF-expressing lentiviral vector into several muscles of $SOD1^{G93A}$ mice delayed the onset as well as the progression of the disease even at onset of paralysis (Azzouz et al., 2004). Interestingly, mouse models in which the hypoxia-response element in the VEGF gene was deleted showed a decrease in VEGF expression in normoxia and under hypoxic conditions. This model resulted in a progressive motor neuron degeneration disease that resembles ALS (Oosthuyse, et al., 2001). A meta-analysis of over 900 individuals from Sweden and over 1,000 individuals from Belgium and England with a specific haplotype for VEGF associated with reduced circulating VEGF and VEGF gene transciption showed a two-fold increase in the risk of developing ALS for these individuals (Lambrechts et al., 2003). In another study, $SOD1^{G93A}$ mice crossed with VEGF haplotype mice showed a much more severe motor neuron degeneration. VEGF probably has neuronal direct and indirect neuroprotective effects preventing ischemic changes while regulating vascular perfusion.

Additionally, VEGF-B, a homolog of VEGF with minimal angiogenetic activity, was shown to be protective for cultured primary motor neurons. In addition, transgenic mice with deletion of the VEGF-B gene were implicated in an ALS-like pathogenesis, as shown crossing a VEGF-B knockout mouse with transgenic mice expressing human mutant SOD1 ($mSOD1/VEGF\text{-}B^{-/-}$) (Poesen et al., 2008). $mSOD1/VEGF\text{-}B^{-/-}$ mice showed an earlier death and more severe motor neuron degeneration compared with mutant SOD1 transgenic mice. Intracerebroventricular administration of VEGF-B in a $SOD1^{G93A}$ rat model of ALS prolonged the survival of mutant SOD-expressing rats, suggesting that VEGF is neuroprotective by a mechanism independent of angiogenesis (Poesen et al., 2008).

Other beneficial growth factors are innsuline growth factor-1, glial cell line –derived neurotrophic factor, and brain derived neurotrophic factor.

8. RNA metabolism disorders

Ubiquinated intracytoplamsmatic inclusions containing trans-activation response DNA-binding protein of 43 KDa (TDP-43), encoded by the TARDBP gene in chromosome-1, had been identified in motor neurons of patients with sALS and frontal lobar degeneration (FTLD) linked to TDP-43 pathology (FTLD-TDP) (Neumann et al., 2006). TDP-43 positive inclusions were also identified in patients with non-SOD1 fALS. Gene mutations of the TDP-43 gene probably accounts for 5% of patients with fALS. All the cases of sALS and SOD1 negative fALS have neural and glial inclusions immunoreactive to both ubiquitin and TDP-43 whereas positive SOD1 mutations in fALS were absent of TDP-43 immunoreactivity. (MacKenzie et al., 2007; Tran et al., 2007). TDP-43 inclusions were also identified in patients with Guamanian parkinsonism-dementia complex, and familial British dementia (Sreedharan et al., 2008; Kabashi et al., 2008; Van Deerlin et al., 2008; Yokoseki et al., 2008; Rutherford et al., 2008; Del Bo et al., 2009; Hasegawa et al., 2007; Schwab et al., 2009). TDP-43 is a nuclear protein expressed in almost all tissues that binds to mRNA and DNA and regulates mRNA processing processes such as splicing, translation, and gene transcription. TDP-43 structure consists of two RNA recognition motifs (RRMs) that bind to nucleic acids, and a glycine rich domain containing the majority of ALS associated mutations (Cohen et al., 2012; Buratti et al., 2001). Genetic mutation of another RNA processing protein, fused in sarcoma /translated in liposarcoma (FUS/TLS), has been also associated with ALS (Kwiatkowski et al., 2009; Vance et al., 2009). The FUS/TLS has a similar structure to TDP-43 with RRM and glycin rich domains. FUS/TLS, also a nuclear protein, accumulates in intracytoplasmatic tau- and TDP-43 negative inclusions in patients with fALS, sALS, and frontal lobar degeneration FTLD-FUS (Mackenzie et al., 2010). TDP-43 and FUS/TLS stabilized mRNA encoding histone deacetylase 6 (HDAC6) involved in clearance of misfolded protein aggregates (Kim et.al, 2010, Fiesel, et al., 2010; Lee et al., 2010; Kawaguchi et al., 2003). TDP-43 binds to a wide range of RNA targets and promotes the synthesis of several proteins implicated in the neuronal development and integrity (Tollervey et al., 2011). TDP-43 expression is carefully controlled by a tightly autoregulated mechanism (Winton et al., 2008). Thus, TDP-43 abnormalities in RNA binding and autoregulation, and FUS/TLS may have a essential role in neuronal integrity. TDP-43 also has a protective effect on mitochondrial function; abnormal expression of mitochondrial fission/fusion proteins in transgenic mice expressing human wild-type TDP-43 transgene driven by mouse prion promoter had been reported (Xu et al., 2010). In cultured cells, exposure to stress caused TDP-43 to be relocated into stress granules (SGs). This abnormal localization of TDP-43 could start a pathological TDP-43 aggregation or TDP-43 interaction with other SGs-proteins. A similar process may occur with FUS/TLS protein (Bosco et al., 2010; Dormann et al., 2010). The formation of SGs may lead to pathological inclusion aggregations resulting in neuronal and glial cell damage. Hyperphosphorilated TDP-43 aggregates were identified in ALS spinal cord and FTLP-TDP brain tissue. TDP-43 glycin-rich domain, where most of the mutations had been identified, seems to be required for TDP-43 association with SGs. Expression of insoluble aggregates of TDP-43 terminal fragment was implicated in the generation of SGs (Liu-Yesucevitz et al., 2010). In addition, TDP-43 interacts with cytoplasmatic Ataxin-2 protein resulting in TDP-43 accumulation in misfolded aggregates. Mutant polyglutamine expansions within ataxin-2 enhanced the binding to TDP-43 facilitating the formation of aggregates in ALS patients (Elden,AC et al., 2010). The formation of these aggregates seems to be implicated in neuronal death, but the mechanism remains elusive.

9. Non-cell autonomous mechanisms

Evidence is accumulating indicating that motor neuron degeneration in ALS is not only restricted to neuronal autonomous cell death but it is rather a more complex process involving inflammatory neurotoxicity from non-neuronal glial cells such as astrocytes and microglia (Phani et al., 2012). Support for non-autonomous evidence comes from several studies in transgenic mutant SOD1 mice. The expression of mutant SOD1 restricted to motor neurons *in vivo* was not enough or caused a mild neurodegeneration (Jaarsma et. al.; 2008). Indeed, when mutant SOD1 expression was reduced in microglia and macrophages there was a reduction in motor neuron degeneration (Boillee 2006, Wang 2009). In addition, mutant SOD1 expression in astrocytes is required to cause neurodegeneration by release of toxic factors (Gong et. al., 2000; Nagai et al. 2007). Co-cultures of healthy motor neurons with astrocytes expressing mutant SOD1 resulted in more than 50% motor neuron death (Marchetto et al, 2008), while astrocytes obtained from postmortem tissue from patients with fALS and sALS were both toxic to motor neurons (Haidet-Phillips et al., 2011). In agreement, mutant SOD1 knockdown in astrocytes attenuated toxicity towards motor neurons, suggesting that the mutant enzyme plays a role in both fALS and sALS (Phillips et al., 2011). $SOD1^{G93A}$ glial-restricted precursor cells transpanted into the cervical spinal cord of wild type rats survived and differentiated efficiently into astrocytes. These graft-derived $SOD1^{G93A}$ astrocytes induced host ubiquitination and death of motor neurons, reactive astrocytosis, and reduction of the glial glutamate transporter GLT-1 expression that was associated with animal limb weakness and respiratory dysfunction (Papadeas et al., 2011). The $SOD1^{G93A}$ astrocyte-induced motor neuron death may be madiated by host microglial activation (Papadeas et al., 2011).

Abnormalities in the immune system have also been observed in ALS patients. Blood samples of ALS patients have increased levels of $CD4^+$ cells and reduced levels of $CD8^+$ T lymphocytes. However, early in the disease when motor features are still mild there is a reduction in $CD4^+$/$CD25^+$ T-regulatory cells (T-reg) and $CD14^+$ monocytes. These observations suggest that the reduction in circulating T-reg cells could be due to the relocation of the cells into the central nervous system. Upon relocation, the T-reg cells would activate the innate immune cells like microglia, leading to the release of anti-inflammatory cytokines such as interleukin-10 and transforming growth factor-β to protect the affected area (Kipnis et al., 2004 and Mantonavi, et al., 2009). Indeed, immunostaining for the astrocytic marker glial fibrillary acid protein (GFAP) showed a significantly increased presence of astrocytes in the precentral gyrus of patients with both fALS and sALS. In addition, staining for activated microglia and macrophages markers such as leukocyte common antigen (LCA), lymphocytes function associate molecule (LFA-1), complementary receptors CR3 (CD11b), and CR4 (CD11c) was also increased in motor cortex, brainstem, and corticospinal tract (Kawamata, et al., 1992; Papidimitriou et al., 2010). Samples from brain and spinal cord from animal models and patient with ALS also showed a significant increase in activated or reactive astrocytes, an indication of neuroinflammation (Sta et al., 2011).

Astrocytes and microglia play an essential role in immune surveillance and response in the central nervous system. Reactive astrocytes recruited to the injured area reestablish the blood-brain-barrier (BBB), release neurotrophins and growth factors (IGF-1), clear debri, and isolate the injured region through the formation of a glial scar (Papadimitriou et al 2010; Dong and Benviste 2001). Microglia are also activated in the presence of antigens exposed during neurodegeneration leading to the phagocytosis of cellular debri and the secretion of several neurotrophic factors, neurotrophins, and cytokines. However, a poor regulation of these factors could be harmful to motor neurons. Microglia seems to protect motor neurons from neurodegeneration, but is activated in the first steps of neurodegeneration. An increase in the immunostaining for GFAP and CD11 suggests the presence of reactive astrocytes and microglia in SOD1 transgenic mice (Fischer et. al, 2004). Increase in NGF, a sign of reactive atrocytes, leads to aptoptosis in ALS through a pathway involving activation of p75 (Pehar et al., 2004). Additionally, in ALS animal models mutant SOD1-expressing astrocytes are neurotoxic to motor neurons, and reducing mutant SOD1 expression decreases motor neuron degeneration and increases animal life span (Lepore at al., 2008, Barbeito et al., 2010). The release of pro-inflammatory cytokines, oxidative stressors such as prostanglandins, leukotrienes, and reactive nitrogen species (RNS) is toxic to motor neurons (Henkel, et al., 2009). In *in vitro* studies, normal motor neurons die through a pro-apoptotic Bax pathway when co-cultured with astrocytes expressing mutant SOD1 (Nagai at al., 2007). In *in vivo* studies, microglia releases pro-inflammatory cytokines such us TNF-α and IL-1β as well as ROS (Henkel 2009) whereas in ALS patients, there is an increase of pro-inflammatory cytokines and prostranglandin E2 (Papadimitou, 2010). Media obtained from activated microglia causes motor neuron death by activation of TNF-α and NMDA receptors (Moisee and Strong 2006). In mouse model of ALS, a reduction in the expression of mutant SOD1 by microglia does not change age of symptoms onset, but slowed down disease progression (Boillee et al. 2006b). Motor neurons expressing mutant SOD1 are more susceptible to Fas ligand and NO-triggered cell death (Raoul et al., 2002), suggesting that in the context of ALS progression, motor neurons expressing mutant SOD1 are more vulnerable to external stimuli such as ROS, RNS and toxic factors release by surrounding cells.

10. Apoptosis

Apoptosis is a programmed cell death cascade involved in several physiological processes during development and aging. Cell death by apoptosis sustains the homeostasis of cell population in tissues including cell turnover, hormone dependent- and chemical induced-cell death, and immune system development. The programmed cell death also functions as a defense when cells are damaged by disease or noxious stimuli (Elmore, S; 2007). Thereby, inappropriate apoptosis is a potential mechanism implicated in the pathogenesis of several neurodegenerative disorders, including ALS (Elmore, S; 2007). There are two main apoptotic pathways, the extrinsic or death receptor pathway and the intrinsic or mitochondrial pathway (Igney and Krammer, 2002). The extrinsic pathway involves transmembrane receptor-mediated interactions between ligands and death receptors resulting in transmission of death signals from cell surface to the intracellular signaling pathways (Locksley et al., 2001). The most studied ligand and death receptor association are Fas ligand and Fas receptor (FasL/FasR) and tumor necrosis factor (TNF) and its receptor (TNFL/TNFR) (Hsu et al 1995; Wajant, 2002). The intrinsic pathway consists of non-receptor-mediated stimuli that cause changes in the inner mitochondrial membrane. These changes include the opening of mitochondrial membrane pores leading to loss of transmembrane potential and released of pro-apoptotic proteins such as cytochrome c, Smac/DIABLO, HtrA2/Omi, and others ending with the activation of caspases (Sealens, et al., 2004; Du et al., 2000; Van Loo et al., 2002; Garrido at al., 2005). The

Bcl-2 family of proteins regulates the intrinsic apoptotic pathway (Cory and Adams 2002) and these proteins in turn are regulated by the tumor suppressor protein p53 (Schuler and Green, 2001). The Bcl-2 family includes pro-apoptotic and anti-apoptotic proteins. Some of the anti-apoptotic proteins comprise Bcl2, Bcl-x, Bcl XL, Bcl-XS, Bcl-w, BAG, whereas the pro-apoptotic proteins include Bcl-10, BAX, Balk, Bid, Bad, Bim, Bik, and Blk. Both the intrinsic and extrinsic pathways require a specific stimuli to activate its own caspase initiator (caspase -2,-8,-9,-10). These two pathways, once activated, convey in the activation of a final execution pathway with cleavage of caspase-3, resulting in DNA fragmentation, cytoskeletal and nuclear protein cleavage, protein cross-linking, apoptotic bodies formation, expression of ligands for phagocytic recognizion, and final uptake by phagocytic cells (Martinvalet, et al, 2005). There is compelling evidence in ALS, at least in mutant SOD1-ALS, that toxicity is mediated by apoptosis. In transgenic SOD1 mice there are numerous apoptotic findings such as DNA fragmentation, caspase activation, and altered expression of the anti-apoptotic protein Bcl-2 (Durham HD, et al. 1997; Spooren WP et al. 2000). Motor neuron degeneration in ALS structurally resembles apoptosis. The neuronal death progression is divided in 3 sequential stages: chromatolysis, somatodendritic attrition, and apoptosis. In ALS, in the spinal cord anterior horn and motor cortex there is DNA fragmentation and increased in caspase-3 activity. Vulnerable central nervous system regions affected by ALS show elevation of pro-apoptotic proteins Bax and Bak and reduction of the antiapoptotic protein Bcl-2 in mitochondrial-enriched membrane compartment. Co-immunoprecipitation experiments show greater Bax-Bax interactions and lower Bax-Bcl-2 interactions in the mitochondrial-enriched membrane compartment of ALS motor cortex compared with controls, (Martin LJ, 1999). In mutant SOD1 mice apoptotic signals are activated in sequence, caspase 1, an inflammatory caspase, is activated at disease onset while activated caspase-3 is detected later in the curse of the disease (Pasinelli, P, et al. 2000). In SOD1 mice, intracerebroventricular injection of a broad caspase-inhibitor reduces caspase 1 and caspase 3 mRNA levels resulting in spear motor neurons at the spinal cord and delay in disease onset and progression compared with vehicle-infused mice (Li M, et al.; 2000). Overexpression of the antiapoptotic protein Bcl-2 and deletion of the pro-apoptotic protein Bax preserve motor function and prolong life in a $SOD1^{G93A}$ model. Genetic deletion of mitochondrial pro-apoptotic Bak and Bax proteins in a mouse model of ALS prevent neuronal loss and axonal degeneration, and delayed onset of disease (Reyes et al., 2012).

In $SOD1^{G93A}$ transgenic mice, cytosolic release of cytochrome c was observed (Pasinelli, et al., 2004; Kirkinezos et al., 2005; Takeuchi et al., 2002), and levels of pro-apoptotic proteins Bad and Bax were increased while those of anti-apoptotic proteins Bcl2, Bcl-xL and XIAP were decreased (Guegan et al., 2001; Vukosavic et al., 1999; Ishigaki et al., 2002). Caspase 1 and caspase 3 were also sequentially activated in motor neurons and astrocytes in $SOD1^{G93A}$, $SOD1^{G37R}$, and $SOD1^{G85R}$ mice (Li et al., 2000; Pasinelli et al., 1998; Pasinelli et al., 2000). Intraventricular administration of minocycline, which inhibits cytochrome c release from mitochondria, was shown to delay disease onset and extend survival (Zhu et al., 2002). However minocycline failed in human ALS patients (Gordon et al, 2007). Similar results were observed upon intraventricular administration of the broad-spectrum caspase inhibitor zVAD-fmk (Li et al., 2000). Additionally, over-expression of anti-apoptotic protein Bcl-2 delayed activation of the caspases, attenuated neuron degeneration and delayed disease onset and mortality (Vukosavic et al., 1999, Kostic et al., 1997).

11. Conclusion

The research in the ALS field encounters many limitations, what is clearly reflected in the little progress accomplished in the therapy of this neurodegenerative disorder. Most of the studies describe the mechanisms involved in the pathogenesis of the familial form of ALS, which accounts for a minority of all the ALS cases. However, some of the hypothesis currently under investigation may also explain how the pathology develops in the sporadic forms of ALS. In the last two decades several experimental models *in vitro* and *in vivo* have shaded light into the pathogenesis of the disease. Several potential mechanisms have been implicated in ALS onset and progression including oxidative stress, excitotoxicity, mitochondrial dysfunction, glial activation, RNA-processing, and growth factor abnormalities. Whether these mechanisms intertwine, work in parallel or in sequence to cause neuronal death remains to be investigated.

Author details

Fabian H. Rossi[1,2], Maria Clara Franco[1,2] and Alvaro G. Estevez[1,2]

1 Orlando VA Healthcare System, Orlando, USA

2 Burnett School of Biomedical Sciences, College of Medicine, University of Central Florida, Orlando, USA

References

[1] Al-chalabi, A, Andersen, P. M, Nilsson, P, Chioza, B, Andersson, J. L, Russ, C, Shaw, C. E, Powell, J. F, & Leigh, P. N. Deletions of the heavy neurofilament subunit tail in amyotrophic lateral sclerosis. Hum Mol Genet (1999).

[2] Al-chalabi, A, & Leigh, P. N. (2000). Recent advances in amyotrophic lateral sclerosis. Current Opinion in Neurology; , 13(4), 397-405.

[3] Alexianu, M. E, Ho, B. K, & Mohamed, A. H. La Bella V, Apple SH. The role of calcium-binding protein in selective motor neuron vulnerability in Amyotrophic Lateral Sclerosis. Annals of Neurology (1994).

[4] Arisato, T, Okubo, R, Arata, H, Abe, K, Fukada, K, Sakoda, S, Shimizu, A, Qin, X. H, Izumo, S, Osame, M, & Nakagawa, M. Clinical and pathological studies of familial

amyotrophic lateral sclerosis (FALS) with SOD1 H46R mutation in large Japanese families. Acta Neuropathol (2003).

[5] Barbeito, A. G, Mesci, P, & Boilee, S. (2010). Motor neuron-immune interactions: the vicious circle of ALS. J. Neural Transm.; , 117, 981-1000.

[6] Barbeito, L. H, Pehar, M, Cassina, P, Vargas, M. R, Peluffo, H, Viera, L, Estévez, A. G, & Beckman, J. S. (2004). A role for astrocytes in motor neuron loss in amyotrophic lateral sclerosis. Brain Res Brain Res Rev.; 47(1-3):263-74.

[7] Beckman, J. S, Carson, M, Smith, C. D, & Koppenol, W. H. (1993). ALS, SOD and peroxynitrite. Nature 364:584.

[8] Boeve, B. F, Boylan, K. B, Graff-radford, N. R, Dejesus-hernandez, M, Knopman, D. S, Pedraza, O, Vemuri, P, Jones, D, Lowe, V, Murray, M. E, Dickson, D. W, Josephs, K. A, Rush, B. K, Machulda, M. M, Fields, J. A, Ferman, T. J, Baker, M, Rutherford, N. J, Adamson, J, Wszolek, Z. K, Adeli, A, Savica, R, Boot, B, Kuntz, K. M, Gavrilova, R, Reeves, A, Whitwell, J, & Kantarci, K. Jack CR Jr, Parisi JE, Lucas JA, Petersen RC, Rademakers R. (2012). Characterization of frontotemporal dementia and/or amyortrophic lateral sclerosis associated with the GGGGcc repeat expansion in C9ORF72. Brain.; , 135(3), 765-783.

[9] Bogaert, E, Ydewalle, d, & Van Den, C. Bosch L. (2010). Amyotrophic lateral sclerosis and excitotoxicity: from pathological mechanism to therapeutic target. CNS Neurol Disord Drug Targets Jul; , 9(3), 297-304.

[10] Boillée, S, Yamanaka, K, Lobsiger, C. S, Copeland, N. G, Jenkins, N. A, Kassiotis, G, Kollias, G, & Cleveland, D. W. (2006). Onset and progression in inherited ALS determined by motor neurons and microglia. Science; , 312, 1389-1392.

[11] Boillee, S, & Cleveland, D. W. (2008). Revisiting oxidative damage in ALS: microglia, Nox, and mutant SOD1. J Clin Invest , 118, 474-478.

[12] Borthwick, G. M, Johnson, M. A, Ince, P. G, Shaw, P. J, & Turnbull, D. M. (1999). Mitochondrial enzyme activity in amyotrophic lateral sclerosis: implications for the role of mitochondria in neuronal cell death. Ann Neurol.; , 46, 787-790.

[13] Bosco, D. A, Lemay, N, Ko, H. K, Zhou, H, & Burke, C. Kwiatkowski TJ Jr, Sapp P, McKenna-Yasek D, Brown RH Jr, Hayward LJ. (2010). Mutant FUS proteins that cause amyotrophic lateral sclerosis incorporate into stress granules. Hum. Mol. Genet. , 19, 4160-4175.

[14] Bowling, A. C, Schulz, J. B, & Brown, R. H. Jr., Beal MF. (1993). Superoxide dismutase activity, oxidative damage, and mitochondrial energy metabolism in familial and sporadic amyotrophic lateral sclerosis. J Neurochem.; , 61, 2322-2325.

[15] Breuer, A. C, & Atkinson, M. B. (1988). Fast axonal transport alterations in amyotrophic lateral sclerosis (ALS) and in parathyroid hormone (PTH)-treated axons. Cell Motil Cytoskeleton; , 10, 321-330.

[16] Breuer, A. C, Lynn, M. P, Atkinson, M. B, Chou, S. M, Wilbourn, A. J, Marks, K. E, Culver, J. E, & Fleegler, E. J. (1987). Fast axonal transport in amyotrophic lateral sclerosis: an intra-axonal organelle traffic analysis. Neurology; , 37, 738-748.

[17] Brownell B Oppenheimer DRHughes JT. (1970). The central nervous system in the motor neuron disease. J Neurol Neurosurg Psychiatry; , 33, 338-357.

[18] Bruijin, L. I, Becher, M. W, & Lee, M. K. (1997). ALS-linked SOD1 mutant G85R mediates damage to astrocytes and promotes rapidly progressive disease with SOD1 containing inclusions. Neuron; , 18, 327-338.

[19] Bruijn, L. I, Miller, T. M, & Cleveland, D. W. (2004). Unraveling the mechanisms involved in motor neuron degeneration in ALS. Annu Rev Neurosci.; , 27, 723-749.

[20] Buratti, E, & Baralle, F. E. (2001). Characterization and functional implicatios of the RNA binding properties of the nuclear factor TDP-43, a novel splicing regulator of CFTR exon 9. J. Biol. Chem.; , 276, 36337-36343.

[21] Cagnin, A, Brooks, D. J, Kennedy, A. M, Gunn, R. N, Myers, R, Turkheimer, F. E, Jones, T, & Banati, R. B. (2001). In vivo measurement of activated microglia in dementia. Lancet , 358, 461-467.

[22] Carri, M. T, Ferri, A, Battistoni, A, Famhy, L, Gabbianelli, R, Poccia, F, & Rotilio, G. (1997). Expression of a Cu,Zn superoxide dismutase typical of familial amyotrophic lateral sclerosis induces mitochondrial alteration and increase of cytosolic Ca2+ concentration in transfected neuroblastoma SH-SY5Y cells. FEBS Lett.; , 414, 365-368.

[23] Cassina, P, Cassina, A, Pehar, M, Castellanos, R, Gandelman, M, De Leon, A, & Radi, R. (2008). Mitochondrial dysfunstion in SODG93A-bearing astrocyres promoters motor neuron degeneration: prevention of mitochondrial target antioxidants. J Neurosci.; (28)16:4115-4122.

[24] Celio, M. R. K and Parvalbumin in the rat nervous system. Neuroscience; (35)2:375-475

[25] Choi, D. W, Koh, J, & Peters, S. (1988). Pharmacology of glutamate neurotoxicity in cortical cell cultures: attenuation by NMDA antagonists. J. Neurosci., , 8, 185-196.

[26] Cohen, T. J. Lee VMY, and Trojanowski Q. (2011). TDP-43 functions and pathogenic mechanisms implicated in TDP-43 proteinopathies. Trends In Molecular Medicine; , 17(11), 659-667.

[27] Collard, J. F, Cote, F, & Julien, J. P. (1995). Defective axonal transport in a transgenic mouse model of amyotrophic lateral sclerosis. Nature; , 375, 61-64.

[28] Corbo, M, & Hays, A. P. (1992). Peripherin and neurofilament protein coexist in spinal spheroids of motor neuron disease. J. Neuropathol Exp Neurol , 51(5), 531-7.

[29] Cory, S, & Adams, J. M. (2002). The Bcl2 family: regulators of the cellular life-or-death switch. Nat Rev Cancer. , 2, 647-56.

[30] Côté, F, Collard, J. F, & Julien, J. P. (1993). Progressive neuronopathy in transgenic mice expressing the human neurofilament heavy gene: a mouse model of amyotrophic lateral sclerosis. Cell; 73:35.

[31] Crow, J. P, Strong, M. J, Zhuang, Y, Ye, Y, & Beckman, J. S. (1997b). Superoxide dimutase catalyzes nitration of tyrosines by peroxinitrite in the rod and head domains of neurofilament L. J Neurochem , 69, 1945-1953.

[32] Damiano, M, Starkov, A. A, Petri, S, Kipiani, K, Kiaei, M, & Mattiazzi, M. Flint Beal M, Manfredi G. (2006). Neural mitochondrial Ca2+ capacity impairment precedes the onset of motor symptoms in G93A Cu/Zn-superoxide dismutase mutant mice. J Neurochem.; , 96, 1349-1361.

[33] De Vos, K. J, Chapman, A. L, Tennant, M. E, Manser, C, Tudor, E. L, Lau, K. F, Brownlees, J, Ackerley, S, Shaw, P. J, Mcloughlin, D. M, Shaw, C. E, Leigh, P. N, Miller, C. C, & Grierson, A. J. (2007). Familial amyotrophic lateral sclerosis-linked SOD1 mutants perturb fast axonal transport to reduce axonal mitochondria content. Hum Mol Genet.;, 16, 2720-2728.

[34] Del Bo RGhezzi S, Corti S, Pandolfo M, Ranieri M, Santoro D, Ghione I, Prelle A, Orsetti V, Mancuso M, Sorarù G, Briani C, Angelini C, Siciliano G, Bresolin N, Comi GP. (2009). TARDBP (TDP-43) sequence analysis in patients with familial and sporadic ALS: identification of two novel mutations. Eur J Neurol., 16(6), 727-732.

[35] Dong, Y, & Benveniste, E. N. (2001). Immune function of astrocytes. Glia; , 36, 180-190.

[36] Dormann, D, Rodde, R, Edbauer, D, Bentmann, E, Fischer, I, Hruscha, A, Than, M. E, Mackenzie, I. R, Capell, A, Schmid, B, Neumann, M, & Haass, C. (2010). ALS- associated fused in sarcoma (FUS) mutation disrupt Transportin-mediated nuclear import. EMBO J. , 29, 2841-2857.

[37] Du, C, Fang, M, Li, Y, Li, L, & Wang, X. (2000). Smac, a mitochondrial protein that promotes cytochrome c-dependent caspase activation by eliminating IAP inhibition. Cell; , 102, 33-42.

[38] Dunlop, J. Beal McIlvain H, She Y, Howland DS. (2003). Impaired spinal cord glutamate transport capacity and reduced sensitivity to riluzole in a transgenic superoxide dismutase mutant rat model of amyotrophic lateral sclerosis. J Neurosci; 23:1688.

[39] Durham, H. D, Roy, J, Dong, L, & Figlewicz, D. A. (1997). Aggregation of mutant Cu/Zn superoxide dismutase proteins in a culture model of ALS. J Neuropathol Exp Neurol; 56:523.

[40] Elden, A. C, Kim, H. J, Hart, M. P, Chen-plotkin, A. S, Johnson, B. S, Fang, X, Armakola, M, Geser, F, Greene, R, Lu, M. M, Padmanabhan, A, Clay-falcone, D, Mccluskey, L, Elman, L, Juhr, D, Gruber, P. J, Rüb, U, Auburger, G, Trojanowski, J. Q, Lee, V. M, Van Deerlin, V. M, Bonini, N. M, & Gitler, A. D. (2010). Ataxin-2 intermediate-

length polyglutamine expansions are associated with increased risk for ALS. Nature 466. , 1069-1075.

[41] Elmore, S. (2007). Apoptosis: a review of Programmed Cell Death. Toxicol Pathol. , 35(4), 495-516.

[42] Estévez, A. G, Spear, N, Manuel, S. M, Barbeito, L, Radi, R, & Beckman, J. S. (1998). Role of endogenous nitric oxide and peroxinitrite formation in the survival and death of motor neurons in culture. Progress in Brain Research; , 118, 269-280.

[43] Estévez, A. G, Crow, J. P, Sampson, J. B, Reiter, C, Zhuang, Y. X, Richardson, G. J, Tarpey, M. M, Barbeito, L, & Beckman, J. S. (1999). Induction of nitric oxide-dependent apoptosis in motor neurons by zinc-deficient superoxide dismutase. Science , 286, 2498-2500.

[44] Ferri, A, Cozzolino, M, Crosio, C, Nencini, M, Casciati, A, Gralla, E. B, Rotilio, G, Valentine, J. S, & Carri, M. T. Familial ALS-superoxide dismutases associate with mitochondria and shift their redox potentials. (2006). Proc Natl Acad Sci U S A.; , 103, 13860-13865.

[45] Fiesel, F. C, Voigt, A, & Weber, S. S. Van den Haute C, Waldenmaier A, Görner K, Walter M, Anderson ML, Kern JV, Rasse TM, Schmidt T, Springer W, Kirchner R, Bonin M, Neumann M, Baekelandt V, Alunni-Fabbroni M, Schulz JB, Kahle PJ. (2010). Knockdown of transactive response DNA-binding protein (TDP-43) downregulate histone deacetylase 6. EMBO J. , 29, 209-221.

[46] Figlewicz DA, Krizus A, Martinoli MG, Meininger V, Dib M, Rouleau GA, Julien JP. 1994. Variants of the heavy neurofilament subunit are associated with the development of amyotrophic lateral sclerosis. Hum Mol Genet 3:1757-1761.

[47] Fischer, L. R, Culver, D. G, Tennant, P, Davis, A. A, Wang, M, Castellano-sanchez, A, Khan, J, Polak, M. A, & Glass, J. D. (2004). Amyotrophic lateral sclerosis is a distal axonopathy: evidence in mice and man. Exp. Neurol. , 185, 232-240.

[48] Geser, F, Martinez-lage, M, Robinson, J, Uryu, K, Neumann, M, Brandmeir, N. J, Xie, S. X, Kwong, L. K, Elman, L, Mccluskey, L, Clark, C. M, Malunda, J, Miller, B. L, Zimmerman, E. A, Qian, J, Van Deerlin, V, Grossman, M, Lee, V. M, & Trojanowski, J. Q. (2009). Clinical and pathological continuum of multisystem TDP-43 proteinopathies. Arch Neurol. , 66(2), 180-9.

[49] Ghatak, N. R, Campbell, W. W, Lippman, R. H, & Hadfield, M. G. (1986). Anterior horn changes of motor neuron disease associated with demyelinating radiculopathy. J Neuropathol Exp Neurol Jul;, 45(4), 385-95.

[50] Gong, Y. H, Parsadanian, A. S, Andreeva, A, Snider, W. D, & Elliott, J. L. (2000). Resticted expression of G86R Cu/Zn superoxide dismutase in astrocytes results in astrocytosis but does cause motor neuron degeneration. J Neurosci , 20, 660-665.

[51] Gould, T. W, & Oppenheim, R. W. (2011). Motor neuron trophic factors: therapeutic use in ALS? Brain Res Rev , 67, 1-39.

[52] Gordon, P.H, Moore, D.H, Miller, R.G, Florence, J.M, Verheijde, J.L, Doorish, C, Hilton, J.F, Spitalny, G.M, & Mac, R.B. . Barohn, R. Tandan. 2007. Efficacy of minocycline in patients with amyotrophic lateral sclerosis: a phase III randomised trial. Lancet Neurol.6:1045-1053.

[53] Grosskreutz, J, Haaztert, K, Dewil, M, Van Damme, P, & Calleweart, G. van Den Bosh. (2007). Role of mitochondria in kainate induced fast calcium transient in culture of spinal motor neurons. Cell Calcium; (42)1:56-59.

[54] Guegan, C, Vila, M, Rosoklija, G, Hays, A. P, & Przedborski, S. (2001). Recruitment of the mitochondrial-dependent apoptotic pathway inamyotrophic lateral sclerosis. J Neurosci. , 21, 6569-6576.

[55] Guo, H, Lai, L, & Butchbach, M. E. (2003). Increased expression of the glial glutamate transporter EAAT2 modulates excitotoxicity and delays the onset of but not the outcome of ALS in mice. Hum Mol Genet; , 12, 2119-2532.

[56] Gurney, M. E, Cutting, F. B, Zhai, P, Doble, A, Taylor, C. P, Andrus, P. K, & Hall, E. D. (1996). Benefit of vitamin E, riluzole, and gabapentin in the transgenic model of familial amyotrophic lateral sclerosis. Ann Neurol; , 39, 147-157.

[57] Haidet-phillips, A. M, Hester, M. E, Miranda, C. J, Meyer, K, Braun, L, Frakes, A, Song, S, Likhite, S, Murtha, M. J, Foust, K. D, Rao, M, Eagle, A, Kammesheidt, A, Christensen, A, Mendell, J. R, Burghes, A. H, & Kaspar, B. K. (2011). Astrocytes from familial and sporadic ALS patients are toxic to motor neurons. Nature biotechnology , 29, 824-828.

[58] Hasegawa, M, Arai, T, Akiyama, H, Nonaka, T, Mori, H, Hashimoto, T, Yamazaki, M, & Oyanagi, K. (2007). TDP-43 is deposited in the Guam parkinsonism- dementia complex brains. Brain. , 130, 1386-1394.

[59] He, C. Z, & Hays, A. P. (2004). Expression of peripherin in ubiquinated inclusions of amyotrophic lateral sclerosis. J Neurol Sci 15;, 217(1), 47-54.

[60] Heath and Shaw(2002). Update on the glutaminergic neurotransmitter system and the role of excitotoxicity in amyothrophic lateral sclerosis Muscle Nerve; , 26, 438-458.

[61] Henkel, J. S, Beers, D. R, Zhao, W, & Appel, S. H. (2009). Microglia in ALS: the good, the bad, and the resting. J. Neiroimmune Pharmacol. , 4, 389-398.

[62] Higgins, C. M, Jung, C, Ding, H, & Xu, Z. (2002). Mutant Cu, Zn superoxide dismutase that causes motoneuron degeneration is present in mitochondria in the CNS. J Neurosci.; 22:RC215.

[63] Hirano, A, Nakano, I, Kurland, L. T, Mulder, D. W, Holley, P. W, & Saccomanno, G. (1984). Fine structural study of neurofibrillary changes in a family with amyotrophic lateral sclerosis. J Neuropathol Exp Neurol.; , 43, 471-480.

[64] Hollenbeck, P. J, & Saxton, W. M. (2005). The axonal transport of mitochondria. J Cell Sci.; , 118, 5411-5419.

[65] Howland, D. S, Liu, J, & She, Y. (2002). Focal loss of the glutamate transporter EAAT2 in transgenic rat model of SOD1 mutant mediated amyotrophic lateral sclerosis (ALS). Proc Natl Acad Sci USA; , 99, 1604-1609.

[66] Hsu, H, Xiong, J, & Goeddel, D. V. (1995). The TNF receptor 1-associated protein TRADD signals cell death and NF-kappa B activation. Cell. , 81, 495-504.

[67] Hughes, J. T. (1982). Pathology of amyotrophic lateral sclerosis. Adv Neurol.; , 36, 61-74.

[68] Igney, F. H, & Krammer, P. H. (2002). Death and anti-death: tumour resistance to apoptosis. Nat Rev Cancer. , 2, 277-88.

[69] Ince, G. I, & Wharton, S. B. Cytopathology of motor neuron. Handbook of clinical neurology. Eisen AA and Shaw PJ (eds.) Elesevier , 89-119.

[70] Ince, P, Stout, N, Shaw, P, Slade, J, Hunziker, W, Heizman, C. W, & Bainbridge, K. G. (1993). Parvalbumine and Calbidin D-28 K in human motor system and in motor neuron disease. Neuropathology and Applied Neurobiology (19)4:291-299.

[71] Ince PG Evans JKnopp M. (2003). Corticospinal tract degeneration in the progressive muscular atrophy variant of ALS. Neurology; , 60, 1525-1258.

[72] Ince, P. G. Neuroapthology. In Brown RJ, Meininger V, Swash M (eds) Amyotrophic lateral sclerosis. Martin Dunitz, London, , 83-112.

[73] Ischiropoulos, H, Zhu, L, Chen, J, Tsai, M, Martin, J. C, Smith, C. D, & Beckman, J. S. (1992). Peroxynitrite-mediated tyrosine nitration catalyzed by superoxide dismutase. Archives of Biochemistry and Biophysics , 298, 431-437.

[74] Ishigaki, S, Liang, Y, Yamamoto, M, Niwa, J, Ando, Y, Yoshihara, T, Takeuchi, H, Doyu, M, & Sobue, G. (2002). X-Linked inhibitor of apoptosis protein is involved in mutant SOD1-mediated neuronal degeneration. J Neurochem. , 82, 576-584.

[75] Jaarsma, D, Teuling, E, Haasdijk, E, et al. (2008). Neuron-specific expression of mutant superoxide dismutase is sufficient to induce amyotrophic lateral sclerosis in transgenic mice. J. Neurosci. , 28, 2075-2088.

[76] Jaiswal, M. K, Zech, W. D, Goos, M, Leutbecher, C, Ferri, A, Zippelius, A, Carri, M. T, Nau, R, & Keller, B. U. (2009). Impairment of mitochondrial calcium handling in a mtSOD1 cell culture model of motoneuron disease. BMC Neurosci.; 10:64.

[77] Jung, C, Higgins, C. M, & Xu, Z. (2002). A quantitative histochemical assay for activities of mitochondrial electron transport chain complexes in mouse spinal cord sections. J Neurosci Methods.; , 114, 165-172.

[78] Kabashi, E, Valdmanis, P. N, Dion, P, Spiegelman, D, & Mcconkey, B. J. Vande Velde C, Bouchard JP, Lacomblez L, Pochigaeva K, Salachas F, Pradat PF, Camu W, Meininger V, Dupre N, Rouleau GA. (2008). TARDBP mutations in individuals with sporadic and familial amyotrophic lateral sclerosis. Nat Genet. , 40(5), 572-574.

[79] Kamo, H, Haebara, H, Akiguchi, M, et al. (1987). A distinctive pattern of reactive gliosis in the precental cortex in amyothophic lateral sclerosis. Acta Neuropathol , 74, 33-38.

[80] Kawaguchi, Y, Kovacs, J. J, Mclaurin, A, Vance, J. M, Ito, A, & Yao, T. P. (2003). The deacetylase HDAC6 regulates aggresome formation and cell viability in response to misfolded protein stress. Cell; , 115, 727-738.

[81] Kawahara, Y, Ito, K, Sun, H, Aizawa, H, Kanazawa, I, & Kwak, S. (2004). Glutamate receptors: RNA editing and death of motor neurons. Nature 427 (6977): 801.

[82] Kawamata, H, & Manfredi, G. (2008). Different regulation of wild-type and mutant Cu,Zn superoxide dismutase localization in mammalian mitochondria. Hum Mol Genet.; , 17, 3303-3317.

[83] Kawamata, T, Akiyama, H, Yamada, T, & Mc Greer, P. L. (1992). Immunologic reaction in amyotrophic lateral sclerosis brain and spinal cord tissue. Am. J. Pathol. , 140, 691-707.

[84] Kim, S. H, Shanware, N. P, Bowler, M. J, & Tibbetts, R. S. (2010). Amyotrophic lateral sclerosis-associated proteins TDP-43 and FUS/TLS function in common biochemical complex to co-regulate HDAC6 mRNA. J. Biol. Chem. , 285, 34097-34105.

[85] Kirkinezos, I. G, Bacman, S. R, Hernandez, D, Oca-cossio, J, Arias, L, & Morales, C. T. (2005). Cytochrome c association with the inner mitochondria membrane is impaired in central nervous system of G93ASOD1 mice. J Neurosci (25)1:164-172.

[86] Kobayashi, S, Ishigaki, M, & Doyu, G. Sobue. (2002). Mitochondrial localization of mutant superoxide dismutase 1 triggers caspase-dependent cell death in a cellular model of familia amyotrophic lateral sclerosis. J Biol Chem. , 277, 50966-50972.

[87] Kong, J, & Xu, Z. (1998). Massive mitochondrial degeneration in motor neurons triggers the onset of amyotrophic lateral sclerosis in mice expressing a mutant SOD1. J Neurosci.; , 18, 3241-3250.

[88] Kostic, V, Jackson-lewis, V, De Bilbao, F, Dubois-dauphin, M, & Przedborski, S. (1997). Bcl-2: prolonging life in a transgenic mouse model of familial amyotrophic lateral sclerosis. Science. , 277, 559-562.

[89] Kruman, I. I, Pedersen, W. A, Springer, J. E, & Mattson, M. P. (1999). ALS-linked Cu/Zn-SOD mutation increases vulnerability of motor neurons to excitotoxicity by a

mechanism involving increased oxidative stress and perturbed calcium homeostasis. Exp Neurol.; , 160, 28-39.

[90] Kwiatkowski TJ JrBosco DA, Leclerc AL, Tamrazian E, Vanderburg CR, Russ C, Davis A, Gilchrist J, Kasarskis EJ, Munsat T, Valdmanis P, Rouleau GA, Hosler BA, Cortelli P, de Jong PJ, Yoshinaga Y, Haines JL, Pericak-Vance MA, Yan J, Ticozzi N, Siddique T, McKenna-Yasek D, Sapp PC, Horvitz HR, Landers JE, Brown RH Jr. (2009). Mutations in the FUS/TLS gene on chromosome 16 cause familial amyotrophic lateral sclerosis. Science. , 323(5918), 1205-1208.

[91] Lacomblez, L, Bensimon, G, Leigh, P. N, Guillet, P, & Maininger, V. Dose-ranging study of riluzole in Amyotrophic Lateral Sclerosis. Amyotrophic Lateral Sclerosis/ Riluzole Study Group II. Lancet , 347, 1425-1431.

[92] LaMonte BHWallace KE, Holloway BA, Shelly SS, Ascaño J, Tokito M, Van Winkle T, Howland DS, Holzbaur EL. (2002). Disruption of dynein/dynactin inhibits axonal transport in motor neurons causing late-onset progressive degeneration. Neuron , 34, 715-727.

[93] Lepore, A. C, Rauck, B, Dejea, C, Pardo, A. C, Rao, M. S, Rothstein, J. D, & Maragakis, N. J. (2008). Focal transplantation of astrocytes replacement is neuroprotective in a model of motor neuron disease. Nat. Neurosci. , 11, 1294-1301.

[94] Lee, J. Y, Nagano, Y, Taylor, J. P, Lim, K. L, & Yao, T. P. (2010). Disease-causing mutations in parkin impair mitochondrial ubiquitination, aggregation, and HDAC6-dependent mitophagy. J. Cell Biol. , 189, 671-679.

[95] Leigh, P. N, & Garofolo, O. (1995). The molecular pathology of motor neurone disease. In Motor neurone disease. M. Swash and P.N. Leigh, editors. Springer Verlag, London. , 139-161.

[96] Li, L, Prevette, D, Oppenheim, R. W, & Milligan, C. E. (1998). Involvement of specific caspases in motoneuron cell death in vivo and in vitro following trophic factor deprivation. Mol Cell Neurosci , 12, 157-167.

[97] Li, L, Oppenheim, R. W, Lei, M, & Houenou, L. J. (1994). Neurotrophic agents prevent motoneuron death following sciatic nerve section in the neonatal mouse. J Neurobiol , 25, 759-766.

[98] Li, M, Ona, V. O, Guegan, C, Chen, M, Jackson-lewis, V, Andrews, L. J, Olszewski, A. J, Stieg, P. E, Lee, J. P, Przedborski, S, & Friedlander, R. M. (2000). Functional role of caspase-1 and caspase-3 in an ALS transgenic mouse model. Science. , 288, 335-339.

[99] Li, M, Ona, V. O, Guégan, C, Chen, M, Jackson-lewis, V, Andrews, L. J, Olszewski, A. J, Stieg, P. E, Lee, J. P, Przedborski, S, & Friedlander, R. M. (2000). Functional role of caspase-1 and caspase-3 in an ALS transgenic mouse model. Science., 288, 335-339.

[100] Ligon, L. A. LaMonte BH, Wallace KE, Weber N, Kalb RG, Holzbaur EL. (2005). Mutant superoxide dismutase disrupts cytoplasmic dynein in motor neurons. Neuroreport.; , 16, 533-536.

[101] Lin CL, Bristol LA, Jin L, Dykes-Hoberg M, Crawford T, Clawson L, Rothstein JD. 1998. Aberrant RNA processing in a neurodegenerative disease: the cause for absent EAAT2, a glutamate transporter, in amyotrophic lateral sclerosis. Neuron 1998; 20:589.

[102] Lin, H, & Schlaepfer, W. W. (2006). Role of neurofilament aggregation in motor neuron disease. Ann Neurol; 60:399.

[103] Ling, S. C, Albuquerque, C. P, Han, J. S, Lagier-tourenne, C, Tokunaga, S, Zhou, H, & Cleveland, D. W. (2010). ALS-associated mutations in TDP-43 increase its stability and promote TDP-43 complexes with FUS/TLS. Proc Natl Acad Sci U S A 107:13318.

[104] Liu-yesucevitz, L, et al. (2010). Tar DNA binding protein-43 (TDP-43) associates with stress granules: analysis of cultured cells and pathological brain tissue. PLos ONE 5, e13250.

[105] Locksley, R. M, Killeen, N, & Lenardo, M. J. (2001). The TNF and TNF receptor superfamilies: integrating mammalian biology. Cell; , 104, 487-501.

[106] Mackenzie, I. R, Rademakers, R, & Neumann, M. (2010). TDP43 and FUS in amyotrophic lateral sclerosis and frontotemporal dementia. Lancet Neurol. , 9, 995-1007.

[107] Mackenzie, I. R, Bigio, E. H, Ince, P. G, Geser, F, Neumann, M, Cairns, N. J, Kwong, L. K, Forman, M. S, Ravits, J, Stewart, H, Eisen, A, Mcclusky, L, Kretzschmar, H. A, Monoranu, C. M, Highley, J. R, Kirby, J, Siddique, T, Shaw, P. J, Lee, V. M, & Trojanowski, J. Q. (2007). Pathological TDP-43 distinguishes sporadic amyotrophic lateral sclerosis from amyotrophic lateral sclerosis with SOD1 mutations. , 61(5), 427-434.

[108] Mackenzie, I. R, Bigio, E. H, Ince, P. G, Geser, F, Neumann, M, Cairns, N. J, Kwong, L. K, Forman, M. S, Ravits, J, Stewart, H, Eisen, A, Mcclusky, L, Kretzschmar, H. A, Monoranu, C. M, Highley, J. R, Kirby, J, Siddique, T, Shaw, P. J, Lee, V. M, & Trojanowski, J. Q. (2007). Pathological TDP-43 distinguishes sporadic amyotrophic lateral sclerosis from amyotrophic lateral sclerosis with SOD1 mutations. Ann Neurol. , 61(5), 427-34.

[109] Magrane, J, & Manfredi, G. (2009). Mitochondrial function, morphology, and axonal transport in amyotrophic lateral sclerosis. Antioxidants & Redox Signaling; , 11(7), 1615-1626.

[110] Manfredi, G, & Xu, Z. (2005). Mitochondrial dysfunction and its role in motor neuron degeneration in ALS. Mitochondrion; , 5, 77-87.

[111] Mantovani, S, Garbelli, S, Pasini, A, Alimonti, D, Perotti, C, Melazzini, M, Bendotti, C, & Mora, G. (2009). Immune system alteration is sporadic amyotrophic lateral scle-

rosis patients suggest an ongoing neuroinflammatory process. J. Neuroimmunol. 210., 73-79.

[112] Maragakis, N. J, & Galvez-jimenez, N. (2012). Epidemiology and pathogenesis of amyotrophic lateral sclerosis. UpToDate;, 1-16.

[113] Marchetto MCNMuotri A, Mu Y, Smith AM, Gage FH. (2008). Non-Cell-Autonomous effect on human SODG37r astrocytes on motor neurons derived from human embryonic stem cells. Stem Cell;, 3, 649-657.

[114] Martin, L. J, Gertz, B, Pan, Y, Price, A. C, Molkentin, J. D, & Chang, Q. (2009). The mitochondrial permeability transition pore in motor neuron involvement in the pathobiology of ALS mice. Experimental Neurology; (218)2:333-346

[115] Martin, L. J. (1999). Neuronal death in amyotrophic lateral sclerosis is apoptosis: possible contribution of a programmed cell death mechanism. 2000. J Neuropathol Exp Neurol ; 58:459.

[116] Martin, L. J. (1999). Neuronal death in amyotrophic lateral sclerosis is apoptosis: possiblecontribution of a programmed cell death mechanism. J Neuropathol Exp Neurol , 58, 459-471.

[117] Martinvalet, D, Zhu, P, & Lieberman, J. (2005). Granzyme A induces caspase- independent mitochondrial damage, a required first step for apoptosis. Immunity; , 22, 355-70.

[118] Matsumoto, S, Goto, S, Kusaka, H, Imai, T, Murakami, N, Hashizume, Y, Okazaki, H, & Hirano, A. (1993). Ubiquitin-positive inclusion in anterior horn cells in subgroups of motor neuron diseases: a comparative study of adult-onset amyotrophic lateral sclerosis, juvenile amyotrophic lateral sclerosis and Werdnig-Hoffmann disease. J Neurol Sci;, 115(2), 208-13.

[119] Mattiazzi, M, Aurelio, D, Gajewski, M, Martushova, C. D, Kiali, K, Beal, M, & Manfredi, M. F. G. (2002). Mutated human SOD1 caused dysfunction of oxidative phosphorilation in mitochondrial of transgenic mice. The Journal of Biological Chemistry; (277)33:29626-29633

[120] Menzies, F. M, Cookson, M. R, Taylor, R. W, Turnbull, D. M, Chrzanowska-lightowlers, Z. M, Dong, L, Figlewicz, D. A, & Shaw, P. J. (2002). Mitochondrial dysfunction in a cell culture model of familial amyotrophic lateral sclerosis. Brain; , 125, 1522-1533.

[121] Milligan, C. E, Oppenheim, R. W, & Schwartz, L. M. (1994). Motoneurons deprived of trophic support in vitro require new gene expression to undergo programmed cell death. J Neurobiol , 25, 1005-1016.

[122] Moisse, K, & Strong, M. J. (2006). Innate immunity in amyotrophic lateral sclerosis Biochim. Biophys. Acta;, 1762, 1083-1093.

[123] Morrison, B. M, Morrison, J. H, & Gordon, J. W. Superoxide dismutase and neurofilament transgenic models of amyotrophic lateral sclerosis. J Exp Zool (1998).

[124] Nagai, M, Re, D. B, Nagata, T, Chalazonitis, A, Jessell, T. M, Wichterle, H, & Przedborski, S. (2007). Astrocytes expressing ALS-Linked mutated ALS release factors selectively toxic to motor neurons. Nat. Neurosci. , 10, 615-622.

[125] Nangaku, M, Sato-yoshitake, R, Okada, Y, Noda, Y, Takemura, R, Yamazaki, H, & Hirokawa, N. a novel microtubule plus end-directed monomeric motor protein for transport of mitochondria. Cell; , 79, 1209-1220.

[126] Neumann, M, Kwong, L. K, Sampathu, D. M, Trojanowski, J. Q, & Lee, V. M. (2007). TDP-43 proteinopathy in frontotemporal lobar degeneration and amyotrophic lateral sclerosis: protein misfolding diseases without amyloidosis. Arch Neurol. , 64(10), 1388-94.

[127] Neumann, M, Sampathu, D. M, Kwong, L. K, Truax, A. C, Micsenyi, M. C, Chou, T. T, Bruce, J, Schuck, T, Grossman, M, Clark, C. M, Mccluskey, L. F, Miller, B. L, Masliah, E, Mackenzie, I. R, Feldman, H, Feiden, W, Kretzschmar, H. A, Trojanowski, J. Q, & Lee, V. M. (2006). Ubiquitinated TDP-43 in frontotemporal lobar degeneration and amyotrophic lateral sclerosis. Science; , 314(5796), 130-133.

[128] Nicholls, D. G, Vesce, S, Kirk, L, & Chalmers, S. (2003). Interaction between mitochondrial bioenergetics and cytoplasma calcium in cultured cerebellar granule cells. Cell Calcium; (34)4-5:407-424.

[129] Niwa, J, Ishigaki, S, Hishikawa, N, Yamamoto, M, Doyu, M, Murata, S, Tanaka, K, Taniguchi, N, & Sobue, G. (2002). Dorfin ubiquitylates mutant SOD1 and prevents mutant SOD1-mediated neurotoxicity. J Biol Chem.; , 277(39), 36793-8.

[130] Oppenheim, R. W. (1997). Related mechanisms of action of growth factors and antioxidants in apoptosis: an overview. Adv Neurol , 72, 69-78.

[131] Okado-matsumoto, A, & Fridovich, I. (2001). Subcellular distribution of superoxide dismutases (SOD) in rat liver: Cu,Zn-SOD in mitochondria. J Biol Chem.; , 276, 38388-38393.

[132] Okamoto, K, Hirai, S, Amari, M, Watanabe, M, & Sakurai, A. (1993). Bunina bodies in amyotrophic lateral sclerosis immunostained with rabbit anti-cystatin C serum. Neurosci Lett; , 1962, 125-128.

[133] Okamoto Y, Ihara M, Urushitani M, Yamashita H, Kondo T, Tanigaki A, Oono M, Kawamata J, Ikemoto A, Kawamoto Y, Takahashi R, Ito H. 2011. An autopsy case of SOD1-related ALS with TDP-43 positive inclusions. Neurology 2011; 77:1993.

[134] Papadeas, S. T, Kraig, S. E, Banion, C. O, Lepore, A. C, & Nagarkis, N. J. (2011). Astrocytes carrying the superoxide dismutase 1 (SOD1G93A) mutation induce wild-type motor neuron degeneration in vivo. Proc Natl Acad Sci U S A; (108)43:1703-17808.

[135] Papadimitriou, D, Le, V, & Verche, A. Jacquier et al. (2010). Inflammatory in ALS and SMA: sorting out the good from the evil. Neurobiol. Dis.; , 37, 493-502.

[136] Pasinelli, P, & Brown, R. H. (2006). Molecular Biology of amyothrophic lateral sclerosis: insights from genetics. Nature; , 7, 710-723.

[137] Pasinelli, P, Belford, M. E, Lennon, N, Bacskai, B. J, Hyman, B. T, & Trotti, D. Brown, Jr. RH. (2004). Amyotrophic lateral sclerosis-associated SOD1 mutant proteins bind and aggregate with Bcl-2 in spinal cord mitochondria. Neuron; , 43, 19-30.

[138] Pasinelli, P, Borchelt, D. R, Houseweart, M. K, & Cleveland, D. W. Brown Jr. RH. (1998). Caspase-1 is activated in neural cells and tissue with amyotrophic lateral sclerosis-associated mutations in copper-zinc superoxide dismutase. Proc Natl Acad Sci U S A; , 95, 15763-15768.

[139] Pasinelli, P, & Houseweart, M. K. Brown Jr. RH, Cleveland DW. (2000). Caspase-1 and-3 are sequentially activated in motor neuron death in Cu,Zn superoxide dismutase-mediated familial amyotrophic lateral sclerosis. Proc Natl Acad Sci U S A. , 97, 13901-13906.

[140] Pehar, M, Cassina, P, Vargas, M. R, Castellanos, R, Viera, L, Beckman, J. S, Estévez, A. G, & Barbeito, L. (2004). Astrocytic production of nerve growth factor in motor neuron disorder apoptosis: implications for amyotrophic lateral slcerosis. J. Neurochem. , 89, 464-473.

[141] Phani, S, Re, D. B, & Przedborski, S. (2012). The role of the immune system in ALS. Frontiers in Pharmacology; (3)150:1-6.

[142] Philips, T, & Robberecht, W. (2011). Neuroinflammation in amyotrophic lateral sclerosis: role of glial activation in motor neuron disease. Lancet Neurol; 10:253.

[143] Piao, Y. S, Wakabayashi, K, Kakita, A, Yamada, M, Hayashi, S, Morita, T, Ikuta, F, Oyanagi, K, & Takahashi, H. (2003). Neuropathology with clinical correlation of sporadic amyotrophoic lateral sclerosis: 102 autopsy cases examined between 1962 and 2000. Brain Pathol , 12, 10-22.

[144] Pioro, E. P, Majors, A. W, Mitsumoto, H, Nelson, D. R, & Ng, T. C. (1999). H-MRS evidence of neurodegeneration and excess glutamate + glutamine in ALS medulla. Neurology. , 53(1), 71-9.

[145] Puls, I, & Jonnakuty, C. LaMonte BH, Holzbaur EL, Tokito M, Mann E, Floeter MK, Bidus K, Drayna D, Oh SJ, Brown RH Jr, Ludlow CL, Fischbeck KH. (2003). Mutant dynactin in motor neuron disease. Nat Genet. , 33(4), 455-6.

[146] Puls, I, Oh, S. J, Sumner, C. J, Wallace, K. E, Floeter, M. K, Mann, E. A, Kennedy, W. R, Wendelschafer-crabb, G, Vortmeyer, A, Powers, R, Finnegan, K, Holzbaur, E. L, Fischbeck, K. H, & Ludlow, C. L. (2005). Distal spinal and bulbar muscular atrophy caused by dynactin mutation. Ann Neurol. , 57, 687-694.

[147] Raimondi, A, Mangolini, A, Rizzardini, M, Tartari, S, Massari, S, Bendotti, C, Francolini, M, Borgese, N, Cantoni, L, & Pietrini, G. (2006). Cell culture models to investigate the selective vulnerability of motoneuronal mitochondria to familial ALS-linked G93ASOD1. Eur J Neurosci.; , 24, 387-399.

[148] Raoul, C, Estévez, A. G, Nishimune, H, Cleveland, D. W, Delapeyrière, O, Henderson, C. E, Haase, G, & Pettmann, B. (2002). Motoneuron death triggered by a specific pathway downstream of Fas: potentiation by ALS-linked SOD1 mutations. Neuron , 35, 1067-1083.

[149] Reiner, A, Medina, L, Figueredo-cardenas, G, & Anfinson, S. (1995). Brainstem motoneuron pools that are selectively resistant in amyotrophic lateral sclerosis are preferentially enriched in parvalbumin: evidence from monkey brainstem for a calcium-mediated mechanism in sporadic ALS. Exp Neurol.; , 131, 239-250.

[150] Reyes, N. A, Fisher, J. K, & Austgen, K. VandenBerg S, Huang EJ, Oakes SA. (2010). Blocking the mitochondrial apoptotic pathway preserves motor neuron viability and function in a mouse model of amyotrophic lateral sclerosis. J Clin Invest 120:3673.

[151] Robberecht, W, & Philips, T. (2013). The changing scene of amyotrophic lateral sclerosis. Nat Rev Neurosci , 14, 248-264.

[152] Rothstein, J. D. (2009). Current hypotheses for the underlying biology of amyotrophic lateral sclerosis. Ann Neurol 65 Suppl 1, S, 3-9.

[153] Rothstein JD Dunlop JBeal McIlvain H, She Y, Howland DS. (2003). Impaired spinal cord glutamate transport capacity and reduced sensitivity to riluzole in a transgenic superoxide dismutase mutant rat model of amyotrophic lateral sclerosis. J Neurosci; 23:1688.

[154] Rothstein, J. D, Dykes-hoberg, M, & Pardo, C. A. (1996). Knockout of glutamate transporters reveals a major role of astroglial transport in excitotoxicity and clearance of glutamate. Neuron; , 16, 675-686.

[155] Rothstein, J. D, Martin, L. J, & Kuncl, R. W. (1992). Decreased glutamate transport by the brain and spinal cord in amyotrophic lateral sclerosis. N Engl J Med; , 326, 1464-1468.

[156] Rothstein, J. D, Tsai, G, Kuncl, R. W, Clawson, L, Cornblath, D. R, Drachman, D. B, Pestronk, A, Stauch, B. L, & Coyle, J. T. (1990). Abnormal excitatory amino acid metabolism in amyotrophic lateral sclerosis. Ann Neurol. , 28(1), 18-25.

[157] Rothstein, J. D, Van Kammen, M, Levey, A. I, Martin, L. J, & Kuncl, R. W. (1995). Selective loss of glial glutamate transporter GLT-1 in amyotrophic lateral sclerosis. Ann Neurol , 38, 73-84.

[158] Rothstein, J. D, Van Kammen, M, & Levey, A. I. (1995). Selective loss of glial glutamate transporter GLT-1 in amyotrophic lateral sclerosis. Ann Neurol; , 38, 73-84.

[159] Rowland, K. C, Irby, N. K, & Spirou, G. A. (2000). Specialized synapse-associated structures within the calyx of Held. J Neurosci.; , 20, 9135-9144.

[160] Rutherford, N. J, Zhang, Y. J, Baker, M, Gass, J. M, Finch, N. A, Xu, Y. F, Stewart, H, Kelley, B. J, Kuntz, K, Crook, R. J, Sreedharan, J, Vance, C, Sorenson, E, Lippa, C, Bigio, E. H, Geschwind, D. H, Knopman, D. S, Mitsumoto, H, Petersen, R. C, Cashman, N. R, Hutton, M, Shaw, C. E, Boylan, K. B, Boeve, B, Graff-radford, N. R, Wszolek, Z. K, Caselli, R. J, Dickson, D. W, Mackenzie, I. R, Petrucelli, L, & Rademakers, R. (2008). Novel mutations in TARDBP (TDP-43) in patients with familial amyotrophic lateral sclerosis. PloS Genet. 4(9):e1000193

[161] Saelens, X, Festjens, N, Vande, L, Walle, M, & Van Gurp, G. van Loo, P. Vandenabeele. (2004). Toxic proteins released from mitochondria in cell death. Oncogene; , 23, 2861-74.

[162] Sasaki, S, & Iwata, M. (1996). Impairment of fast axonal transport in the proximal axons of anterior horn neurons in amyotrophic lateral sclerosis. Neurology.; , 47, 535-540.

[163] Sasaki, S, & Iwata, M. (1996). Ultrastructural study of synapses in the anterior horn neurons of patients with amyotrophic lateral sclerosis. Neurosci Lett.; , 204, 53-56.

[164] Sasaki, S, & Maruyama, S. (1994). Immunocytochemical and ultrastructural studies of the motor cortex in amyotrophic lateral sclerosis. Acta Neuropathol; , 87(6), 578-85.

[165] Schuler, M, & Green, D. R. (2001). Mechanisms of apoptosis. Biochem Soc Trans. 29:684-8., 53.

[166] Schwab, C, Arai, T, Hasegawa, M, Akiyama, H, Yu, S, & Mcgeer, P. L. (2009). TDP-43 pathology in familial British dementia. Acta Neuropatol.; , 118(2), 303-11.

[167] Shaw PJ, Forrest V, Ince PG, Richardson JP, Wastell HJ. 1995. CSF and plasma amino acid levels in motor neuron disease: elevation of CSF glutamate in a subset of patients. Neurodegeneration 1995; 4:209.

[168] Shepherd, G. M, & Harris, K. M. (1998). Three-dimensional structure and composition of CA3-->CA1 axons in rat hippocampal slices: implications for presynaptic connectivity and compartmentalization. J Neurosci.; , 18, 8300-8310.

[169] Shibata, N, Hirano, A, Kobayashi, M, Siddique, T, Deng, H. X, Hung, W. Y, Kato, T, & Asayama, K. (1996). Intense superoxide dismutase-1 immunoreactivity in intracytoplasmatic hyaline inclusions of familial amyotrophic lateral sclerosis with posterior column involvement. J Neuropathol Exp Neurol , 55, 481-490.

[170] Shook, S. J, & Pioro, E. P. (2009). Racing against the clock: recognizing, differenciating, diagnosisng, and referring the amyotrophic lateral sclerosis patient. Ann Neurol; , 65, 10-16.

[171] Silani, V, Braga, M, & Ciammola, V. Cardin, Scarlato G. (2000). Motor neuron in culture as model to study ALS. Journal of Neurology ; (247)1:128-136.

[172] Sitte, H, Wanschitz, J, & Berger, M. (2001). Autoradiography with [3H] PK11195 of spinal tract degeneration in amyotrophic lateral sclerosis. Acta Neuropathologica; , 101, 75-78.

[173] Sotelo-silveira, J. R, Lepanto, P, Elizondo, M. V, Horjales, S, & Palacios, F. Martinez Palma L, Marin M, Beckman JS, Barbeito L. (2009). Axonal mitochondrial clusters containing mutant SOD1 in transgenic models of ALS. Antioxid Redox Signal.

[174] Spooren, W. P, & Hengerer, B. DNA laddering and caspase like activity in the spinal cord of a mouse model of familial amyotrophic lateral sclerosis. Cell Mol Biol (Noisy-le-grand) 46:63., 3.

[175] Spreux-veroquaux, O, Bensomon, G, & Lacomblez, l. (2002). Glutamate levels in cerebrospinal fluid in amyotrophic lateral sclerosis :reappraisal using a new HPLC method with coulometric detection in large cohort of patients. J Neurol Sci; , 193, 73-78.

[176] Sreedharan, J, Blair, I. P, Tripathi, V. B, Hu, X, Vance, C, Rogelj, B, Ackerley, S, Durnall, J. C, Williams, K. L, Buratti, E, Baralle, F, De Belleroche, J, Mitchell, J. D, Leigh, P. N, Al-chalabi, A, Miller, C. C, Nicholson, G, & Shaw, C. E. (2008). TDP-43 mutation in familial and sporadic amyotrophic lateral sclerosis. Science. , 319(5870), 1668-1672.

[177] Sta, M, Sylva-steeland, R. M, Casula, M, et al. (2011). Innate and adaptive immunity in amyotrophic lateral sclerosis : evidence of complement activation. Neurobiol. Dis.; , 42, 211-220.

[178] Sterneck, E, Kaplan, D. R, & Johnson, P. F. (1996). Interleukin-6 induces expression of peripherin and cooperates with Trk receptor signaling to promote neuronal differentiation in PC12 cells. J Neurochem.; 67:1365.

[179] Sturtz, L. A, Diekert, K, Jensen, L. T, Lill, R, & Culotta, V. C. (2001). A fraction of yeast Cu,Zn-superoxide dismutase and its metallochaperone, CCS, localize to the intermembrane space of mitochondria. A physiological role for SOD1 in guarding against mitochondrial oxidative damage. J Biol Chem.; , 276, 38084-38089.

[180] Sumi, H, Kato, S, Mochimaru, Y, Fujimura, H, Etoh, M, & Sakoda, S. (2009). Nuclear TAR DNA binding protein 43 expression in spinal cord neurons correlates with the clinical course in amyotrophic lateral sclerosis. J Neuropathol Exp Neurol 2009; 68:37.

[181] Tan, C. F, Eguchi, H, Tagawa, A, Onodera, O, Iwasaki, T, Tsujino, A, Nishizawa, M, Kakita, A, & Takahashi, H. (2007). TDP-43 immunoreactivity in neuronal inclusions in familial amyotrophic lateral sclerosis with and without SOD1 gene mutation. Acta Neuropathol. 113, (5): 535-542.

[182] Tan, C. F, Eguchi, H, Tagawa, A, Onodera, O, Iwasaki, T, Tsujino, A, Nishizawa, M, Kakita, A, & Takahashi, H. (2007). TDP-43 immunoreactivity in neuronal inclusions

in familial amyotrophic lateral sclerosis with or without SOD1 gene mutation. Acta Neuropathol. , 113, 535-542.

[183] Tanaka, Y, Kanai, Y, Okada, Y, Nonaka, S, Takeda, S, Harada, A, & Hirokawa, N. (1998). Targeted disruption of mouse conventional kinesin heavy chain, kif5B, results in abnormal perinuclear clustering of mitochondria. Cell; , 93, 1147-1158.

[184] Tollervey, J. R, Curk, T, Rogelj, B, Briese, M, Cereda, M, Kayikci, M, König, J, Hortobágyi, T, Nishimura, A. L, Zupunski, V, Patani, R, Chandran, S, Rot, G, Zupan, B, Shaw, C. E, & Ule, J. (2011). Characterizing the RNA targets and position-dependent splicing regulation by TDP-43. Nat. Neurosci. , 14, 452-458.

[185] Troost, D. Sillevis Smitt PA, de Jong JM, Swaab DF. (1992). Neurofilament and glial alterations in the cerebral cortex in amyotrophic lateral sclerosis. Acta Neuropathol; , 84(6), 664-73.

[186] Trotti, D, Rolfs, A, & Danbolt, N. C. (1999). SOD1 mutant linked to amyotrophic lateral sclerosis selectively inactivate a glial glutamate transporter. Nat Neurosci.; , 2, 427-433.

[187] Van Deerlin, V. M, Leverenz, J. B, Bekris, L. M, Bird, T. D, Yuan, W, Elman, L. B, Clay, D, Wood, E. M, Chen-plotkin, A. S, Martinez-lage, M, Steinbart, E, Mccluskey, L, Grossman, M, Neumann, M, Wu, I. L, Yang, W. S, Kalb, R, Galasko, D. R, Montine, T. J, Trojanowski, J. Q, Lee, V. M, Schellenberg, G. D, & Yu, C. E. (2008). TARDBP mutations in amyotrophic lateral sclerosis.with TDP-43 neuropathology: a genetic and histopathological analysis. Lancet Neurol. , 7(5), 409-416.

[188] Van Den Bosch LVandenbergerghe W, Klaassen H, Van Houtte E, Robberecht W. (2000). Ca (+2) permeable AMPA receptors and selective vulnerability of motor neurons. J Neurol Sci,; , 180, 29-34.

[189] Van Loo, G, Saelens, X, van Gurp, M, & Mac, M. . Martin, P. Vandenabeele. 2002. The role of mitochondrial factors in apoptosis: a Russian roulette with more than one bullet. Cell Death Differ.; 9:1031-42.

[190] Vance, C, Rogelj, B, Hortobágyi, T, De Vos, K. J, Nishimura, A. L, Sreedharan, J, Hu, X, Smith, B, Ruddy, D, Wright, P, Ganesalingam, J, Williams, K. L, Tripathi, V, Al-saraj, S, Al-chalabi, A, Leigh, P. N, Blair, I. P, Nicholson, G, De Belleroche, J, Gallo, J. M, Miller, C. C, & Shaw, C. E. (2009). Mutations in FUS, a RNA processing protein cause familial amyotrophic lateral sclerosis type 6. Science. , 323(5918), 1208-12011.

[191] Vande Velde CMiller TM, Cashman NR, Cleveland DW. (2008). Selective association of misfolded ALS-linked mutant SOD1 with the cytoplasmic face of mitochondria. Proc Natl Acad Sci U S A.; , 105, 4022-4027.

[192] Varadi, A, Johnson-cadwell, L. I, Cirulli, V, Yoon, Y, Allan, V. J, & Rutter, G. A. (2004). Cytoplasmic dynein regulates the subcellular distribution of mitochondria by

controlling the recruitment of the fission factor dynamin-related protein-1. J Cell Sci.; , 117, 4389-4400.

[193] Vijayvergiya, C, Beal, M. F, Buck, J, & Manfredi, G. (2005). Mutant superoxide dismutase 1 forms aggregates in the brain mitochondrial matrix of amyotrophic lateral sclerosis mice. J Neurosci.; , 25, 2463-2470.

[194] Vukosavic, S, Dubois-dauphin, M, Romero, M, N, & Przedborski, S. (1999). Bax and Bcl-2 interaction in a transgenic mouse model of familial amyotrophic lateral sclerosis. J Neurochem.; , 73, 2460-2468.

[195] Wajant, H. (2002). The Fas signaling pathway: more than a paradigm. Science; , 296, 1635-6.

[196] Wang, L, Sharma, K, Grisotti, K, G, & Roos, R. P. (2009). The effect of mutant SOD1 dismutase activity on non-cell autonomous degeneration in familial amyotrophic lateral sclerosis. Neurobiol. Dis. , 35, 234-240.

[197] Williams, T. L, Day, N. C, Ince, P. G, Kamboj, R. K, & Dhaw, P. J. (1997). Calcium permeable alpha-3hydroxy-5-methyl-4-isoxazole propionic acid receptors: a molecular determinant of selective vulnerability in amyotrophic lateral sclerosis. Ann Neurol; , 43, 200-207.

[198] Williamson, T. L, & Cleveland, D. W. (1999). Slowing of axonal transport is a very early event in the toxicity of ALS-linked SOD1 mutants to motor neurons. Nat Neurosci.; , 2, 50-56.

[199] Winton, M. J, Igaz, L. M, Wong, M. M, Kwong, L. K, Trojanowski, J. Q, & Lee, V. M. (2008). Disturbance of nuclear and cytoplasmatic TAR DNA-binding protein (TDP-43) induces disease-like redistribution, sequestration, and aggregrate formation. J. Biol. Chem. , 283, 13302-13309.

[200] Wong, N. K, He, B. P, & Strong, M. J. (2000). Characterization of neuronal intermediate filament protein expression in cervical spinal motor neurons in sporadic amyotrophic lateral sclerosis (ALS). J Neuropathol Exp Neurol; 59:972.

[201] Wong, P. C, Pardo, C. A, Borchelt, D. R, Lee, M. K, Copeland, N. G, Jenkins, N. A, Sisodia, S. S, Cleveland, D. W, & Price, D. L. (1995). An adverse property of a familial ALS-linked SOD1 mutation causes motor neuron disease characterized by vacuolar degeneration of mitochondria. Neuron.; , 14, 1105-1116.

[202] Xu, Y. F, Gendron, T. F, Zhang, Y. J, Lin, W. L, Alton, D, Sheng, S, Casey, H, Tong, M. C, Knight, J, Yu, J, Rademakers, X, Boylan, R, Hutton, K, Mcgowan, M, Dickson, E, Lewis, D. W, & Petrucelli, J. L. (2010). Wild type human TDP-43 expression causes TDP-43 phosphorylation, mitochondrial aggregation, motor deficits, and early mortality in transgenic mice. J. Neurosci. , 30, 10851-10859.

[203] Yaginuma, H, Sato, N, Homma, S, & Oppenheim, R. W. (2001). Roles of caspases in the programmed cell death of motoneurons in vivo. Arch Histol Cytol , 64, 461-474.

[204] Yokoseki, A, Shiga, A, Tan, C. F, Tagawa, A, Kaneko, H, Koyama, A, Eguchi, H, Tsujino, A, Ikeuchi, T, Kakita, A, Okamoto, K, Nishizawa, M, Takahashi, H, & Onodera, O. (2008). TDP-43 mutation in familial amyotrophic lateral sclerosis. Ann Neurol. , 63(4), 538-42.

[205] Zhang, B, Tu, P, Abtahian, F, Trojanowski, J. Q, & Lee, V. M. (1997). Neurofilaments and orthograde transport are reduced in ventral root axons of transgenic mice that express human SOD1 with a G93A mutation. J Cell Biol.; , 139, 1307-1315.

[206] Zhang, Y, Oko, R, & Van Der Hoorn, F. A. (2004). Rat kinesin light chain 3 associates with spermatid mitochondria. Dev Biol.; , 275, 23-33.

[207] Zhu, S, Stavrovskaya, I. G, Drozda, M, Kim, B. Y, Ona, V, Li, M, Sarang, S, Liu, A. S, Hartley, D. M, Wu, D. C, Gullans, S, Ferrante, R. J, Przedborski, S, Kristal, B. S, & Friedlander, R. M. (2002). Minocycline inhibits cytochrome c release and delays progression of amyotrophic lateralsclerosis in mice. Nature; , 417, 74-78.

Chapter 2

Multiple Routes of Motor Neuron Degeneration in ALS

Jin Hee Shin and Jae Keun Lee

Additional information is available at the end of the chapter

http://dx.doi.org/10.5772/56625

1. Introduction

Amyotrophic lateral sclerosis (ALS) is an adult-onset neurological disorder with higher selectivity in the degeneration of the upper and lower motor neurons, which leads to progressive paralysis of voluntary muscles. Although most cases fall under sporadic ALS (sALS), 10% of cases are inherited and known as familial ALS (fALS). The etiology of most ALS cases remains unknown, but mutations of ALS-linked Cu/Zn superoxide dismutase 1 (SOD1) are the most common causes of fALS and are responsible for its neurotoxicity and disease propagation due to the acquired toxic gain-of-function [1-2]. Studies in both human ALS patients and the transgenic ALS mouse model have delineated multiple pathological mechanisms of neuronal death that include genetic mutations, excitotoxicity, free radicals, apoptosis, inflammation, and protein aggregation. Targeting the multiple routes of the motor neuron degeneration is likely to contribute to the development of novel therapeutics for ALS patients.

2. Excitotoxicity

2.1. Glutamate neurotoxicity

Glutamate mediates excitatory synaptic transmission by activating the ionotropic glutamate receptors that are sensitive to N-methyl-D-aspartate (NMDA), α-amino-3-hydroxy-5-methyl-4-isoxazolepropionic acid (AMPA), or kainate. While the ionotropic glutamate receptors constitute fast excitatory synapses in the brain and the spinal cord, the glutamate receptors are excessively activated under pathological conditions such as hypoxic ischemia, trauma, and epilepsy, which triggers degeneration of neurons and oligodendrocytes. Extensive evidence supports the causative role of Ca^{2+}-permeable ionotropic glutamate receptors in motor neuron degeneration in ALS patients. Intracellular Ca^{2+} overload causes catastrophic neuronal death by impairing mitochondria or activating proteases, cytosolic phospholipase A2, kinases, endonucleases, and nuclear factor kappa B [3].

2.1.1. Abnormal glutamate re-uptake in ALS

Glutamate transporter 1 (GLT-1), also known as excitatory amino acid transporter 2 (EAAT2), and glutamate-aspartate transporter (GLAST), the primary transporters of glutamate into astrocytes, plays a central role in regulating the extracellular levels of glutamate [4-5]. The expression of GLT-1 was markedly reduced in the motor cortex and the spinal cord of sporadic and familial ALS patients [6]. In mutant SOD1 mice, the levels and the activity of EAAT2 were reduced in the spinal cord [7-8]. The levels of extracellular glutanmate increased in the plasma and the cerebrospinal fluid of ALS patients [9-10] and of mutant SOD1-expressing rodent models [7,11-12]. Reducing the expression of EAAT2 with antisense oligonucleotide reduced transporter activity induces neuronal death in vitro and in vivo [13]. Crossing transgenic mice that overexpress EAAT2 with SOD1G93A mice caused delayed motor deficit [14]. In addition, increasing the expression of GLT-1 significantly extended the survival of mutant SOD1 mice [15]. More recently, a sumoylated fragment of EAAT2 cleaved to by activating caspase-3 was shown to cause motor neuron death [16]. This implies that reduced glutamate uptake into astrocytes mediates degeneration of spinal motor neurons in ALS.

2.1.2. Mediation of motor neuron degeneration by the Ca^{2+} permeability of AMPA receptors

Ca^{2+}-permeable AMPA glutamate receptors appear to mediate chronic motor neuron degeneration in ALS. AMPA receptors consist of heteromeric combinations of four sub-units, GluR1-4 [17]. The glutamate (Q)/arginine (R)-editing of the GluR2 mRNA provides a positively charged form of GluR2 protein with arginine, which is responsible for Ca^{2+} impermeability [18]. When AMPA receptors contain reduced levels of Q/R-edited GluR2, the AMPA receptor complex becomes more permeable to Ca^{2+} [18]. The motor neuron of ALS patients showed evidence of defective editing of the pre-mRNA of GluR2 [19]. While lack of GluR2 accelerated motor neuron degeneration and shortened the life span of the SOD1 mice, overexpression of GluR2 delayed the disease onset and reduced the mortality of mutant SOD1 mice [20-21]. Moreover, the GluR2-N transgenic mice that expressed GluR2 gene encoding a asparagine at the Q/R site showed late-onset degeneration of the spinal motor neurons and motor function deficit [22]. Crossbreeding GluR2-N mice with mutant SOD1 mice aggravated motor neuron degeneration and shortened the survival time.

2.1.3. Therapies related to glutamate-mediated excitotoxicity

Although riluzole, the only approved disease-modifying therapy available to ALS patients since 1995, has been shown to inhibit glutamate release, subsequent studies demonstrated that riluzole inhibited AMPA receptors and presynaptic NMDA receptors [23-24]. Administration of riluzole significantly improved the motor neuron survival, motor function, and life expectancy of mutant SOD1 mice [25]. Similar beneficial effects of AMPA receptor antagonists such as memantine, 1,2,3,4-tetrahydro-6-nitro-2,3-dioxo-benzo[f]quinoxaline-7-sulfonamide (NBQX), and talampanel have been verified in mutant SOD1 mice [26-28]. The B-lactam antibiotic cefriaxone increased GLT-1 expression in spinal cord culture and in normal rats. The cefriaxone treatment delayed motor deficits with marginal survival in SOD1G93A mice [15]. An adaptive design Phase II/III study revealed good tolerability over 20 weeks [29]. The extened phase III of this study is ongoing.

3. Oxidative stress

3.1. Homeostasis and generation of free radicals in cells

Free radicals, including reactive oxygen species (ROS) and reactive nitrogen species (RNS), are characterized by unpaired electrons in their outer orbit. The most common cellular free radicals are hydroxyl (OH) radicals, superoxide (O_2^-) anions, and nitric monoxide (NO). Although hydrogen peroxide (H_2O_2) and peroxynitrite (ONOO-) are literally not free radicals, they are deemed to generate free radicals through various chemical reactions in many cases. Free radicals are cleared through several defense mechanisms, as follows: (1) catalytic removal of reactive species by enzymes such as superoxide dismutase, catalase, and peroxidase; (2) scavenging of reactive species by low-molecular-weight agents that were either synthesized in vivo (including glutathione, α-keto acids, lipoic acid, and coenzyme Q) or obtained from the diet [including ascorbate (vitamin C) and α-tocopherol (vitamin E)]; and (3) minimization of the availability of pro-oxidants such as transition metals [30]. CNS, which is mainly composed of polyunsaturated fatty acids (PUFAs), is readily susceptible to oxidative damage because the system demands a high metabolic oxidative rate with limited anti-oxidants and has a high transition metal content that acts as a potent pro-oxidant through the Haber-Weiss reaction or the Fenton reaction [51]. Upon shifting to pro-oxidants, CNS is promptly attacked by ROS that includes H_2O_2, NO, O_2^- , and highly reactive OH and NO and undergoes serious functional abnormality that is directly related to the demise of the course of neurons.

3.2. Evidence of oxidative stress in ALS

There is extensive evidence of the causative role of oxidative stress in motor neuron degeneration in ALS. The 3-nitrotyrosine(3-NT) level was elevated in subjects with both sporadic and familial cases of ALS, and the immunoreactivity of 3-NT became more evident within large motor neurons in the ventral horn of the lumbar spinal cord [31-32]. Higher carbonylation of proteins with the use of 2,4-dinitrophenylhydrazine (DNPH) was detected in the spinal cord in sporadic ALS [33]. Elevation of 8-hydroxy-2-deoxyguanosine (8-OHdG) was found in the CSF, serum, and urine of ALS patients [34]. The 4-hydroxynonenal level increased in the serum of ALS patients [35]. Transgenic ALS mice overexpression of the human mutant SOD1 revealed oxidative damage to proteins, lipids, and DNA [36-37].

3.2.1. Role of mitochondria in oxidative stress

Mitochondria produce ATP using about 90% of the O_2 that is taken up by neurons. During electron transfer in the inner membrane of the organelle, electrons spontaneously leak from the electron transport chain and react with available O_2 to produce superoxide, which makes mitochondria the major cellular sources of ROS. Mitochondria exist in the motor neurons due to the high rate of metabolic demand, which makes motor neurons more vulnerable to cumulative oxidative stress. Free radicals that accumulate over time decrease mitochondrial efficacy and increase the production of mutated mitochondrial DNA related to the aging process, although mitochondria have their own specific anti-oxidants that consist of SOD1, SOD2, glutathioneperoxidase, and peroxiredoxin 3 and can usually combat the high rate of ROS production [38]. Morphological abnormality in the organelle, which includes a fragmented network and swelling, and increased cristae have been observed in the soma and proximal axons of ventral motor neurons of sporadic ALS (sALS) patients [39]. In the axon and soma of motor neurons of mice that expressed $SOD1^{G93A}$ and $SOD1^{G37R}$ [40-41], membrane vacuoles derived from degenerating mitochondria were reported. Morphological alteration in mitochondria was also illustrated in NSC34 motor-neuron-like cells that expressed $SOD1^{G93A}$ [42-43]. Mutant SOD1 that was localized in mitochondria was associated with increased oxidative damage, decreased respiratory activity of the mitochondria, and architectural change. The interaction of mutant SOD1 and mitochondria was enough to result in motor neuron death in neuroblastoma cells [44]. Mitochondrial SOD1 and its chaperone protein named copper chaperone for SOD1 (CCS) are co-localized in the mitochondrial inter-membrane space [45]. The aggregates of mutant SOD1 were shown within the mitochondria in the spinal cord of $SOD1^{G93A}$ mice before the onset of the symptoms [46-47] and were implicated in increased oxidative damage, decreased respiratory activity of mitochondria [48], and mitochondrial swelling and vacuolization [47].

3.2.2. Role of transition metals in oxidative stress

Redox-active transition metals are useful but harmful trace elements. Copper and iron are abundant (~0.1-0.5 mM) in the brain and have been implicated in the generation of ROS in various neurodegenerative diseases that include Alzheimer's disease and Parkinson's disease [49-50]. These transition metals mediate the formation of a hydroxyl radical through the iron-catalyzed or copper-catalyzed Haber-Weiss reactions [51]. Once copper ions are transported into the cell, they must be delivered to specific targets (e.g., SOD1 and cytochrome c oxidase) or stored in copper scavenging systems (e.g., GSH and metallothioneins) [52-53]. When these events are out of control, the cells have an uncomfortable abundance of toxic and radical-generating metal ions. FALS-linked SOD1 mutation has weaker binding affinity to copper ions, which are readily libertated to increase oxidative stress in cells expressed with fALS-SOD1 [54]. The detrimental role of copper in fALS pathogenesis was supported by several experiments that used copper chelators, which delayed the disease onset and prolonged the survival of fALS-G93A mice [55], prevented peroxidase activity by expressing fALS-SOD1 A4V and G93A in vitro [56], and reduced elevated ROS production in the lymphoblasts of fALS patients [57]. Iron is vital for all living organisms because it has an essential role in oxygen transport and electron transfer, and is a cofactor in many enzyme systems that include DNA synthesis. Iron homeostasis and its regulatory system [58] was readily disrupted in the development and progress of neurodegenerative diseases such as AD or PD [59-60]. Recently, several pieces of evidence supported the concept that iron is dysregulated in ALS. An increased ferritin level

http://dx.doi.org/10.5772/56625

was observed in the serum of sporadic ALS patients, which suggests a possible risk factor and the disturbance of iron homeostasis [61-62]. Ferritin was upregulated just prior to the end-stage disease in SOD1-G93A mice, which supports increased Fe levels [63]. In the same animal model, increased iron was evident in the spinal cord at the ages of 90 and 120 days, with the onset of the symptoms and in the late stage, due to the disease progress. The increased iron levels were attenuated by iron chelators, which improved the motor function and the survival [64]. mRNAs associated with iron homeostasis (e.g., DMT1, TfR1, the iron exporter Fpn, and CP) also increased with a caudal-to-rostral gradient, with the highest levels rostrally in the cervical region in SOD1G37R [65]. HFE protein is a membrane protein that can influence cellular iron uptake, and mutated HFE is well recognized in haemochromatosis, a genetic disorder due to the irregular accumulation of free forms of Fe in parenchymal tissue. In studies of sporadic ALS patients, both the prevalence of HFE mutation and its polymorphisms (e.g., H63D) were evident [66-67]. Therefore, HFE polymorphisms in ALS may be associated with the altered Fe homeostasis and oxidative stress in this disease. Although abnormal iron homeostasis was evident, the iron regulation mechanisms for motor neuron death must be explained.

3.2.3. *Possible mechanisms related to oxidative stress in ALS*

Human SOD1 mutation has a toxic gain-of-function that may be due to loss of the active site of copper binding that converts the SOD1 itself to pro-oxidant proteins and participates in ROS generation [68]. Several pieces of evidence have been suggested to show that higher interaction of mutant SOD1 with mitochondria may induce mitochondrial dysfunction and selectively lead to excessive oxidative stress in motor neurons [46]. Reduced transcription factor nuclear erythroid 2-related factor 2 (Nrf2) mRNA and protein expression has been reported in the spinal cord of ALS patients [69]. Crossbreeding SOD1G93A mice with overexpressed Nrf2 extended their survival [70], which suggests that increasing the Nef2 activity may be a novel therapeutic target. Nrf2 activation increases the expression of anti-oxidant proteins due to its interaction with the anti-oxidant-response element (ARE) after its translocation to the nucleus. In another reported mechanism of oxidative stress, the activity of NADPH oxidase (Nox) increased in both sALS patients and mutant SOD1 mice. Expressed Nox in activated microglia may influence motor neuron death. Deletion of either Nox1 or Nox2 prolonged the survival of mutant SOD1G93A mice [71-72]. Protein aggregation is a common pathological feature in ALS patients and animal ALS models. TAR DNA-binding protein-43 (TDP-43) or mutant SOD1 is a constituent of inclusions in ALS patients and mutant SOD1 mice [73-74]. Mutant SOD1 itself caused oxidative damage of proteins in mutant SOD1 mice [37].

3.2.4. *Therapeutic drugs for oxidative stress in ALS*

Several anti-oxidants have been tested using animal ALS models (Table 1). Completed, ongoing, or planned trials explored, are exploring, or will explore the value of anti-oxidants. Vitamin E, the most potent natural scavenger of ROS and RNS, delayed their clinical onset and slowed the disease progression in mutant SOD1 mice [25]. Long-term vitamin E supplements reduced the risk of death from ALS in ALS-free subjects [75-76]. Unfortunately, two vitamin

E clinical trials failed to show the vitamin's efficacy in ALS patients due to impermeable BBB penetration [77]. Creatine, N-acetylcysteine, AEOL-10150, and edarabone have successfully improved the motor function and survival of mutant SOD1 mice [78-81]. Creatine and N-acetylcystein were not effective in the clinical trial phase II.

4. Apoptosis

4.1. Evidence of apoptosis in ALS

Kerr et al. (1972)[82] reported electron microscopic features of shrinkage necrosis or apoptosis that are expected to play a role in the regulation of the number of cells under physiological and pathological conditions. The apoptotic cells were accompanied by condensation of the nucleus and the cytoplasm, nuclear fragmentation, and aggregated condensation of nuclear chromatin. Interestingly, apoptosis is prevented by inhibitors of protein and mRNA synthesis, and thus, appears to require the expression and activation of death-regulating proteins in neurons and non-neuronal cells [83-84]. The morphological and molecular features of apoptosis have been reported in the nervous system during the development of various neurological diseases. Apoptosis is probably correlated with the demise of motor neurons in ALS. Degenerating motor neurons in the spinal cord and the motor cortex are illustrated by the dark and shrunken cytoplasm and nuclei, chromatin condensation, and apoptotic bodies in the cells. Various pro-apoptosis proteins are activated in the ALS-injured area, and protein synthesis inhibitors attenuate ALS-related neuronal death.

4.1.1. Death receptor Fas

The death receptor Fas (CD95 or APO-1) belongs to the tumor necrosis factor (TNF) receptor superfamily and functions as a key determinant of cell fate under physiological and pathological conditions [86-87]. The Fas ligand (Fas-L) activates Fas in an autocrine or paracrine manner, which leads to the trimerization of Fas with Fas-associating protein within the death domain (FADD) and procaspase-8. Fas activation has been shown as an obligatory step in apoptosis in neurons deprived of trophic factors [88-90]. Fas antibodies were more frequently found in the serum of sporadic or familial ALS patients than in that of the normal controls [91], which also induced apoptosis in the human neuroblastoma cell line and in neuron-glia co-cultured cells of the spinal cord of rat embryos [92]. Primary motor neurons of mouse embryos that expressed mutant SOD1 were susceptible to Fas-induced death [93]. Continuous silencing of the Fas receptor on the motor-neuron-ameliorated motor function and survival of SOD1G93A mice using small interfering RNA-mediated interference supported the role of Fas-linked motor neuron degeneration in ALS [94]. In SOD1G93A mice, a Fas pathway is required to allow Fas interaction with FADD, which in turn recruits caspase-8 as one of the downstream effectors. In addition, TIMP-3 controls Fas-mediated apoptosis by inhibiting the MMP-3-mediated shedding activity in the Fas ligand on the cell surface [95]. The FASS/FADD-mediated motor neuron degeneration was attenuated by Lithium treatment in SOD1G93A

http://dx.doi.org/10.5772/56625

mice [96]. A Fas/NO feedback loop with downstream Daxx and P38 was proposed as another Fas pathway of motor neuron death in mutant SOD1 mice [97].

4.1.2. Pro-apoptotic family of Bcl-2

The physiological and pathological roles of the Bcl-2 family have been extensively reviewed [98-99]. The physical balance between anti-apoptotic and pro-apoptotic members of the Bcl-2 family generally appears to determine the fate of developing and mature cells. Anti- and pro-apoptotic proteins are separated by the presence or absence of Bcl-2 homology (BH) domains. There are four domains: BH1-BH4. Bcl-2 and Bcl-xL contain all four domains and are anti-apoptotic. The pro-apoptotic Bcl-2 family includes Bax, Bcl-x_s, Bak, Bad, and Bid and participates in the neuronal death process. Unbalanced pro- or anti-apoptotic proteins activate caspase-realted apoptosis by releasing cytochrome c into cytosol. Bax is oligomerized, inserted into the outer membrane of mitochondria, and shown to induce cytochrome c release [100-101]. The ratio of the apoptotic cell death genes Bax to Bcl-2 increases at both the mRNA and protein levels in the spinal motor neurons of ALS patients and SOD1G93A mice [102-104]. Interestingly, mutant SOD1 was highly associated with Bcl-2 in the mitochondria, which resulted in conformational or phenotypic change of Bcl-2 that weakened the mitochondria in the spinal cord [105]. Blunt Bcl-2 may contribute to the activation of the mitochondrial apoptosis machinery such as caspase-9, caspase 3, and cytochrome c in the spinal motor neurons of ALS transgenic mice and humans with ALS [106-107]. To support this idea, Bcl-2 overexpression or Bax depletion crossbred with SOD1G93A mice delayed the onset of symptoms and extended the life expectancy [108-109].

4.1.3. Caspase cascade

Caspases, a family of cysteine-dependent aspartate-directed proteases, mediate the propagation and execution of apoptosis. They can be classified into initiator caspases and effector caspases [110]. Caspase-9 is an initiator caspase and is proteolytically activated by apaf-1, a cytoplasmic protein that is homologous to ced-4, and by cytochrome c. The latter is located in the intermembrane space of the mitochondria and released into the cytoplasm by the pro-apoptotic Bcl-2 (e.g., Bax) that is transported from the cytoplasm into the mitochondria in the early phase of apoptosis. Caspase-8, which is known as another initiator caspase, is activated through the interaction of procaspase-9 with the Fas receptor and the FADD adapter. Activated caspase-8 and caspase-9 can activate downstream caspases such as caspase-3, 6, and 7 that can cleave to a number of proteins that are essential to the structure, signal transduction, and cell cycle and terminate the overall apoptosis process. Under the ER (endoplasmic reticulum) stress, caspase-12 is activated with the cleavage (activation) of caspase-9 and caspase-3, regardless of the release of cytochrome c. Marginally, ER stress triggers caspase-8 activation, which results in a mitochondria-mediated pathway via Bid cleavage. The caspase-1, -3, and -9 activities were higher in the motor neurons of the spinal cord or the motor cortex of ALS patients than in those of the control [107,111]. Caspase-1 truncated Bid to be highly reactive [106]. The orderly activation of caspase-1 and -3 was evident, and their mRNAs were abundant in animal ALS models [111-112]. The sequential activation of caspase-9 to caspase-7 was required for the mitochondria-dependent apoptosis pathway in a rodent ALS model [107]. Moreover, caspase-9 was simultaneously activated with a death receptor pathway that contained Fas, FADD, caspase-8, and caspase-3 in the ALS mice after their motor neuron death began [95-96]. Cleaved forms of caspase-12 were expressed presymptomatically in animal models, which shows evidence of ER stress [113]. A more advanced mechanism than that with caspases revealed that caspases such as caspase-3 or caspase-7 mediated TDP-43 cleavage [114], which was observed immunologically in an aggregated form in the cytoplasmic inclusions in ALS. Intraventricular administration of zVAD-fmk, a broad-spectrum caspase inhibitor, prolonged the survival of G93ASOD1 mice [111], which supports the causative role of caspase cascade in motor neuron death.

4.1.4. Anti-apoptotic drugs served as therapy for ALS

Even though minocycline has anti-inflammatory effects that prevent microglia proliferation, the drug prevented apoptotic motor neuron death by inhibiting cytochrome c release in mutant SOD1 mice [115]. The beneficial effects were proven in several studies to prolong survival and ameliorate the motor function [115-117]. Minocycline accelerated disease progression in a clinical trial, though [118]. TCH-346, a molecule that binds to glyceraldehyde 3-phosphate dehydrogenase (GAPDH), was used in small samples in a Phase II/III randomized trial, but it did not show beneficial effects [119].

5. Inflammation

5.1. Microglia and astrocyte

Microglia activation is an early event in all forms of pathology. Thus, activated microglia was initially considered a sensitive marker to identify sites that were predestined for tissue. The classical bone-marrow-derived microglial cells dwell in the gray matter and have ramified (highly branched) structures with a small portion of perinuclear cytoplasm and a small, dense, and heterochromatic nucleus. In many CNS pathologies, the cells increase, and this may arise from either local proliferation or recruitment from the blood, or both. The morphology of microglia becomes reactive under pathological conditions that were determined as infiltration of blood-derived cells, local BBB [120], or presence of damaged neurons. Microglia near areas of neuronal injury tend to have more amoeboid features with intense cell bodies and reduced numbers of shortened and thick processes [121] that lead to a structural morphology similar to that of macrophages. A shift in the active style of microglia affects neural, vascular, and blood-borne cells due to several secretions that include pro-inflammatory cytokines and chemokines, nitric oxide, and reactive oxygen intermediates. Astrocytes have many essential physiological functions in the CNS such as provision of trophic support for neurons, conduct of synaptic formation and plasticity, and regulation of the cerebral blood flow. Due to their strategic structure, they are in close contact with CNS resident cells and blood vessels [122-123]. An inflammatory insult causes proliferation of astrocytes and morphological changes. Astroglial activation is recognized via increased expression of the intermediate filament glial fibrillary acidic protein (GFAP) and the marker aldehyde dehydrogenase 1 family, member L1 (ALDH1L1). Although astrocytes are not immune cells, they can contribute to the immune response in pathological conditions. Microgliosis and astrocytosis are promient features of neurodegenerative diseases that include AD, PD, and ALS.

5.2. Evidence of inflammation in ALS

Several studies have shown the possibility that glial cells adjacent to degenerating motor neurons, mainly primed microglia and astrocytes, have causative roles in the course of disease propagation in ALS. Massive gliosis is apparent in pathologically vulnerable departments of CNS in both human ALS patients and ALS animal models [124-125]. Microglia antibodies have also been found in the CSF of an ALS patient [126]. Recently, the presence of activated microglia was visualized via positron emission tomography (PET), using [^{11}C](R)-PK11195, in the motor cortex, dorsolateral prefrontal cortex, thalamus, and pos of living patients [127]. In the presymptomatic stage of the disease, TNF-α and M-CSF expression increased in a transgenic ALS model. Interestingly, the increase in the expressed TNF-α was found to be correlated to the severity of motor neuron loss [128]. The elevation of TNF-α and of its two receptors [TNFRI (p55TNF) and TNFRII (p75TNF)] was observed in the serum of ALS patients, unlike in those of healthy controls [129]. To date, primed microglia-sensitive intracellular signaling that affectas ALS is authorized by the activation of p38 mitogen-activated protein kinase (p38MAPK), the translocation of the transcription factor NF-κB into the nucleus, and the upregulation of COX-2. The activation of NF-κB regulates the transcription of a wide range of inflammation-related genes that include inducible nitric oxide synthesis (iNOS), COX-2, MCP-1, MMP-9, IL-2, IL-6, IL-8, IL-12p40, IL-2 receptor, ICAM-1, TNF-α, and IFN-γ [130], which leads to the secretion of many inflammatory mediators. The aforementioned genes were shown to have changed in the tissues of ALS patients and hSOD1 transgenic mice [128,131-133]. COX-2 is inducible and is a rate-limiting enzyme of the synthesis pathways of the prostaglandins (PG) PGD_2, PGE_2, PGF_2a, and PGI_2 and thromboxane (TXA_2). Prostaglandins play a role in various cellular effectors that include the instigation of inflammatory responses, the re-arrangement of cytoskeletons, and gene transcription changes [134]. COX-2 expression was significantly elevated in motor neuron and glial cells in the spinal cord of ALS patients [135-136], and the COX-2 activity increased in the spinal cord of ALS patients [137]. In addition, the PGE_2 levels jumped up in the CSF of ALS patients by two to 10 times, compared with the controls [137]. The deletion of the prostaglandin E(2) EP2 receptor in SOD1G93A mice improved their motor function and prolonged their survival, which suggests that PGE2 signalling via the EP2 receptor acts as an inflammatory mediator in motor neuron degeneration [138].

5.2.1. Non-cell-autonomous neurotoxicity in ALS

Aside from degenerating motor neurons, microglia and astrocytes concomitantly play a role in disease progression in ALS model mice. Recent reports emphasized the potential role of non-cell-autonomous mechanisms, which are harmonious with and critical in SOD1G93A-induced cell-autonomous death signals [139-140]. Either neuron-specific or glia-specific expression of SOD1 mutation in mice led to the ALS phenotype, with marginal effects [141-142]. Specific expression of mutant SOD1 within neurons using *Nefl* (neurofilament light chain) promoters did not cause motor neuron degeneration in transgenic mice [142]. Consistently, selective expression of mutant SOD1 in microglia or astrocytes did not kill motor neurons [141,143].These non-cell-autonomous deaths of motor neurons were supported by an analysis of chimeric mice that had mixed populations of normal cells and cells that expressed mutant SOD1 [144]. Conditional knockout of mutant SOD1 in motor neurons using an *Isl1* promoter-driven *Cre* transgene that is expressed in the spinal cord delayed the disease onset in and prolonged the survival of mutant SOD1 transgenic mice. On the other hand, however, selective removal from cells of the myeloid lineage that included microglia using a *Cd11b* promoter-driven *Cre* transgene did not delay the disease onset but extended its progress [139]. In the same lineages, selective viral vector-mediated delivery of small interfering RNAs against human SOD1 in motor neurons delayed the disease onset but did not modify the disease progression once it started [145], whereas silencing of mutant SOD1 within myeloid cells or astrocytes slowed the disease progression rather than the disease onset [139-140]. After all the bone marrow of mutant-SOD1-expressing $PU^{-/-}$ mice, which lacked myeloid and lymphoid cells, were replaced with wild-type-SOD1 bone marrow, their disease progression and survival improved [143], which suggests that microglia and astrocytes were not sufficient for the initiation of motor neuron death, but hastened the disease progression.

5.2.2. Systemic inflammation

Damaged or aged brains continuously suffer from systemic inflammation connected with peripheral factors, regardless of the presence of innate inflammation in the CNS [146-147]. Three critical components are directly correlated with the synthesis of cytokines and inflammatory mediators in the brain parenchyma to communicate an inflammatory signal to the brain and to trigger tissue injury. First, inflammatory responses in the thoracic-abdominal cavity are transduced into the brain via vagal-nerve sensory afferents, and then the outflow of a vagal efferent seems to manipulate these events through acetylcholine secretion, which acts on alpha 7 nicotinic receptors of macrophages [148]. Second, cytokines and inflammatory mediators from the specific area of the inflammation are put into the blood and communicate with macrophages and other cells in the circumventricular organs, which lack a patent blood-brain barrier [149]. Third, the cytokines or inflammatory mediators themselves might directly communicate with the brain endothelium via receptors expressed on the endothelium [150]. Several pieces of evidence showed that a systemic immune response is related to a clinically symptomatic feature of a neurodegenerative disease such as AD. In accordance with frequently circulating cytokines in the blood or CSF of AD patients, the abundance of pro-inflammatory factors preceded the clinical onset of dementia in the subjects [151]. Aged people with systemic infections have a double risk of developing AD. Similarly, the correlation of clinical events with systemic immunity was experimentally evaluated in an animal that was challenged with systemic stimulation. Infection of aged rats with LPS revealed neuronal loss in the brain and the memory deficits [152]. Thus, it can be said that systemic inflammation contributes to the onset and progression of neurodegenerative diseases. In recent clinical and pathological studies, ALS patients revealed dysregulation of their systemic inflammatory components, which belonged to alterations in their microglia/macrophage activation profiles [153]; elevated levels of complementary proteins in their sera [154]; increased IL-13-producing T cells and circulating neutrophils [155-156]; and higher production of $CD8^+$ T cells in the lymphocytes [157]. Monocyte chemoattractant protein (MCP)-1 and RANTES were abundant in the cerebrospinal fluid and sera of ALS patients [158-161]. Increased MCP-1 was shown in the microglia of mutant SOD1 mice [162-163]. Moreover, the higher LPS level in the plasma of ALS patients was proportional to the total abnormally activated monocyte/macrophage contents of the peripheral blood [164]. Long-term exposure to LPS also furthered the disease progression in animal ALS models, which implies that systemic inflammation connected to peripheral factors and innate immunity in the CNS concurrently influences the disease course [165]. With aging, the blood-brain barrier (BBB) is less tight and thus, more vulnerable to systemic inflammation. The collapse of BBB or of the blood-spinal cord barrier (BSCB) was shown in animal ALS models or human ALS patients using evans blue leakage and immunohistochemistry against the anti-CD44 antibody, respectively [166-167]. Under these conditions, peripheral-inflammation-inducing factors were very apparent in the CNS and thereby affected the neurodegeneration.

5.2.3. *Therapies for inflammation in ALS*

Minocycline, which is believed to attenuate microglia activation, or celecoxib, a cox-2 inhibitor, showed beneficial effects in mutant SOD1 mice [115-117,168-169]. Clinical studies on the two drugs did not disprove, however, their therapeutic property in ALS patients. Thalidomide, glatiramer acetate, and ONO-2506 also supported the causative role of the inflammation in the pathology in ALS mice that showed improved motor function and survival [170-171], but their beneficial effects were not linked to the ALS patients.

6. Mitochondrial pathology in ALS

Mitochondria constitute approximately 25% of the cytoplasmic volume in most eukaryotic cells and produce cellular energy in the form of ATP via electron transport and oxidative phosphorylation. During electron transfer in the inner membrane of the organelle, electrons spontaneously leak from the electron transport chain and react with available O_2 to produce superoxide, which makes mitochondria the major cellular sources of ROS. Mitochondria have been recognized as target organelles for the regulation and execution of cell death under pathological conditions [172-173]. There are many mitochondria in the motor neurons because of the high rate of metabolic demand therein, which implies that motor neurons are susceptible to functional or morphological alteration in mitochondria. Mtochondrial abnormality may play a crucial role in the pathologic mechanism of motor neuron diseases and of ALS. Studies with ALS patients and animal ALS models have been performed to examine both the morphologic and functional abnormalities of the mitochondria [174]. Morphological abnormality in the organelle that includes a fragmented network, swelling, and increased cristae has been observed in the soma and proximal axons of ventral motor neurons of sporadic ALS (sALS) patients [39]. In ALS patients, a reduction in complex IV of the electron transport chain activity was evident and has been associated with mutations in mitochondrial DNA [175-176]. Although SOD1 is mainly localized in cytosols, it is also resilient in other subcellular compartments such as the mitochondria [45,177-178] and even the endoplasmic reticulum [182]. The aggregates of mutant SOD1 were shown within the mitochondria of the spinal cord of $SOD1^{G93A}$ mice before the onset of symptoms [46-47] and were implicated in increased oxidative damage, decreased respiratory activity of mitochondria [48], and the appearance of mitochondrial swelling and vacuolization [47]. Dissociated cytochrome c from the interaction of mitochondria with mutant SOD1 activates apoptosis [44]. Mitochondria function as reservoirs of intracellular Ca^{2+}, as ER. Once overloaded in cytosol, the accumulated Ca^{2+} in the mitochondria prepares the organelle to undergo permeability transition, and then swells and ruptures in their outermembrane, which in turn produces free radicals from them and oxidizes their lipids and DNA [179-180]. Ca^{2+}-induced mitochondrial damage can also result in mitochondrial release of cytotoxic substances such as cytochrome c [181] and can affect caspase cascade. The homeostasis at the intracellular Ca^{2+} level was also disturbed in motor neurons of SOD1G93A mice [182]. Moreover, increased Ca^{2+} uptake into the mitochondria of motor neurons easily occurred after exposure to the glutamate agonist AMPA or kinate, and triggered increased ROS generation [183]. ALS-linked SOD1 has been shown to slow down fast axonal transport of mitochondria. The axonal mitochondria transport was primarily reduced in the anterograde direction, which suggests that the energy supply in the presynaptic terminals of the motor endplates is compromised [184]. Multiple functions of the mitochondria over cellular injury and the apearance of mitochondrial dysfunction in the presymptomatic stage may contribute to various routes of neuronal death in ALS. More recently, in mice that expressed human TDP-43 only in neurons that included motor neurons, massive accumulation of mitochondria in TDP-43-negative cytoplasmic inclusions in the motor neurons were reported and the lack of mitochondria in the motor axon terminal was observed [185]. In addition, the transgenic mice that overexpressed human TDP-43 driven by the mouse prion promoter demonstrated motor deficits, early mortality, and mitochondrial aggregation [186]. These results imply that TDP-43 is indirectly involved in mitochondrial dysfunction in neurodegenerative diseases such as ALS.

7. Autophagy in ALS

Autophagy is a degradative mechanism that is involved in the recycling and turnover of long-life proteins and organelles [187]. Autophagy is basically induced by lack of nutrients and energy or by various toxicants. Although its primary role is adaptation to scarcity, this degradative process is also critical for the normal turnover of cytoplasmic contents that include neurons. Genetic ablation of autophagy-related genes provokes neurodeneration even with lack of disease-like mutant proteins [188]. Recent studies verified the importance of the autophagy pathway in various pathological conditions that include neurodegenerative diseases [189]. Interestingly, the catabolic process is both beneficial and detrimental to cells, depending on its context and specific stimuli. The lethality of mutated SOD1 is the result of abnormal protein aggregates, which impair the degradation machinery such as the ubiqutinproteasome system and the autophay-lysosome pathway [190-191]. Enhancing the latter with physiological characteristics prevents motor neuron dysfunction in vivo [192-193]. Defects in the autophagy pathway have a principal disease-causing role in human pathologies that include neurodegeneration [189,194]. Studies of the spinal motor neurons of ALS patients [195] and ALS transgenic mice [196] have delineated the abnormality in autophagy, which is probably correlated with the pathogenesis of the disease [192-193,197]. A growing number of studies support the concept that autophagy makes diseased motor neurons healthy by clearing the aggregated mutant SOD1, which was accomplished by inducing autophagy, as illustrated by the increased number of autophagosomes and the higher level of autophagy markers such as Beclin-1, ATG5-ATG12 complex, and LC3-II [192-193]. It is also possible, however, that blunt autophagy in neurodegenerative conditions was accompanied by the abnormal accumulation of autophagosomes and excessive markers, which might have killed the neurons [197-198] and which indicates the compensatory role of autophagy in inherited ALS. Thus, the detailed molecular mechanism of the development of autophagy-mediated diseases must be explained.

8. Therapeutic strategy for ALS

8.1. Separate routes of motor neuron degeneration in ALS

The parallel pathway of oxidative stress and Fas-mediated apoptosis in motor neuron death in SOD1G93A mice was previously focused on [96]. This study provided the first evidence that combination therapy that targets oxidative stress and apoptosis together also delays the onset and progression of motor dysfunction and extends the survival time of ALS transgenic mice. Evidence was accumulated that shows that oxidative stress and apoptotic insults cause neuronal death through distinctive pathways and with unique morphological changes. The neurotrophins' nerve growth factor, the brain-derived neurotrophic factor (BDNF), neurotrophin 3 (NT-3), and NT-4/5, and the insulin-like growth factors IGF-I and IGF-II, promote neuronal survival by preventing programmed cell death or apoptosis, but they significantly enhance necrotic degeneration of neurons exposed to oxidative stress or deprived of oxygen and glucose [199-200]. Neurotrophins can induce oxidative stress by upregulating NADPH oxidase, which leads to neuronal cell necrosis [201]. Surprisingly, the insulin-like growth factor 1 (IGF-1) prevented neuronal cell apoptosis and protected spinal motor neurons in ALS mice [199,202], but markedly potentiated neuronal cell necrosis induced by hydroxyl radicals or glutathione depletion [203]. Given that oxidative stress and apoptosis play a central role in motor neuron degeneration and can contribute to neuronal death through distinctive routes in ALS, it was hypothesized that a therapeutic approach that targets both oxidative stress and apoptosis would have additive effects on neuronal survival and the motor function. To pharmacologically prevent oxidative stress and apoptosis, Neu2000, a novel anti-oxidant, and Li^+, a well-known anti-apoptosis agent, were used. The former, a chemical derivative of aspirin and sulfasalazine, was developed to protect neurons from oxidative stress with greater potency and safety, and has been shown to be a potent and secure anti-oxidant in vitro and in animal models of hypoxic ischemia [204]. Li^+ has been shown to prevent apoptosis through mecha-

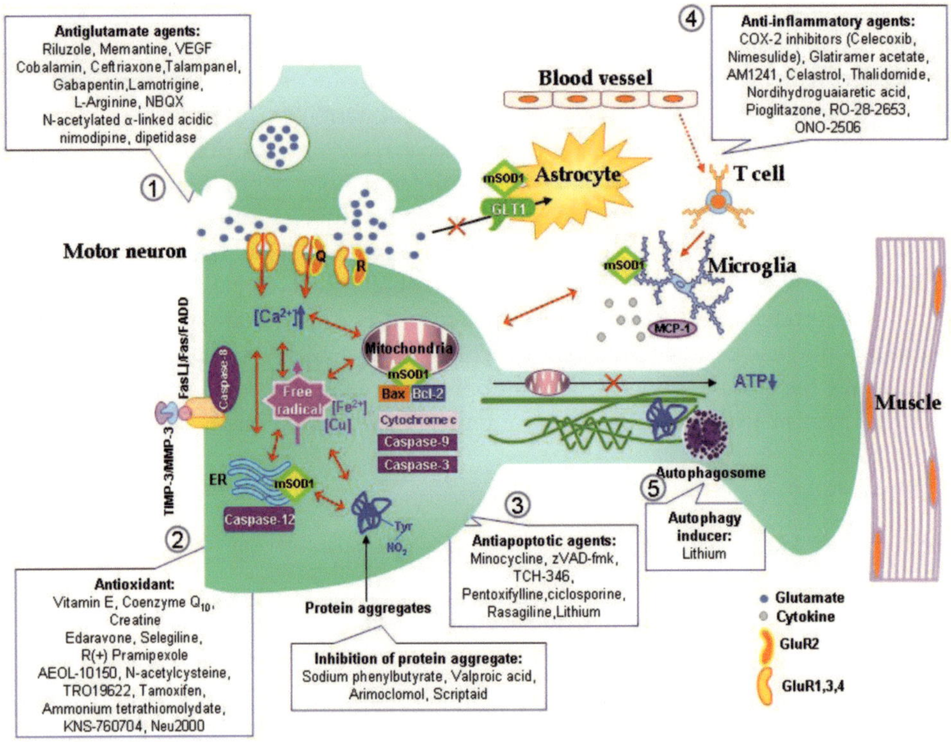

Figure 1. Multiple pathways of motor neuron degeneration and their therapeutic drugs in ALS: (1) increased Ca^{2+} in the motor neuron: dysfunction or downregulation of glutamate transporters such as GLT1 on the astrocytes, elevation of the Ca^{2+} permeable AMPA receptor via downregulation of or a deficit in the post-transcriptional edition of GluR2 sub-units, and mitochondrial dysfunction; (2) oxidative damage of the motor neuron: increased intracellular Ca^{2+} contents, high levels of mitochondria due to high energy demand, and increase in free metal ions such as copper and iron; (3) apoptosis in the motor neuron: activation of the Fas-mediated pathway, alteration of Bcl-2 family proteins via mitochondrial interaction with mSOD1, and initiation, propagation, or execution of caspase cascade; (4) inflammation: non-cell-autonomous motor neuron death (the disease progression is coordinated by mSOD1 expression in all neuronal and non-neuronal cells) and concurrent activation of the innate immune system and systemic inflammation (BBB breakdown may induce a vicious cycle of inflammation); and (5) autophagy: increased autophagosome formation.Current therapeutic drugs were developed basically against a specific route of ALS disease progression.

nisms that involve Bcl-2 upregulation, glycogen synthase kinase-3 beta inhibition, and activation of phosphatidylinositol 3-kinase that activates serine/threonine kinase Akt-1 and phospholipase C gamma [205-206]. An additional benefit of Li+ was recently demonstrated the induction of an autophagy pathway at a low dose, clears altered mitochondria and protein aggregates [192]. In the results of this study, the concurrent administration of Neu2000 and Li $^{+}$, which block free-radical-mediated necrosis and Fas-mediated apoptosis, respectively, significantly delayed the onset and progression of motor neuron degeneration and motor function deficits. Thus, targeting both oxidative stress and the Fas apoptosis pathway with concurrent treatment with Neu2000 and Li^{+} may further improve the neurological function

Compound	Dose	Administration route	Hypothetical mechanism	Survival	Reference
Creatine	1%	diet	Antioxidant	9%	Klivenyi P et al., 1999 [78]
	2%	diet	Antioxidant	17%	
Creatine	2%	diet	Antioxidant	20%	Klivenyi P et al., 2004 [169]
creatine	2%	diet	Antioxidant	12%	Zhang W et al., 2003 [117]
Vitamin E	200 IU	chow	Antioxidant	No effect	Gurney ME et al., 1996 [125]
Edaravone	5 mg/kg	ip	Antioxidant	12.4%	Ito H et al., 2008 [81]
	15 mg/kg	ip		17%	
AEOL-10150	2.5 mg/kg	ip	Antioxidant	26%	Crow JP et al., 2005 [80]
	2.5 mg/kg	sc		22%	
N-acetylcysteine	2 mg/kg/d	drinking water	Antioxidant	7%	Andreassen OA et al., 2000 [79]
TRO19622 (Olesoxime)	3 mg/kg	sc	Antioxidant	10%	Bordet T et al., 2007 [209]
	30 mg/kg	sc		8%	
Ammonium tetrathiomolybdate	5 mg/kg	not described	Antioxidant	25%	Tokuda E et al., 2008 [210]
Neu2000	30 mg/kg	diet	Antioxidant	15%	Shin et al., 2007 [96]
zVAD			Antiapoptotic	22%	Li et al., 2000 [111]
Cyclosporin A	18mg/kg	intrathecal	Antiapoptotic	12%	Keep M et al., 2001 [211]
Minocycline	25 mg/kg	ip	Antiapoptotic/Anti-inflammator	10%	Van Den Bosch L et al., 2002 [116]
	50 mg/kg	ip		15.8%	
Minocycline	11 mg/kg		Antiapoptotic/Anti-inflammator	9%	Zhu S et al., 2002 [115]
Minocycline	22mg/kg/d	ip	Antiapoptotic/Anti-inflammator	13%	Zhang W et al., 2003 [117]
Lithium	1 mEq/kg	ip	Antiapoptotic/Autophagy induce	36%	Fornai F et al., 2007 [192]
Lithium	60 mg/kg	ip	Antiapoptotic/Autophagy induce	8%	Feng H et al., 2008 [212]
Lithium	2%	diet	Antiapoptotic/Autophagy induce	10%	Shin et al., 2007 [96]
Celecoxib	1500ppm	chow	Anti-inflammatory	25%	Drachman DB et al., 2002 [168]
Celecoxib	0.012%	diet	Anti-inflammatory	21%	Klivenyi P et al., 2004 [169]
Thalidomide	50 mg/kg		Anti-inflammatory	12%	Kiaei M et al., 2006 [213]
	100 mg/kg			16%	
Glatiramer acetate	7ug/0.1 ml PBS	immunization	Anti-inflammatory	1.4%	Banerjee R et al., 2008 [171]
AM1241	1 mg/kg	ip	Anti-inflammatory	3%	
Celastrol	8 mg/kg	diet	Anti-inflammatory	13%	Kiaei M et al., 2005 [213]
	2 mg/kg			9.4%	
Nordihydroguaiaretic acid	2500ppm	po	Anti-inflammatory	10%	West M et al., 2004 [214]
RO-28-2653	100 mg/kg	po	Anti-inflammatory	11%	Lorenzl S et al., 2006 [215]
Riluzole	100ug/ml	drinking water	Antiglutamatergic	10%	Gurney ME et al., 1996 [117]
Riluzol	30 mg/kg	drinking water	Antiglutamatergic	11%	Waibel et al., 2004 [224]
Gabapentin	3%	chow	Antiglutamatergic	5%	Gurney ME et al., 1996 [117]
Memantine	10 mg/kg	subcutaneus	Antiglutamatergic	7%	Wang et al., 2005 [216]
Memantine	30 mg/kg	drinking water	Antiglutamatergic	5%	Joo IS et al., 2007 [26]
	90 mg/kg	drinking water		1%	
vegf	1.0 ug/kg	ip	Antiglutamatergic	8%	Zheng C et al., 2004 [217]
		Lentiviral vecor	Antiglutamatergic	30%	Azzouz M et al., 2004 [218]
Ceftriaxone	200 mg/kg	ip	Antiglutamatergic	10%	Rothstein JD et al., 2005 [219]
L-Arginine	6%	drinking water	Antiglutamatergic	20%	Lee J et al., 2009 [220]
N-acetylated a-linked acidic dipetidase	30 mg/kg	po	Antiglutamatergic	15%	Ghadge GD et al., [221]

Table 1. List of drugs tested with ALS mice

and neuronal survival in ALS and possibly other neurological diseases such as stroke, Alzheimer's disease, and Parkinson's disease. The authors' hypothesis was supported by other experiments in which a cocktail of neuroprotective drugs with different modes of action more significantly improved survival and the motor function than did monotherapy in transgenic mouse ALS models [117,207].

8.2. Current treatment and new approach of ALS medications

Riluzole, the only therapeutic drug approved for ALS, extends life expectancy to up to 3 months in human patients. The symptomatic drug potentially targets gluatamate- or oxidative-stress-induced neurodegeneration with marginal apoptosis effects [25]. As mentioned,

Compound	Dose	Survival	Reference
Creatine	2%	12%	Zhang W et al., 2003 [117]
Minocycline	22mg/kg	13%	
Creatine/Minocycline		25%	
Creatine	2%	20%	Klivenyi P et al., 2004 [169]
Celecoxib	0.012%	21%	
Rofecoxib	0.005%	19%	
Creatine/Celecoxib		29%	
Creatine/Rofecoxib		31%	
Rasagiline	2 mg/kg	14%	Waibel et al., 2004 [224]
Riluzol	30 mg/kg	11%	
Rasagiline/Riluzol		20%	
Neu2000	30 mg/kg	15%	Shin et al., 2007 [96]
Lithium	2%	10%	
Neu2000/Lithium	2%	22%	
Lithium	60 mg/kg	8%	Feng H et al., 2008 [212]
Valproic acid	300 mg/kg	10%	
Lithium/ VPA		15%	
Riluzole		7.5%	Del Signore Sj et al., 2009 [222]
Sodium phenylbutyrate		12.8%	
Riluzole/Sodium phenylbutyrate		21.5%	
Minocycline/ Riluzole/ Nimodipine	80 + 40 +30 (mg/kg)	13%	Kriz et al., 2003 [223]

Table 2. Additive effect of combination therapy in ALS mice

therapeutic strategies and drugs developed based on them, as shown in Figure 1, explain the multiple-disease-causing process of ALS. As shown in Table 1, many drugs were evaluated in mice that expressed mutant SOD1. Most of the drugs were beneficial to the motor function and survival in the tests with the mice. Several drugs (such as creatine, celecoxib, gabapentin, topiramate, lamotrigine, minocycline, thalidomide, valproate, vitamin E, and even lithium) showed beneficial effects in animal ALS models, but none of them significantly prolonged the survival or improved the quality of life of human ALS patients. The therapeutic effects on the animal models and the human patients significantly differed due to the following translational mismatch issues: first, the methological inappropriateness of the drug screening with the use of animals that had biological confounding variables such as sex and differences in the treatment initiation time point; second, the lack of correct pharmacokinetics, which were considered in a dose-ranging study of safety/toxicity and BBB penetration; and finally, the methodological pitfall of ALS clinical trials due to the insufficiency of the number of patients, the inclusion of heterogeneous populations, the short duration of the trial, and the inadequate analysis of the efficacy. It should be noted that the combination of creatine and celecoxib improved the motor function in a randomized clinical phase II trial of ALS patients and SOD1G93A mice, although single treatment with either creatine or celecoxib failed to show beneficial effects in human ALS trials [208], which suggests the greater efficacy of combined anti-oxidant and NSAID therapy than those of monotherapy. Several pieces of evidence support the notion that therapeutic combinations are more effective than individual agents in animal ALS models (Table2). More recently, the authors reported that a single agent named

AAD-2004, which has a dual mode of action as an anti-oxidant and an mPGES-1 inhibitor, had better efficacy on the motor function and survival than those of riluzole and ibuprofen.

In support of such a notion, a phase II clinical trial was recently conducted, which showed that the suggested strategy may be feasible and efficient.

9. Conclusion

In ALS, knowledge of the contribution of multiple pathways to the degeneration of motor neurons has expanded greatly and has challenged clinical trials of drugs that target the processes. Better understanding of the detrimental processes that cause neurodegeneration will help define its medical importance and clarify the therapeutic potential of interfering with them.

Author details

Jin Hee Shin[1*] and Jae Keun Lee[2]

*Address all correspondence to: ppzini@hanmail.net

1 GNT Pharma, South Korea

2 School of Life Science and Biotechnology, Korea University, South Korea

References

[1] Rosen, D.R. Sapp, P. O'Regan, J. McKenna-Yasek, D. Schlumpf, K.S. Haines, J.L. Gusella, J.F. Horvitz, H.R. & Brown, R.H. Jr. Genetic linkage analysis of familial amyotrophic lateral sclerosis using human chromosome 21 microsatellite DNA markers. Am J Med Genet. 1994 May;15(51): 61-69.

[2] Gurney, M.E. Transgenic-mouse model of amyotrophic lateral sclerosis. N Engl J Med. 1994 Dec 22;331(25):1721-1722.

[3] Won SJ, Kim DY, Gwag BJ. Cellular and molecular pathways of ischemic neuronal death. J Biochem Mol Biol. 2002 Jan 31;35(1):67-86

[4] Nicholls D, Attwell D. The release and uptake of excitatory amino acids. Trends Pharmacol Sci. 1990 Nov;11(11):462-468.

[5] Barbour B, Brew H, Attwell D. Electrogenic glutamate uptake in glial cells is activated by intracellular potassium. Nature. 1988 Sep 29;335(6189):433-435.

[6] Rothstein, J.D. Van Kammen, M. Levey, A.I. Martin, L.J. & Kuncl, RW. Selective loss of glial glutamate transporter GLT-1 in amyotrophic lateral sclerosis. Ann Neurol. 1995 Jul; 38(1):73-84.

[7] Bendotti, C. Tortarolo, M. Suchak, S.K. Calvaresi, N. Carvelli, L. Bastone, A. Rizzi, M, Rattray M. & Mennini, T. Transgenic SOD1 G93A mice develop reduced GLT-1 in spinal cord without alterations in cerebrospinal fluid glutamate levels. J Neurochem. 2001 Nov;79(4):737-746.

[8] Canton, T. Pratt, J. Stutzmann, J.M. Imperato, A. & Boireau, A. Glutamate uptake is decreased tardively in the spinal cord of FALS mice. Neuroreport. 1998 Mar;309(5): 775-778.

[9] Rothstein, J.D. Tsai, G. Kuncl, R.W. Clawson, L. Cornblath, D.R. Drachman, D.B. Pestronk, A. Stauch, B.L. & Coyle, J.T. Abnormal excitatory amino acid metabolism in amyotrophic lateral sclerosis. Ann Neurol. 1990 Jul;28(1):18-25.

[10] Shaw, P.J. Forrest, V. Ince, P.G. Richardson, J.P. & Wastell, H.J. CSF and plasma amino acid levels in motor neuron disease: elevation of CSF glutamate in a subset of patients. Neurodegeneration. 1995 Jun;4(2):209-216.

[11] Bruijn, L.I. Becher, M.W. Lee, M.K. Anderson, K.L. Jenkins, N.A. Copeland, N.G. Sisodia, S.S. Rothstein, J.D. Borchelt, D.R. Price, D.L. & Cleveland, D.W. ALS-linked SOD1 mutant G85R mediates damage to astrocytes and promotes rapidly progressive disease with SOD1-containing inclusions. Neuron. 1997 Feb;18(2):327-338.

[12] Howland, D.S. Liu, J. She, Y. Goad, B. Maragakis, N.J. Kim, B. Erickson, J. Kulik, J. DeVito, L. Psaltis, G. DeGennaro, L.J. Cleveland, D.W. & Rothstein, J.D. Focal loss of the glutamate transporter EAAT2 in a transgenic rat model of SOD1 mutant-mediated amyotrophic lateral sclerosis (ALS). Proc Natl Acad Sci U S A. 2002 Feb 5;99(3): 1604-1609.

[13] Rothstein JD, Dykes-Hoberg M, Pardo CA, Bristol LA, Jin L, Kuncl RW, Kanai Y, Hediger MA, Wang Y, Schielke JP, Welty DF. Knockout of glutamate transporters reveals a major role for astroglial transport in excitotoxicity and clearance of glutamate. Neuron. 1996 Mar;16(3):675-686.

[14] Guo H, Lai L, Butchbach ME, Stockinger MP, Shan X, Bishop GA, Lin CL. Increased expression of the glial glutamate transporter EAAT2 modulates excitotoxicity and delays the onset but not the outcome of ALS in mice. Hum Mol Genet. 2003 Oct 1;12(19):2519-2532.

[15] Rothstein, J.D. Patel, S. Regan, M.R. Haenggeli, C. Huang, Y.H. Bergles, D.E. Jin, L. Dykes Hoberg, M. Vidensky, S. Chung, D.S. Toan, S.V. Bruijn, L.I. Su, Z.Z. Gupta, P. & Fisher, P.B. Beta-lactam antibiotics offer neuroprotection by increasing glutamate transporter expression. Nature. 2005 Jan 6433 ; 7021 : 73-77.

[16] Foran E, Bogush A, Goffredo M, Roncaglia P, Gustincich S, Pasinelli P, Trotti DMotor neuron impairment mediated by a sumoylated fragment of the glial glutamate transporter EAAT2. Glia. 2011 Nov;59(11):1719-1731.

[17] Hollmann, M. & Heinemann, S. Cloned glutamate receptors. Annu. Rev. Neurosci. 1994;17:31-108.

[18] Burnashev, N. Monyer, H. Seeburg, P.H. & Sakmann, B. Divalent ion permeability of AMPA receptor channels is dominated by the edited form of a single subunit. Neuron. 1992 Jan; 8(1):189-198.

[19] Kawahara, Y. Ito, K. Sun, H. Aizawa, H. Kanazawa, I. & Kwak, S. Glutamate receptors: RNA editing and death of motor neurons. Nature. 2004 Feb;26427(6977): 801.

[20] Van Damme P. Braeken, D. Callewaert, G. Robberecht, W. & Van Den Bosch, L. GluR2 deficiency accelerates motor neuron degeneration in a mouse model of amyotrophic lateral sclerosis. Neuropathol Exp Neurol. 2005 Jul;64(7):605-612.

[21] Tateno, M. Sadakata, H. Tanaka, M. Itohara, S. Shin, RM. Miura, M. Masuda, M. Aosaki, T. Urushitani, M. Misawa, H. & Takahashi, R. Calcium-permeable AMPA receptors promote misfolding of mutant SOD1 protein and development of amyotrophic lateral sclerosis in a transgenic mouse model. Hum Mol Genet. 2004 Oct;113(19): 2183-2196.

[22] Kuner, R. Groom, A.J. Müller, G. Kornau, H.C. Stefovska, V. Bresink, I. Hartmann, B. Tschauner, K. Waibel, S. Ludolph, A.C. Ikonomidou, C. Seeburg, P.H. & Turski, L. Mechanisms of disease: motoneuron disease aggravated by transgenic expression of a functionally modified AMPA receptor subunit. Ann N Y Acad Sci. 2005 Aug; 1053:269-286.

[23] Lamanauskas N and Nistri A. Riluzole blocks persistent Na+ and Ca2+ currents and modulates release of glutamate via presynaptic NMDA receptors on neonatal rat hypoglossal motoneurons in vitro.Eur J Neurosci. 2008 May;27(10):2501-2514.

[24] Albo F, Pieri M, Zona C. Modulation of AMPA receptors in spinal motor neurons by the neuroprotective agent riluzole. J Neurosci Res. 2004 Oct 15;78(2):200-207.

[25] Gurney ME, Cutting FB, Zhai P, Doble A, Taylor CP, Andrus PK, Hall ED. Benefit of vitamin E, riluzole, and gabapentin in a transgenic model of familial amyotrophic lateral sclerosis. Ann Neurol. 1996 Feb;39(2):147-157.

[26] Joo IS, Hwang DH, Seok JI, Shin SK, Kim SU. Oral administration of memantine prolongs survival in a transgenic mouse model of amyotrophic lateral sclerosis. J Clin Neurol. 2007 Dec;3(4):181-186.

[27] Van Damme P, Leyssen M, Callewaert G, Robberecht W, Van Den Bosch L. The AMPA receptor antagonist NBQX prolongs survival in a transgenic mouse model of amyotrophic lateral sclerosis. Neurosci Lett. 2003 Jun 5;343(2):81-84.

[28] Paizs M, Tortarolo M, Bendotti C, Engelhardt JI, Siklós L. Talampanel reduces the level of motoneuronal calcium in transgenic mutant SOD1 mice only if applied presymptomatically. Amyotroph Lateral Scler. 2011 Sep;12(5):340-384.

[29] Gutteridge, J.M. & Halliwell, B. Free radicals and antioxidants in the year 2000. A historical look to the future. Ann N Y Acad Sci. 2000;899:136-147.

[30] Halliwell, B & Gutteridge, J.M. Oxygen toxicity, oxygen radicals, transition metals and disease. Biochem. J. 1984 Apr 1;219(1):1-14.

[31] Beal, M.F. Ferrante, R.J. Browne, S.E. Matthews, R.T. Kowall, N.W. & Brown, R.H. Jr. (1997) Increased 3-nitrotyrosine in both sporadic and familial amyotrophic lateral sclerosis. Ann Neurol. 1997 Oct 42;4:644-654.

[32] Abe, K. Pan, L.H. Watanabe, M. Konno, H. Kato, T. & Itoyama, Y. Upregulation of protein-tyrosine nitration in the anterior horn cells of amyotrophic lateral sclerosis. Neurol Res. 1997 Apr 19;2(12):4-8.

[33] Poon, H.F. Hensley, K. Thongboonkerd, V. Merchant, M.L. Lynn, B.C. Pierce, W.M. Klein, J.B. Calabrese, V. & Butterfield, D.A. Redox proteomics analysis of oxidatively modified proteins in G93A-SOD1 transgenic mice--a model of familial amyotrophic lateral sclerosis. Free Radic Biol Med. 2005 Aug;1539(4):453-462.

[34] Bogdanov M, Brown RH, Matson W, Smart R, Hayden D, O'Donnell H, Flint Beal M, Cudkowicz M. Increased oxidative damage to DNA in ALS patients. Free Radic Biol Med. 2000 Oct 1;29(7):652-658.

[35] Simpson EP, Henry YK, Henkel JS, Smith RG, Appel SH. Increased lipid peroxidation in sera of ALS patients: a potential biomarker of disease burden. Neurology. 2004 May 25;62(10):1758-1765.

[36] Ferrante, R.J. Browne, S.E. Shinobu, L.A. Bowling, A.C. Baik, M.J. MacGarvey, U. Kowall, N.W. Brown, R.H. Jr & Beal, MF. Evidence of increased oxidative damage in both sporadic and familial amyotrophic lateral sclerosis. J Neurochem. 1997 Nov; 69(5):2064-2074.

[37] Andrus PK, Fleck TJ, Gurney ME, Hall ED. Protein oxidative damage in a transgenic mouse model of familial amyotrophic lateral sclerosis. J Neurochem. 1998 Nov;71(5): 2041-2048.

[38] Starkov, A.A. The role of mitochondria in reactive oxygen species metabolism and signaling. Ann N Y Acad Sci. 2008 Dec;1147:37-52.

[39] Sasaki, S. & Iwata, M. Mitochondrial alterations in the spinal cord of patients with sporadic amyotrophic lateral sclerosis. J Neuropathol Exp Neurol. 2007 Jan;66(1): 10-16.

[40] Dal Canto, M.C. & Gurney, M.E. Neuropathological changes in two lines of mice carrying a transgene for mutant human Cu,Zn SOD, and in mice overexpressing wild

type human SOD: a model of familial amyotrophic lateral sclerosis (FALS). Brain Res. 1995 Apr;3676(1):25-40.

[41] Wong, P.C. Pardo, C.A. Borchelt, D.R. Lee, M.K. Copeland, N.G. Jenkins, N.A. Sisodia, S.S. Cleveland, D.W. & Price, D.L. An adverse property of a familial ALS-linked SOD1 mutation causes motor neuron disease characterized by vacuolar degeneration of mitochondria. Neuron. 1995 Jun;14(6):1105-1116.

[42] Menzies, F.M. Cookson, M.R. Taylor, R.W. Turnbull, D.M. Chrzanowska-Lightowlers, Z.M. Dong, L. Figlewicz, D.A. & Shaw, P.J. Mitochondrial dysfunction in a cell culture model of familial amyotrophic lateral sclerosis. Brain. 2002 Jul;125(Pt 7): 1522-1533.

[43] Raimondi, A. Mangolini, A. Rizzardini, M. Tartari, S. Massari, S. Bendotti, C. Francolini, M. Borgese, N. Cantoni, L. & Pietrini, G. Cell culture models to investigate the selective vulnerability of motoneuronal mitochondria to familial ALS-linked G93ASOD1. Eur J Neurosci. 2006 Jul;24(2):387-399.

[44] Takeuchi H, Kobayashi Y, Ishigaki S, Doyu M, Sobue G. Mitochondrial localization of mutant superoxide dismutase 1 triggers caspase-dependent cell death in a cellular model of familial amyotrophic lateral sclerosis. J Biol Chem. 2002 Dec 27;277(52): 50966-50972

[45] Okado-Matsumoto, A. & Fridovich, I. Subcellular distribution of superoxide dismutases (SOD) in rat liver: Cu,Zn-SOD in mitochondria. J Biol Chem. Vol. 19276, No. 42, (Oct 2001), pp.38388-38393.

[46] Liu J, Lillo C, Jonsson PA, Vande Velde C, Ward CM, Miller TM, Subramaniam JR, Rothstein JD, Marklund S, Andersen PM, Brännström T, Gredal O, Wong PC, Williams DS, Cleveland DW. Toxicity of familial ALS-linked SOD1 mutants from selective recruitment to spinal mitochondria. Neuron. 2004 Jul 8;43(1):5-17.

[47] Jaarsma, D. Rognoni, F. van Duijn, W. Verspaget, H.W. Haasdijk, E.D. & Holstege, J.C. CuZn superoxide dismutase (SOD1) accumulates in vacuolated mitochondria in transgenic mice expressing amyotrophic lateral sclerosis-linked SOD1 mutations. Acta Neuropathol. 2001 Oct;102(4):293-305.

[48] Mattiazzi, M. D'Aurelio, M. Gajewski, CD. Martushova, K. Kiaei, M. Beal, MF. & Manfredi, G. Mutated human SOD1 causes dysfunction of oxidative phosphorylation in mitochondria of transgenic mice. J Biol Chem. 2002 Aug;16277(33): 29626-29633.

[49] Deibel, M. A., Ehmann, W. D., and Markesbery, W. R., Copper, iron, and zinc imbalances in severely degenerated brain regions in Alzheimer's disease: possible relation to oxidative stress. 1996 Nov;143(1-2):137-142.

[50] Youdim, M. B., Ben-Shachar, D., and Riederer, P., The possible role of iron in the etiopathology of Parkinson's disease. Mov. Disord., 1993;8(1):1-12.

[51] Haber, F. and Weiss, J., The catalytic descomposition of hydrogen peroxide by iron salts, Proc. R. Soc., London A 147, 332, 1934.

[52] Rae, T.D. Schmidt, P.J. Pufahl, R.A. Culotta, V.C. & O'Halloran, T.V. Undetectable intracellular free copper: the requirement of a copper chaperone for superoxide dismutase. Science.1999 Apr;30284(5415):805-808.

[53] Puig, S. & Thiele, D.J. Molecular mechanisms of copper uptake and distribution. Curr Opin Chem Biol. 2002 Apr;6(2):171-180.

[54] Hayward, L.J. Rodriguez, J.A. Kim, J.W. Tiwari, A. Goto, J.J. Cabelli, D.E. Valentine, J.S. & Brown, R.H. Jr. Decreased metallation and activity in subsets of mutant superoxide dismutases associated with familial amyotrophic lateral sclerosis. J Biol Chem. 2002 May;3277(18):15923-15931.

[55] Hottinger, A.F. Fine, E.G. Gurney, M.E. Zurn, A.D. & Aebischer, P. The copper chelator d-penicillamine delays onset of disease and extends survival in a transgenic mouse model of familial amyotrophic lateral sclerosis. Eur J Neurosci. 1997 Jul;9(7): 1548-1551.

[56] Wiedau-Pazos, M. Goto, J.J. Rabizadeh, S. Gralla, E.B. Roe, J.A. Lee, M.K. Valentine, J.S. & Bredesen, D.E. Altered reactivity of superoxide dismutase in familial amyotrophic lateral sclerosis. Science. 1996 Jan;26271(5248):515-518.

[57] Said Ahmed, M. Hung, W.Y. Zu, J.S. Hockberger, P. & Siddique, T. Increased reactive oxygen species in familial amyotrophic lateral sclerosis with mutations in SOD1. J Neurol Sci. 2000 Jan;15176(2):88-94.

[58] Bishop, G.M. Robinson, S.R. Liu, Q. Perry, G. Atwood, C.S. & Smith, M.A. Iron: a pathological mediator of Alzheimer disease? Dev Neurosci. 2002;24(2-3):184-187.

[59] Zecca, L. Youdim, MB. Riederer, P. Connor, J.R. & Crichton, R.R. Iron, brain ageing and neurodegenerative disorders. Nat Rev Neurosci. 2004 Nov;5(11):863-873.

[60] Berg, D. Gerlach, M. Youdim, M.B. Double, K.L. Zecca, L. Riederer, P. & Becker, G. Brain iron pathways and their relevance to Parkinson's disease. J Neurochem. 2001 Oct;79(2):225-236.

[61] Qureshi, M. Brown, R.H. Jr. Rogers J.T. & Cudkowicz, M.E. Serum ferritin and metal levels as risk factors for amyotrophic lateral sclerosis. Open Neurol J 2008 Sep 12;2:51-54.

[62] Goodall, E.F. Haque, M.S. & Morrison, K.E. Increased serum ferritin levels in amyotrophic lateral sclerosis (ALS) patients. J Neurol. 2008 Nov;255(11):1652-1656.

[63] Olsen, M.K. Roberds, S.L. Ellerbrock, B.R. Fleck, T.J. McKinley, D.K. & Gurne,y M.E. Disease mechanisms revealed by transcription profiling in SOD1-G93A transgenic mouse spinal cord. Ann Neurol. 2001 Dec;50(6):730-740.

[64] Wang, Q. Zhang, X. Chen, S. Zhang, X. Zhang, S. Youdium, M. & Le, W. Prevention of motor neuron degeneration by novel iron chelators in SOD1(G93A) transgenic mice of amyotrophic lateral sclerosis. Neurodegener Dis. 2011;8(5):310-321.

[65] Jeong, S.Y. Rathore, K.I. Schulz, K. Ponka, P. Arosio, P. & David, S. Dysregulation of iron homeostasis in the CNS contributes to disease progression in a mouse model of amyotrophic lateral sclerosis. J Neurosci. 2009 Jan 21;29(3):610-619.

[66] Wang, X.S. Lee, S. Simmons, Z. Boyer, P. Scott, K. Liu, W. & Connor, J. Increased incidence of the Hfe mutation in amyotrophic lateral sclerosis and related cellular consequences. J Neurol Sci. 2004 Dec;15227(1):27-33.

[67] Goodall, E.F. Greenway, M.J. van Marion, I. Carroll, C.B. Hardiman, O. & Morrison, K.E. Association of the H63D polymorphism in the hemochromatosis gene with sporadic ALS. Neurology. 2005 Sep;2765(6):934-937.

[68] Yim HS, Kang JH, Chock PB, Stadtman ER, Yim MB. A familial amyotrophic lateral sclerosis-associated A4V Cu, Zn-superoxide dismutase mutant has a lower Km for hydrogen peroxide. Correlation between clinical severity and the Km value. J Biol Chem. 1997 Apr 4;272(14):8861-8863.

[69] Sarlette A, Krampfl K, Grothe C, Neuhoff N, Dengler R, Petri S. Nuclear erythroid 2-related factor 2-antioxidative response element signaling pathway in motor cortex and spinal cord in amyotrophic lateral sclerosis. J Neuropathol Exp Neurol 2008 Nov;67(11):1055-1062.

[70] Vargas MR, Johnson DA, Sirkis DW, Messing A, Johnson JA. Nrf2 activation in astrocytes protects against neurodegeneration in mouse models of familial amyotrophic lateral sclerosis. J Neurosci. 2008 Dec 10;28(50):13574-13581.

[71] Wu DC, Ré DB, Nagai M, Ischiropoulos H, Przedborski S. The inflammatory NADPH oxidase enzyme modulates motor neuron degeneration in amyotrophic lateral sclerosis mice. Proc Natl Acad Sci U S A. 2006 Aug 8;103(32):12132-12137.

[72] Marden JJ, Harraz MM, Williams AJ, Nelson K, Luo M, Paulson H, Engelhardt JF. Redox modifier genes in amyotrophic lateral sclerosis in mice. J Clin Invest. 2007 Oct; 117(10):2913-2919.

[73] Neumann M, Sampathu DM, Kwong LK, Truax AC, Micsenyi MC, Chou TT, Bruce J, Schuck T, Grossman M, Clark CM, McCluskey LF, Miller BL, Masliah E, Mackenzie IR, Feldman H, Feiden W, Kretzschmar HA, Trojanowski JQ, Lee VM. Ubiquitinated TDP-43 in frontotemporal lobar degeneration and amyotrophic lateral sclerosis. Science. 2006 Oct 6;314(5796):130-133.

[74] Shan X, Vocadlo D, Krieger C. Mislocalization of TDP-43 in the G93A mutant SOD1 transgenic mouse model of ALS. Neurosci Lett. 2009 Jul 17;458(2):70-74.

[75] Wang H, O'Reilly ÉJ, Weisskopf MG, Logroscino G, McCullough ML, Schatzkin A, Kolonel LN, Ascherio A. Vitamin E intake and risk of amyotrophic lateral sclerosis: a

pooled analysis of data from 5 prospective cohort studies. Am J Epidemiol. 2011 Mar 15;173(6):595-602.

[76] Ascherio A, Weisskopf MG, O'reilly EJ, Jacobs EJ, McCullough ML, Calle EE, Cudkowicz M, Thun MJ. Vitamin E intake and risk of amyotrophic lateral sclerosis. Ann Neurol. 2005 Jan;57(1):104-110.

[77] Pappert EJ, Tangney CC, Goetz CG, Ling ZD, Lipton JW, Stebbins GT, Carvey PM. Alpha-tocopherol in the ventricular cerebrospinal fluid of Parkinson's disease patients: dose-response study and correlations with plasma levels. Neurology. 1996 Oct;47(4):1037-1042.

[78] Klivenyi P, Ferrante RJ, Matthews RT, Bogdanov MB, Klein AM, Andreassen OA, Mueller G, Wermer M, Kaddurah-Daouk R, Beal MF. Neuroprotective effects of creatine in a transgenic animal model of amyotrophic lateral sclerosis. Nat Med. 1999 Mar;5(3):347-350.

[79] Andreassen OA, Dedeoglu A, Klivenyi P, Beal MF, Bush AI. N-acetyl-L-cysteine improves survival and preserves motor performance in an animal model of familial amyotrophic lateral sclerosis. Neuroreport. 2000 Aug 3;11(11):2491-2493.

[80] Crow JP, Calingasan NY, Chen J, Hill JL, Beal MF. Manganese porphyrin given at symptom onset markedly extends survival of ALS mice. Ann Neurol. 2005 Aug;58(2): 258-265.

[81] Ito H, Wate R, Zhang J, Ohnishi S, Kaneko S, Ito H, Nakano S, Kusaka H. Treatment with edaravone, initiated at symptom onset, slows motor decline and decreases SOD1 deposition in ALS mice. Exp Neurol. 2008 Oct;213(2):448-455.

[82] Kerr, J. F., Wyllie, A. H., and Currie, A. R. Apoptosis: a basic biological phenomenon with wide-ranging implications in tissue kinetics, Br. J. Cancer, 1972 Aug;26(4): 239-257.

[83] Wyllie, A. H., Morris, R. G., Smith, A. L., and Dunlop, D. Chromatin cleavage in apoptosis: association with condensed chromatin morphology and dependence on macromolecular synthesis, J. Pathol. 1984 Jan;142(1):67-77.

[84] Martin, D. P., Schmidt, R. E., DiStefano, P. S., Lowry, O. H., Carter, J. G., and Johnson, E. M. Inhibitors of protein synthesis and RNA synthesis prevent neuronal death caused by nerve growth factor deprivation, J. Cell Biol. 1988 Mar;106(3):829-844.

[85] Martin, LJ. Neuronal death in amyotrophic lateral sclerosis is apoptosis: possible contribution of a programmed cell death mechanism. J Neuropathol Exp Neurol. 1999 May;58(5):459-471.

[86] Nagata, S. Apoptosis by death factor. Cell. 1997 Feb 7;88(3):355-365.

[87] Strasser, A., O'Connor, L., and Dixit, V. M. Apoptosis signaling, Annu. Rev. Biochem. 2000;69:217-245.

[88] Cheema, Z. F., Wade, S. B., Sata, M., Walsh, K., Sohrabji, F., and Miranda, R. C. Fas/Apo [apoptosis]-1 and associated proteins in the differentiating cerebral cortex: induction of caspase-dependent cell death and activation of NF-kappaB, J. Neurosci. 1999 Mar 1;19(5):1754-1770.

[89] Le-Niculescu, H., Bonfoco, E., Kasuya, Y., Claret, F. X., Green, D. R., and Karin, M. Withdrawal of survival factors results in activation of the JNK pathway in neuronal cells leading to Fas ligand induction and cell death. Mol. Cell Biol. 1999 Jan;19(1): 751-763.

[90] Raoul, C., Henderson, C. E., and Pettmann, B. Programmed cell death of embryonic motoneurons triggered through the Fas death receptor, J. Cell Biol. 1999 Nov 29;147(5):1049-1062.

[91] Sengun, I.S. & Appel, S.H. Serum anti-Fas antibody levels in amyotrophic lateral sclerosis. J Neuroimmunol. 2003 Sep;142(1-2):137-140.

[92] Yi, F.H. Lautrette, C. Vermot-Desroches, C. Bordessoule, D. Couratier, P. Wijdenes, J. Preud'homme, J.L. & Jauberteau, M.O. In vitro induction of neuronal apoptosis by anti-Fas antibody-containing sera from amyotrophic lateral sclerosis patients. J Neuroimmunol. 2000 sep;22109(2):211-220.

[93] Raoul, C. Estévez, A.G. Nishimune, H. Cleveland, D.W. deLapeyrière, O. Henderson, C.E. Haase, G. & Pettmann, B. Motoneuron death triggered by a specific pathway downstream of Fas. potentiation by ALS-linked SOD1 mutations. Neuron.2002 Sep; 1235(6):1067-1083.

[94] Locatelli F, Corti S, Papadimitriou D, Fortunato F, Del Bo R, Donadoni C, Nizzardo M, Nardini M, Salani S, Ghezzi S, Strazzer S, Bresolin N, Comi GP. Fas small interfering RNA reduces motoneuron death in amyotrophic lateral sclerosis mice. Ann Neurol. 2007 Jul;62(1):81-92.

[95] Lee, J.K. Shin, J.H. Suh, J. Choi, I.S. Ryu, K.S. & Gwag, B.J. Tissue inhibitor of metalloproteinases-3 (TIMP-3) expression is increased during serum deprivation-induced neuronal apoptosis in vitro and in the G93A mouse model of amyotrophic lateral sclerosis: a potential modulator of Fas-mediated apoptosis. Neurobiol Dis. 2008 May; 30(2):174-185.

[96] Shin, J.H. Cho, S.I. Lim, H.R. Lee, J.K. Lee, Y.A. Noh, J.S. Joo, I.S. Kim, K.W. & Gwag, B.J. Concurrent administration of Neu2000 and lithium produces marked improvement of motor neuron survival, motor function, and mortality in a mouse model of amyotrophic lateral sclerosis. Mol Pharmacol. 2007 Apr;71(4):965-975.

[97] Raoul C, Buhler E, Sadeghi C, Jacquier A, Aebischer P, Pettmann B, Henderson CE, Haase G. Chronic activation in presymptomatic amyotrophic lateral sclerosis (ALS) mice of a feedback loop involving Fas, Daxx, and FasL. Proc Natl Acad Sci U S A. 2006 Apr 11;103(15):6007-6012.

[98] Merry, D. E. and Korsmeyer, S. J. Bcl-2 gene family in the nervous system, Annu. Rev. Neurosci. 1997;20:245-267.

[99] Chao, D. T. and Korsmeyer, S.J. BCL-2 family: regulators of cell death, Annu. Rev. Immunol. 1998;16:395-419.

[100] Hsu, Y. T., Wolter, K. G., and Youle, R. J. Cytosol-to-membrane redistribution of Bax and Bcl-X(L) during apoptosis, Proc. Natl. Acad. Sci. U.S.A.1997 Apr 15;94(8): 3668-3672.

[101] Gross, A., Jockel, J., Wei, M. C., and Korsmeyer, S. J. Enforced dimerization of BAX results in its translocation, mitochondrial dysfunction and apoptosis, EMBO J 1998 Jul 15;17(14):3878-3885.

[102] Ekegren, T. Grundström, E. Lindholm, D. & Aquilonius, S.M. Upregulation of Bax protein and increased DNA degradation in ALS spinal cord motor neurons. Acta Neurol Scand.1999 Nov;100(5):317-321.

[103] Mu, X. He, J. Anderson, D.W. Trojanowski, J.Q. & Springer, J.E. Altered expression of bcl-2 and bax mRNA in amyotrophic lateral sclerosis spinal cord motor neurons. Ann Neurol. 1996 Sep;40(3):379-386.

[104] Vukosavic, S. Dubois-Dauphin, M. Romero, N. & Przedborski, S. Bax and Bcl-2 interaction in a transgenic mouse model of familial amyotrophic lateral sclerosis. J Neurochem. 1999 Dec;73(6):2460-2468

[105] Pasinelli, P. Belford, M.E. Lennon, N. Bacskai, B.J. Hyman, B.T. Trotti, D. & Brown, R.H. Jr. Amyotrophic lateral sclerosis-associated SOD1 mutant proteins bind and aggregate with Bcl-2 in spinal cord mitochondria. Neuron. 2004 Jul;843(1):19-30.

[106] Guégan, C. Vila, M. Rosoklija, G. Hays, A.P. & Przedborski, S. Recruitment of the mitochondrial-dependent apoptotic pathway in amyotrophic lateral sclerosis. J Neurosci. 2001 Sep;121(17):6569-6576.

[107] Inoue, H. Tsukita, K. Iwasato, T. Suzuki, Y. Tomioka, M. Tateno, M. Nagao, M. Kawata, A. Saido, T.C. Miura, M. Misawa, H. Itohara, S. & Takahashi, R. The crucial role of caspase-9 in the disease progression of a transgenic ALS mouse model. EMBO J. 2003 Dec;1522(24):6665-6674.

[108] Kostic, V. Jackson-Lewis, V. de Bilbao, F. Dubois-Dauphin, M. & Przedborski, S. Bcl-2: prolonging life in a transgenic mouse model of familial amyotrophic lateral sclerosis. Science. 1997 Jul;25277(5325):559-562.

[109] Gould, T.W. Buss, R.R. Vinsant, S. Prevette, D. Sun, W. Knudson, C.M. Milligan, C.E. & Oppenheim, R.W. Complete dissociation of motor neuron death from motor dysfunction by Bax deletion in a mouse model of ALS. J Neurosci. 2006 Aug;2326(34): 8774-8786.

[110] Earnshaw, W. C., Martins, L. M., and Kaufmann, S. H. Mammalian caspases: structure, activation, substrates, and functions during apoptosis, Annu. Rev. Biochem 1999;68:383-424.

[111] Li, M. Ona, V.O. Guégan, C. Chen, M. Jackson-Lewis, V. Andrews, L.J. Olszewski, A.J. Stieg P.E. Lee, J.P. Przedborski, S. & Friedlander, R.M. Functional role of caspase-1 and caspase-3 in an ALS transgenic mouse model. Science. 2000 Apr; 14288(5464):335-339.

[112] Ando, Y. Liang, Y. Ishigaki, S. Niwa, J. Jiang, Y. Kobayashi, Y. Yamamoto, M. Doyu, M. & Sobue, G. Caspase-1 and -3 mRNAs are differentially upregulated in motor neurons and glial cells in mutant SOD1 transgenic mouse spinal cord: a study using laser microdissection and real-time RT-PCR. Neurochem Res. 2003 Jun;28(6):839-846.

[113] Nagata, T. Ilieva, H. Murakami, T. Shiote, M. Narai, H. Ohta, Y. Hayashi, T. Shoji, M. & Abe, K. Increased ER stress during motor neuron degeneration in a transgenic mouse model of amyotrophic lateral sclerosis. Neurol Res. 2007 Dec;29(8):767-771.

[114] Zhang YJ, Xu YF, Dickey CA, Buratti E, Baralle F, Bailey R, Pickering-Brown S, Dickson D, Petrucelli L. Progranulin mediates caspase-dependent cleavage of TAR DNA binding protein-43. J Neurosci. 2007 Sep 26;27(39):10530-10534.

[115] Zhu S, Stavrovskaya IG, Drozda M, Kim BY, Ona V, Li M, Sarang S, Liu AS, Hartley DM, Wu DC, Gullans S, Ferrante RJ, Przedborski S, Kristal BS, Friedlander RM. Minocycline inhibits cytochrome c release and delays progression of amyotrophic lateral sclerosis in mice. Nature. 2002 May 2;417(6884):74-78.

[116] Van Den Bosch L, Tilkin P, Lemmens G, Robberecht W. Minocycline delays disease onset and mortality in a transgenic model of ALS. Neuroreport. 2002 Jun 12;13(8): 1067-1070.

[117] Zhang W, Narayanan M, Friedlander RM. Additive neuroprotective effects of minocycline with creatine in a mouse model of ALS. Ann Neurol. 2003 Feb;53(2):267-270.

[118] Gordon PH, Moore DH, Miller RG, Florence JM, Verheijde JL, Doorish C, Hilton JF, Spitalny GM, MacArthur RB, Mitsumoto H, Neville HE, Boylan K, Mozaffar T, Belsh JM, Ravits J, Bedlack RS, Graves MC, McCluskey LF, Barohn RJ, Tandan R; Western ALS Study Group. Efficacy of minocycline in patients with amyotrophic lateral sclerosis: a phase III randomised trial. Lancet Neurol. 2007 Dec;6(12):1045-1053.

[119] Miller R, Bradley W, Cudkowicz M, Hubble J, Meininger V, Mitsumoto H, Moore D, Pohlmann H, Sauer D, Silani V, Strong M, Swash M, Vernotica E; TCH346 Study Group. Phase II/III randomized trial of TCH346 in patients with ALS. Neurology. 2007 Aug 21;69(8):776-784.

[120] Nimmerjahn A, Kirchhoff F, Helmchen F. Resting microglial cells are highly dynamic surveillants of brain parenchyma in vivo. Science. 2005 May 27;308(5726):1314-318.

[121] Cunningham O, Campion S, Perry VH, Murray C, Sidenius N, Docagne F, Cunningham C. Microglia and the urokinase plasminogen activator receptor/uPA system in innate brain inflammation. Glia. 2009 Dec;57(16):1802-1814.

[122] Venance L, Cordier J, Monge M, Zalc B, Glowinski J, Giaume C. Homotypic and heterotypic coupling mediated by gap junctions during glial cell differentiation in vitro. Eur J Neurosci. 1995 Mar 1;7(3):451-461

[123] Rash JE, Yasumura T, Dudek FE, Nagy JI. Cell-specific expression of connexins and evidence of restricted gap junctional coupling between glial cells and between neurons. J Neurosci. 2001 Mar 15;21(6):1983-2000.

[124] Kawamata T, Akiyama H, Yamada T, McGeer PL. Immunologic reactions in amyotrophic lateral sclerosis brain and spinal cord tissue. Am J Pathol. 1992 Mar;140(3): 691-707.

[125] Hall ED, Oostveen JA, Gurney ME. Relationship of microglial and astrocytic activation to disease onset and progression in a transgenic model of familial ALS. Glia. 1998 Jul;23(3):249-256.

[126] Banati RB, Gehrmann J, Kellner M, Holsboer F. Antibodies against microglia/brain macrophages in the cerebrospinal fluid of a patient with acute amyotrophic lateral sclerosis and presenile dementia. Clin Neuropathol. 1995 Jul-Aug;14(4):197-200

[127] Turner MR, Cagnin A, Turkheimer FE, Miller CC, Shaw CE, Brooks DJ, Leigh PN, Banati RB. Evidence of widespread cerebral microglial activation in amyotrophic lateral sclerosis: an [11C](R)-PK11195 positron emission tomography study. Neurobiol Dis. 2004 Apr;15(3):601-609.

[128] Yoshihara T, Ishigaki S, Yamamoto M, Liang Y, Niwa J, Takeuchi H, Doyu M, Sobue G. Differential expression of inflammation- and apoptosis-related genes in spinal cords of a mutant SOD1 transgenic mouse model of familial amyotrophic lateral sclerosis. J Neurochem. 2002 Jan;80(1):158-167.

[129] Poloni M, Facchetti D, Mai R, Micheli A, Agnoletti L, Francolini G, Mora G, Camana C, Mazzini L, Bachetti T. Circulating levels of tumour necrosis factor-alpha and its soluble receptors are increased in the blood of patients with amyotrophic lateral sclerosis. Neurosci Lett. 2000 Jun 30;287(3):211-214.

[130] Baldwin AS Jr. Series introduction: the transcription factor NF-kappaB and human disease. J Clin Invest. 2001 Jan;107(1):3-6.

[131] Hensley K, Floyd RA, Gordon B, Mou S, Pye QN, Stewart C, West M, Williamson K. Temporal patterns of cytokine and apoptosis-related gene expression in spinal cords of the G93A-SOD1 mouse model of amyotrophic lateral sclerosis. J Neurochem. 2002 Jul;82(2):365-374.

[132] Hensley K, Fedynyshyn J, Ferrell S, Floyd RA, Gordon B, Grammas P, Hamdheydari L, Mhatre M, Mou S, Pye QN, Stewart C, West M, West S, Williamson KS. Message

and protein-level elevation of tumor necrosis factor alpha (TNF alpha) and TNF alpha-modulating cytokines in spinal cords of the G93A-SOD1 mouse model for amyotrophic lateral sclerosis. Neurobiol Dis. 2003 Oct;14(1):74-80.

[133] Henkel JS, Engelhardt JI, Siklós L, Simpson EP, Kim SH, Pan T, Goodman JC, Siddique T, Beers DR, Appel SH. Presence of dendritic cells, MCP-1, and activated microglia/macrophages in amyotrophic lateral sclerosis spinal cord tissue. Ann Neurol. 2004 Feb;55(2):221-235.

[134] Bos CL, Richel DJ, Ritsema T, Peppelenbosch MP, Versteeg HH. Prostanoids and prostanoid receptors in signal transduction. Int J Biochem Cell Biol.2004 Jul;36(7): 1187-1205

[135] Yasojima K, Tourtellotte WW, McGeer EG, McGeer PL. Marked increase in cyclooxygenase-2 in ALS spinal cord: implications for therapy. Neurology.2001 Sep 25;57(6): 952-956.

[136] Maihöfner C, Probst-Cousin S, Bergmann M, Neuhuber W, Neundörfer B, Heuss D. Expression and localization of cyclooxygenase-1 and -2 in human sporadic amyotrophic lateral sclerosis. Eur J Neurosci. 2003 Sep;18(6):1527-1534.

[137] Almer G, Guégan C, Teismann P, Naini A, Rosoklija G, Hays AP, Chen C, Przedborski S. Increased expression of the pro-inflammatory enzyme cyclooxygenase-2 in amyotrophic lateral sclerosis. Ann Neurol. 2001 Feb;49(2):176-185

[138] Liang X, Wang Q, Shi J, Lokteva L, Breyer RM, Montine TJ, Andreasson K. The prostaglandin E2 EP2 receptor accelerates disease progression and inflammation in a model of amyotrophic lateral sclerosis. Ann Neurol. 2008 Sep;64(3):304-314.

[139] Boillée S, Yamanaka K, Lobsiger CS, Copeland NG, Jenkins NA, Kassiotis G, Kollias G, Cleveland DW. Onset and progression in inherited ALS determined by motor neurons and microglia. Science. 2006 Jun 2;312(5778):1389-1392.

[140] Yamanaka K, Chun SJ, Boillee S, Fujimori-Tonou N, Yamashita H, Gutmann DH, Takahashi R, Misawa H, Cleveland DW. Astrocytes as determinants of disease progression in inherited amyotrophic lateral sclerosis. Nat Neurosci. 2008 Mar;11(3):251-253.

[141] Gong YH, Parsadanian AS, Andreeva A, Snider WD, Elliott JL. Restricted expression of G86R Cu/Zn superoxide dismutase in astrocytes results in astrocytosis but does not cause motoneuron degeneration. J Neurosci. 2000 Jan 15;20(2):660-605.

[142] Pramatarova A, Laganière J, Roussel J, Brisebois K, Rouleau GA. Neuron-specific expression of mutant superoxide dismutase 1 in transgenic mice does not lead to motor impairment. J Neurosci. 2001 May 15;21(10):3369-3374.

[143] Beers DR, Henkel JS, Xiao Q, Zhao W, Wang J, Yen AA, Siklos L, McKercher SR, Appel SH. Wild-type microglia extend survival in PU.1 knockout mice with familial amyotrophic lateral sclerosis. Proc Natl Acad Sci U S A 2006 Oct 24;103(43): 16021-16026.

[144] Clement AM, Nguyen MD, Roberts EA, Garcia ML, Boillée S, Rule M, McMahon AP, Doucette W, Siwek D, Ferrante RJ, Brown RH Jr, Julien JP, Goldstein LS, Cleveland DW. Wild-type nonneuronal cells extend survival of SOD1 mutant motor neurons in ALS mice. Science. 2003 Oct 3;302(5642):113-117.

[145] Ralph GS, Radcliffe PA, Day DM, Carthy JM, Leroux MA, Lee DC, Wong LF, Bilsland LG, Greensmith L, Kingsman SM, Mitrophanous KA, Mazarakis ND, Azzouz M. Silencing mutant SOD1 using RNAi protects against neurodegeneration and extends survival in an ALS model. Nat Med. 2005 Apr;11(4):429-433.

[146] Cunningham C, Wilcockson DC, Campion S, Lunnon K, Perry VH. Central and systemic endotoxin challenges exacerbate the local inflammatory response and increase neuronal death during chronic neurodegeneration. J Neurosci. 2005 Oct 5;25(40): 9275-9284.

[147] Godbout JP, Chen J, Abraham J, Richwine AF, Berg BM, Kelley KW, Johnson RW. Exaggerated neuroinflammation and sickness behavior in aged mice following activation of the peripheral innate immune system. FASEB J. 2005 Aug;19(10):1329-1331.

[148] Pavlov VA, Tracey KJ. The cholinergic anti-inflammatory pathway. Brain Behav Immun. 2005 Nov;19(6):493-499.

[149] Lacroix S, Feinstein D, Rivest S. The bacterial endotoxin lipopolysaccharide has the ability to target the brain in upregulating its membrane CD14 receptor within specific cellular populations. Brain Pathol. 1998 Oct;8(4):625-640.

[150] Ek M, Engblom D, Saha S, Blomqvist A, Jakobsson PJ, Ericsson- Dahlstrand A. Inflammatory response: pathway across the blood-brain barrier. Nature. 2001 Mar 22;410(6827):430-431

[151] Tilvis RS, Kähönen-Väre MH, Jolkkonen J, Valvanne J, Pitkala KH, Strandberg TE. Predictors of cognitive decline and mortality of aged people over a 10-year period. J Gerontol A Biol Sci Med Sci. 2004 Mar;59(3):268-274.

[152] Semmler A, Frisch C, Debeir T, Ramanathan M, Okulla T, Klockgether T, Heneka MT. Long-term cognitive impairment, neuronal loss and reduced cortical cholinergic innervation after recovery from sepsis in a rodent model. Exp Neurol. 2007 Apr; 204(2):733-740.

[153] Holmøy T. T cells in amyotrophic lateral sclerosis. Eur J Neurol. 2008 Apr;15(4): 360-366.

[154] Goldknopf IL, Sheta EA, Bryson J, Folsom B, Wilson C, Duty J, Yen AA, Appel SH. Complement C3c and related protein biomarkers in amyotrophic lateral sclerosis and Parkinson's disease. Biochem Biophys Res Commun. 2006 Apr 21;342(4):1034-1039.

[155] Shi N, Kawano Y, Tateishi T, Kikuchi H, Osoegawa M, Ohyagi Y, Kira J. Increased IL-13-producing T cells in ALS: positive correlations with disease severity and progression rate. J Neuroimmunol. 2007 Jan;182(1-2):232-235.

[156] Provinciali L, Laurenzi MA, Vesprini L, Giovagnoli AR, Bartocci C, Montroni M, Bagnarelli P, Clementi M, Varaldo PE. Immunity assessment in the early stages of amyotrophic lateral sclerosis: a study of virus antibodies and lymphocyte subsets. Acta Neurol Scand. 1988 Dec;78(6):449-454.

[157] Rentzos M, Evangelopoulos E, Sereti E, Zouvelou V, Marmara S, Alexakis T, Evdokimidis I. Alterations of T cell subsets in ALS: a systemic immune activation? Acta Neurol Scand. 2012 Apr;125(4):260-264.

[158] Baron P, Bussini S, Cardin V, Corbo M, Conti G, Galimberti D, Scarpini E, Bresolin N, Wharton SB, Shaw PJ, Silani V. Production of monocyte chemoattractant protein-1 in amyotrophic lateral sclerosis. Muscle Nerve. 2005 Oct;32(4):541-544.

[159] Wilms H, Sievers J, Dengler R, Bufler J, Deuschl G, Lucius R. Intrathecal synthesis of monocyte chemoattractant protein-1 (MCP-1) in amyotrophic lateral sclerosis: further evidence for microglial activation in neurodegeneration. J Neuroimmunol. 2003 Nov; 144(1-2):139-142.

[160] Nagata T, Nagano I, Shiote M, Narai H, Murakami T, Hayashi T, Shoji M, Abe K.Elevation of MCP-1 and MCP-1/VEGF ratio in cerebrospinal fluid of amyotrophic lateral sclerosis patients. Neurol Res. 2007 Dec;29(8):772-776.

[161] Rentzos M, Nikolaou C, Rombos A, Boufidou F, Zoga M, Dimitrakopoulos A, Tsoutsou A, Vassilopoulos D. RANTES levels are elevated in serum and cerebrospinal fluid in patients with amyotrophic lateral sclerosis. Amyotroph Lateral Scler. 2007 Oct; 8(5):283-287.

[162] Henkel JS, Beers DR, Siklós L, Appel SH. The chemokine MCP-1 and the dendritic and myeloid cells it attracts are increased in the mSOD1 mouse model of ALS. Mol Cell Neurosci. 2006 Mar;31(3):427-437.

[163] Sargsyan SA, Blackburn DJ, Barber SC, Monk PN, Shaw PJ. Mutant SOD1 G93A microglia have an inflammatory phenotype and elevated production of MCP-1. Neuroreport. 2009 Oct 28;20(16):1450-1455.

[164] Zhang R, Hadlock KG, Do H, Yu S, Honrada R, Champion S, Forshew D, Madison C, Katz J, Miller RG, McGrath MS.Gene expression profiling in peripheral blood mononuclear cells from patients with sporadic amyotrophic lateral sclerosis (sALS). J Neuroimmunol. 2011 Jan;230(1-2):114-123

[165] Nguyen MD, D'Aigle T, Gowing G, Julien JP, Rivest S. Exacerbation of motor neuron disease by chronic stimulation of innate immunity in a mouse model of amyotrophic lateral sclerosis. J Neurosci. 2004 Feb 11;24(6):1340-1349.

[166] Garbuzova-Davis S, Saporta S, Haller E, Kolomey I, Bennett SP, Potter H, Sanberg PR. Evidence of compromised blood-spinal cord barrier in early and late symptomatic SOD1 mice modeling ALS. PLoS One. 2007 Nov 21;2(11):e1205.

[167] Garbuzova-Davis S, Woods RL 3rd, Louis MK, Zesiewicz TA, Kuzmin-Nichols N, Sullivan KL, Miller AM, Hernandez-Ontiveros DG, Sanberg PR. Reduction of circu-

lating endothelial cells in peripheral blood of ALS patients. PLoS One. 2010 May 12;5(5):e10614.

[168] Drachman DB, Frank K, Dykes-Hoberg M, Teismann P, Almer G, Przedborski S, Rothstein JD. Cyclooxygenase 2 inhibition protects motor neurons and prolongs survival in a transgenic mouse model of ALS. Ann Neurol. 2002 Dec;52(6):771-778.

[169] Klivenyi P, Kiaei M, Gardian G, Calingasan NY, Beal MF. Additive neuroprotective effects of creatine and cyclooxygenase 2 inhibitors in a transgenic mouse model of amyotrophic lateral sclerosis. J Neurochem. 2004 Feb;88(3):576-582.

[170] Kiaei M, Petri S, Kipiani K, Gardian G, Choi DK, Chen J, Calingasan NY, Schafer P, Muller GW, Stewart C, Hensley K, Beal MF. Thalidomide and lenalidomide extend survival in a transgenic mouse model of amyotrophic lateral sclerosis. J Neurosci. 2006 Mar 1;26(9):2467-2473.

[171] Banerjee R, Mosley RL, Reynolds AD, Dhar A, Jackson-Lewis V, Gordon PH, Przedborski S, Gendelman HE. Adaptive immune neuroprotection in G93A-SOD1 amyotrophic lateral sclerosis mice. PLoS One. 2008 Jul 23;3(7):e2740.

[172] Budd SL, Nicholls DG. Mitochondria in the life and death of neurons. 1998 Essays Biochem. 1998;33:43-52.

[173] Kroemer G. The mitochondrion as an integrator/coordinator of cell death pathways. Cell Death Differ.1998 Jun;5(6):547.

[174] Sasaki S, Iwata M. Ultrastructural study of synapses in the anterior horn neurons of patients with amyotrophic lateral sclerosis. Neurosci Lett.1996 Feb 2;204(1-2):53-56.

[175] Borthwick GM, Johnson MA, Ince PG, Shaw PJ, Turnbull DM. Mitochondrial enzyme activity in amyotrophic lateral sclerosis: implications for the role of mitochondria in neuronal cell death. Ann Neurol. 1999 Nov;46(5):787-790.

[176] Vielhaber S, Winkler K, Kirches E, Kunz D, Büchner M, Feistner H, Elger CE, Ludolph AC, Riepe MW, Kunz WS. Visualization of defective mitochondrial function in skeletal muscle fibers of patients with sporadic amyotrophic lateral sclerosis. J Neurol Sci. 1999 Oct 31;169(1-2):133-139.

[177] Sturtz LA, Diekert K, Jensen LT, Lill R, Culotta VC. A fraction of yeast Cu,Zn-superoxide dismutase and its metallochaperone, CCS, localize to the intermembrane space of mitochondria. A physiological role for SOD1 in guarding against mitochondrial oxidative damage. J Biol Chem. 2001 Oct 12;276(41):38084-38089.

[178] Higgins CM, Jung C, Ding H, Xu Z. Mutant Cu, Zn superoxide dismutase that causes motoneuron degeneration is present in mitochondria in the CNS. J Neurosci. 2002 Mar 15;22(6):RC215.

[179] Dykens JA. Isolated cerebral and cerebellar mitochondria produce free radicals when exposed to elevated CA2+ and Na+: implications for neurodegeneration. J Neurochem. 1994 Aug;63(2):584-591.

[180] Dugan LL, Sensi SL, Canzoniero LM, Handran SD, Rothman SM, Lin TS, Goldberg MP, Choi DW. Mitochondrial production of reactive oxygen species in cortical neurons following exposure to N-methyl-D-aspartate. J Neurosci. 1995 Oct;15(10): 6377-6388.

[181] Luetjens CM, Bui NT, Sengpiel B, Münstermann G, Poppe M, Krohn AJ, Bauerbach E, Krieglstein J, Prehn JH. Delayed mitochondrial dysfunction in excitotoxic neuron death: cytochrome c release and a secondary increase in superoxide production. J Neurosci. 2000 Aug 1;20(15):5715-5723.

[182] Kawamata H, Manfredi G. Mitochondrial dysfunction and intracellular calcium dysregulation in ALS. Mech Ageing Dev. 2010 Jul-Aug;131(7-8):517-526.

[183] Volterra A, Trotti D, Floridi S, Racagni G. Reactive oxygen species inhibit high-affinity glutamate uptake: molecular mechanism and neuropathological implications. Ann N Y Acad Sci. 1994 Nov 17;738:153-162

[184] De Vos KJ, Chapman AL, Tennant ME, Manser C, Tudor EL, Lau KF, Brownlees J, Ackerley S, Shaw PJ, McLoughlin DM, Shaw CE, Leigh PN, Miller CC, Grierson AJ. Familial amyotrophic lateral sclerosis-linked SOD1 mutants perturb fast axonal transport to reduce axonal mitochondria content. Hum Mol Genet. 2007 Nov 15;16(22):2720-2728.

[185] Shan X, Chiang PM, Price DL, Wong PC. Altered distributions of Gemini of coiled bodies and mitochondria in motor neurons of TDP-43 transgenic mice. Proc Natl Acad Sci U S A. 2010 Sep 14;107(37):16325-16330.

[186] Xu YF, Gendron TF, Zhang YJ, Lin WL, D'Alton S, Sheng H, Casey MC, Tong J, Knight J, Yu X, Rademakers R, Boylan K, Hutton M, McGowan E, Dickson DW, Lewis J, Petrucelli L. Wild-type human TDP-43 expression causes TDP-43 phosphorylation, mitochondrial aggregation, motor deficits, and early mortality in transgenic mice. J Neurosci. 2010 Aug 11;30(32):10851-10859.

[187] Klionsky DJ, Emr SD. Autophagy as a regulated pathway of cellular degradation. Science. 2000 Dec 1;290(5497):1717-17121.

[188] Hara T, Nakamura K, Matsui M, Yamamoto A, Nakahara Y, Suzuki-Migishima R, Yokoyama M, Mishima K, Saito I, Okano H, Mizushima N. Suppression of basal autophagy in neural cells causes neurodegenerative disease in mice. Nature. 2006 Jun 15;441(7095):885-889.

[189] Wong E, Cuervo AM. Autophagy gone awry in neurodegenerative diseases. Nat Neurosci. 2010 Jul;13(7):805-811.

[190] Kabashi E, Durham HD. Failure of protein quality control in amyotrophic lateral sclerosis. Biochim Biophys Acta. 2006 Nov-Dec;1762(11-12):1038-1050.

[191] Pasquali L, Ruffoli R, Fulceri F, Pietracupa S, Siciliano G, Paparelli A, Fornai F. The role of autophagy: what can be learned from the genetic forms of amyotrophic lateral sclerosis. CNS Neurol Disord Drug Targets. 2010 Jul;9(3):268-278.

[192] Fornai F, Longone P, Ferrucci M, Lenzi P, Isidoro C, Ruggieri S, Paparelli A. Autophagy and amyotrophic lateral sclerosis: The multiple roles of lithium. Autophagy. 2008 May;4(4):527-530.

[193] Hetz C, Thielen P, Matus S, Nassif M, Court F, Kiffin R, Martinez G, Cuervo AM, Brown RH, Glimcher LH. XBP-1 deficiency in the nervous system protects against amyotrophic lateral sclerosis by increasing autophagy. Genes Dev. 2009 Oct 1;23(19): 2294-2306.

[194] Banerjee R, Beal MF, Thomas B. Autophagy in neurodegenerative disorders: pathogenic roles and therapeutic implications. Trends Neurosci. 2010 Dec;33(12):541-549.

[195] Sasaki S. Autophagy in spinal cord motor neurons in sporadic amyotrophic lateral sclerosis. J Neuropathol Exp Neurol. 2011 May;70(5):349-359.

[196] Li L, Zhang X, Le W. Altered macroautophagy in the spinal cord of SOD1 mutant mice. Autophagy. 2008 Apr;4(3):290-293.

[197] Zhang X, Li L, Chen S, Yang D, Wang Y, Zhang X, Wang Z, Le W. Rapamycin treatment augments motor neuron degeneration in SOD1(G93A) mouse model of amyotrophic lateral sclerosis. Autophagy. 2011 Apr;7(4):412-425.

[198] Venkatachalam K, Long AA, Elsaesser R, Nikolaeva D, Broadie K, Montell C. Motor deficit in a Drosophila model of mucolipidosis type IV due to defective clearance of apoptotic cells. Cell. 2008 Nov 28;135(5):838-851

[199] Ryu BR, Ko HW, Jou I, Noh JS, Gwag BJ. Phosphatidylinositol 3-kinase-mediated regulation of neuronal apoptosis and necrosis by insulin and IGF-I. J Neurobiol. 1999 Jun 15;39(4):536-546.

[200] Won SJ, Park EC, Ryu BR, Ko HW, Sohn S, Kwon HJ, Gwag BJ. NT-4/5 exacerbates free radical-induced neuronal necrosis in vitro and in vivo. Neurobiol Dis. 2000 Aug; 7(4):251-259.

[201] Kim SH, Won SJ, Sohn S, Kwon HJ, Lee JY, Park JH, Gwag BJ. Brain-derived neurotrophic factor can act as a pronecrotic factor through transcriptional and translational activation of NADPH oxidase. J Cell Biol. 2002 Dec 9;159(5):821-831.

[202] Kaspar BK, Lladó J, Sherkat N, Rothstein JD, Gage FH. Retrograde viral delivery of IGF-1 prolongs survival in a mouse ALS model. Science. 2003 Aug 8;301(5634): 839-842.

[203] Gwag BJ, Koh JY, DeMaro JA, Ying HS, Jacquin M, Choi DW. Slowly triggered excitotoxicity occurs by necrosis in cortical cultures. Neuroscience. 1997 Mar;77(2): 393-401.

[204] Gwag BJ, Lee YA, Ko SY, Lee MJ, Im DS, Yun BS, Lim HR, Park SM, Byun HY, Son SJ, Kwon HJ, Lee JY, Cho JY, Won SJ, Kim KW, Ahn YM, Moon HS, Lee HU, Yoon SH, Noh JH, Chung JM, Cho SI. Marked prevention of ischemic brain injury by Neu2000, an NMDA antagonist and antioxidant derived from aspirin and sulfasalazine. J Cereb Blood Flow Metab. 2007 Jun;27(6):1142-1151.

[205] Chalecka-Franaszek E, Chuang DM. Lithium activates the serine/threonine kinase Akt-1 and suppresses glutamate-induced inhibition of Akt-1 activity in neurons. Proc Natl Acad Sci U S A. 1999 Jul 20;96(15):8745-8750.

[206] Kang HJ, Noh JS, Bae YS, Gwag BJ. Calcium-dependent prevention of neuronal apoptosis by lithium ion: essential role of phosphoinositide 3-kinase and phospholipase Cgamma. Mol Pharmacol. 2003 Aug;64(2):228-234.

[207] Petri S, Kiaei M, Kipiani K, Chen J, Calingasan NY, Crow JP, Beal MF. Additive neuroprotective effects of a histone deacetylase inhibitor and a catalytic antioxidant in a transgenic mouse model of amyotrophic lateral sclerosis. Neurobiol Dis. 2006 Apr; 22(1):40-49.

[208] Gordon PH, Cheung YK, Levin B, Andrews H, Doorish C, Macarthur RB, Montes J, Bednarz K, Florence J, Rowin J, Boylan K, Mozaffar T, Tandan R, Mitsumoto H, Kelvin EA, Chapin J, Bedlack R, Rivner M, McCluskey LF, Pestronk A, Graves M, Sorenson EJ, Barohn RJ, Belsh JM, Lou JS, Levine T, Saperstein D, Miller RG, Scelsa SN; Combination Drug Selection Trial Study Group. A novel, efficient, randomized selection trial comparing combinations of drug therapy for ALS. Amyotroph Lateral Scler. 2008 Aug;9(4):212-222.

[209] Bordet T, Buisson B, Michaud M, Drouot C, Galéa P, Delaage P, Akentieva NP, Evers AS, Covey DF, Ostuni MA, Lacapère JJ, Massaad C, Schumacher M, Steidl EM, Maux D, Delaage M, Henderson CE, Pruss RM. Identification and characterization of cholest-4-en-3-one, oxime (TRO19622), a novel drug candidate for amyotrophic lateral sclerosis. J Pharmacol Exp Ther. 2007 Aug;322(2):709-720.

[210] Tokuda E, Ono S, Ishige K, Watanabe S, Okawa E, Ito Y, Suzuki T. Ammonium tetrathiomolybdate delays onset, prolongs survival, and slows progression of disease in a mouse model for amyotrophic lateral sclerosis. Exp Neurol. 2008 Sep;213(1):122-128.

[211] Keep M, Elmér E, Fong KS, Csiszar K. Intrathecal cyclosporin prolongs survival of late-stage ALS mice. Brain Res. 2001 Mar 16;894(2):327-331.

[212] Feng HL, Leng Y, Ma CH, Zhang J, Ren M, Chuang DM. Combined lithium and valproate treatment delays disease onset, reduces neurological deficits and prolongs survival in an amyotrophic lateral sclerosis mouse model. Neuroscience. 2008 Aug 26;155(3):567-572

[213] Kiaei M, Kipiani K, Petri S, Chen J, Calingasan NY, Beal MF. Celastrol blocks neuronal cell death and extends life in transgenic mouse model of amyotrophic lateral sclerosis. Neurodegener Dis.2005;2(5):246-254.

[214] West M, Mhatre M, Ceballos A, Floyd RA, Grammas P, Gabbita SP, Hamdheydari L, Mai T, Mou S, Pye QN, Stewart C, West S, Williamson KS, Zemlan F, Hensley K. The arachidonic acid 5-lipoxygenase inhibitor nordihydroguaiaretic acid inhibits tumor necrosis factor alpha activation of microglia and extends survival of G93A-SOD1 transgenic mice. J Neurochem. 2004 Oct;91(1):133-143.

[215] Lorenzl S, Narr S, Angele B, Krell HW, Gregorio J, Kiaei M, Pfister HW, Beal MF. The matrix metalloproteinases inhibitor Ro 28-2653 [correction of Ro 26-2853] extends survival in transgenic ALS mice. Exp Neurol. 2006 Jul;200(1):166-171.

[216] Wang R, Zhang D. Memantine prolongs survival in an amyotrophic lateral sclerosis mouse model. Eur J Neurosci. 2005 Nov;22(9):2376-80.

[217] Zheng C, Nennesmo I, Fadeel B, Henter JI. Vascular endothelial growth factor prolongs survival in a transgenic mouse model of ALS. Ann Neurol. 2004 Oct;56(4): 564-567.

[218] Azzouz M, Ralph GS, Storkebaum E, Walmsley LE, Mitrophanous KA, Kingsman SM, Carmeliet P, Mazarakis ND. VEGF delivery with retrogradely transported lentivector prolongs survival in a mouse ALS model. Nature. 2004 May 27;429(6990): 413-417.

[219] Rothstein JD, Patel S, Regan MR, Haenggeli C, Huang YH, Bergles DE, Jin L, Dykes Hoberg M, Vidensky S, Chung DS, Toan SV, Bruijn LI, Su ZZ, Gupta P, Fisher PB. Beta-lactam antibiotics offer neuroprotection by increasing glutamate transporter expression. Nature. 2005 Jan 6;433(7021):73-77.

[220] Lee J, Ryu H, Kowall NW. Motor neuronal protection by L-arginine prolongs survival of mutant SOD1 (G93A) ALS mice. Biochem Biophys Res Commun. 2009 Jul 10;384(4):524-529.

[221] Ghadge GD, Slusher BS, Bodner A, Canto MD, Wozniak K, Thomas AG, Rojas C, Tsukamoto T, Majer P, Miller RJ, Monti AL, Roos RP. Glutamate carboxypeptidase II inhibition protects motor neurons from death in familial amyotrophic lateral sclerosis models. Proc Natl Acad Sci U S A. 2003 Aug 5;100(16):9554-9559

[222] Del Signore SJ, Amante DJ, Kim J, Stack EC, Goodrich S, Cormier K, Smith K, Cudkowicz ME, Ferrante RJ. Combined riluzole and sodium phenylbutyrate therapy in transgenic amyotrophic lateral sclerosis mice. Amyotroph Lateral Scler. 2009 Apr; 10(2):85-94.

[223] Kriz J, Gowing G, Julien JP. Efficient three-drug cocktail for disease induced by mutant superoxide dismutase. Ann Neurol. 2003 Apr;53(4):429-436.

http://dx.doi.org/10.5772/56625

[224] Waibel S, Reuter A, Malessa S, Blaugrund E, Ludolph AC. Rasagiline alone and in combination with riluzole prolongs survival in an ALS mouse model. J Neurol. 2004 Sep;251(9):1080-1084.

Chapter 3

Genetics of ALS and Correlations Between Genotype and Phenotype in ALS — A Focus on Italian Population

L. Diamanti, S. Gagliardi, C. Cereda and M. Ceroni

Additional information is available at the end of the chapter

http://dx.doi.org/10.5772/56547

1. Introduction

Amyotrophic Lateral Sclerosis, generally known as ALS, is a lethal neurodegenerative disease that gradually affects the motor neurons (nerve cells) which control muscle movement. The causes of the disease are as yet unknown and the substantial amount of research currently under way has found that the causes of ALS are multifactorial, such as genetic predisposition. In fact, about the involvement of genetic, ALS is a multigenic disease result from mutations in more than one gene (Table 1). The annual incidence of ALS is 0,4-1,76 per 100000 [1]. The majority of cases of ALS are sporadic (90-95%), called SALS. Around 5-10% of cases are considered to be familial (FALS), where the disease is present in both a proband and first-degree or second-degree relative [2-3]. FALS is usually inherited in an autosomal dominant manner, though there are rare cases of autosomal recessive disease. FALS is genetically heterogeneous, including 15 mapped loci, of which the causative genes are identified for 11. Mutations in several of the known FALS genes have also been described in apparently sporadic cases of ALS at low frequencies. Genetic changes detected in sporadic cases arise both from new mutations and also lack of evidence of inheritance due to the difficulty in recognizing a genetic component to rapidly lethal late-onset disease. The systematic, detailed diagnosis of neurological disease in older people is a modern, and still incomplete, medical phenomenon. For any late-onset disorder both incomplete penetrance and premature death of earlier generations due to other causes attenuates the expression of disease within a family so that in many examples where apparently sporadic ALS is associated with genetic mutation there is limited information about the family rather than a clear demonstration of unequivocally de novo genetic change [4].

ALS type	Onset	Inheritance	Locus	Gene	Protein
ALS1	Adult	AD	21q22.1	*SOD1*	Cu/Zn superoxide dismutase
ALS2	Juvenile	AR	2q33-35	ALS2	Alsin
ALS3	Adult	AD	18q21	Unknown	
ALS4	Juvenile	AD	9q34	*SETX*	Senataxin
ALS5	Juvenile	AR	15q15-21	*SPG11*	Spatacsin
ALS6	Adult	AD	16p11.2	*FUS*	Fused in sarcoma
ALS7	Adult	AD	20p13	Unknown	
ALS8	Adult	AD	20q13.33	*VAPB*	VAMP-associated protein B
ALS9	Adult	AD	14q11	*ANG*	Angiogenin
ALS10	Adult	AD	1q36	*TARDBP*	TAR DNA-binding protein
ALS11	Adult	AD	6q21	*FIG4*	PI(3,5)P(2)5-phosphatase
ALS12	Adult	AR/AD	10p15p14	*OPTN*	Optineurin
ALS-FTD1	Adult	AD	9q21-22	Unknown	
ALS-FTD2	Juvenile	AD	9p13.2-21.3	Unknown	
ALS-FTD3	Adult	AD	9p21	*C9Orf72*	C9Orf72

Table 1. Genes and loci associated with ALS.

Discoveries in the clinical genetics of ALS in particular offer opportunities to deepen understanding of various disease phenotypes that appear to share aspects of pathogenesis, confirm previous hypothesis around the concept of disease spectra, in terms of linkage to a specific proteinopathy, and increase the scope of pathological studies of human motor system disease.

Genetic factors may play a role in determining the range of ALS phenotypes although to date no genes have been shown to have a definite effect on phenotype [4]. In fact the genetic alteration is not the only factor that determines the clinical course of the disease, other factors must also contribute to phenotype and it is not yet possible to predict the evolution of patients based solely on presence of the mutation or rate of progression in other family members.

The diagnosis of ALS is based on the original El Escorial diagnostic criteria, revised from 2000 [5-6].

It is a generally accepted notion that the clinical spectrum of ALS includes different phenotypes marked by a varying involvement of spinal and bulbar upper and lower motor neurons. Accordingly, eight distinctive clinical phenotypes are recognised in the literature: classic, bulbar, flail arm, flail leg, pyramidal, respiratory, pure lower motor neuron, pure upper motor neuron.

a. Classic ALS phenotype is characterised by onset of symptomps in the upper or lower limbs, with clear but not predominant pyramidal signs. It is the commonest phenotype in men and the second in women, with a peak of incidence rate in the seventh decade in both

http://dx.doi.org/10.5772/56547

genders. 0-5% of cases have frontotemporal dementia. Median survival time is 2,5 years [4].

b. Bulbar phenotype starts with dysarthria, dysphagia, tongue wasting, fasciculation and no peripheral spinal involvement for the first 6 months after symptomps onset; pyramidal signs aren't required to be evident in the first period but needs to be evident therafter. This subtype has the same incidence in the two genders, with peak of incidence in the eighth decade. It is the commonest phenotype associated with frontotemporal dementia (10%). Median survival time is 2 years [4]. It is now accepted that FTD and MND are part of the same clinicopathological spectrum. Frontotemporal dementia is characterised clinically by progressive behavioural changes and frontal executive deficits and/or selective language difficulties. The presence of FTD is determined using a screening test, such as FAB (frontal assessment battery), and is based on Neary criteria [7-8]. Frontotemporal dementia is present in about 5-10% of patients, however many ALS patients have evidence of FTD behavioural dysfunction that may not satisfy Neary criteria for FTD. Patients often have bulbar phenotype with muscle atrophy, weakness and fasciculations prominent in the tongue and also in the upper extremities.

c. Flail arm phenotype is characterised by progressive, predominantly proximal, weakness and wasting in the upper limbs and functional involvement has to be confined in this parts for at least 12 months after symptomps onset. This phenotype is relatively rare and more common in men, often benign with a median survival time of 4 years. Frontotemporal dementia is rare in this phenotype [4].

d. Flail leg begins with progressive distal onset of symptomps in lower limbs. Patients with symptomps beginning proximally in the legs without distal involvement at onset are classified as classic ALS. This type of disease has the same incidence in two genders. Mean age of onset is about 65 years and the peak of incidence rate is in the eighth decade. Median survival time is 3 years [4].

In two last categories there are forms with pathological deep tendon reflexes or Hoffmann and Babinski sign but without hypertonia or clonus.

e. Patients with pyramidal phenotype have manifestations dominated by severe spastic para/tertaparesis associated with Babinski or Hoffmann sign, hyperactive reflexes, clonic jaw jerk, dysarthric speech and pseudobulbar affect. Spastic paresis could be present at the beginning or in the fully developed stage of the disease. These patients show at the same time clear-cut signs of lower motor neuron impairment from onset of the disease, as indicated by muscle weakness and wasting and by the presence of chronic and active denervation at the EMG examination in at least two different sites. Patients have a quite young age at onset, under 60 years. Both genders are equally represented. FTD is uncommon and median survival time is 6 years [4].

f. There is a particular and the rarest phenotype with respiratory impairment at onset, defined as orthopnoea or dyspnoea at rest or during exertion, with only mild spinal or bulbar signs in the fisrt 6 months after onset. These patients show signs of upper motor neuron involvement. Median survival time is 1,5 years, with the worst prognosis [4].

g. Pure lower motor neuron phenotype is characterised by clinical and electrophysiological evidence of progressive LMN involvement. Patients with family history of inherited spinal muscular atrophy are excluded. It has a low incidence rate and is twice as frequent in men. Patients with this form are younger than those with any other ALS phenotype, with a peak of incidence rate in the seventh decade among men and in the sixth decade among women. Nobody has FTD and mean survival is the longest (7 years) [4].

h. Patients with pure upper motor neuron have signs of UMN involvement (severe spastic para/tertaparesis associated with Babinski or Hoffmann sign, hyperactive reflexes, clonic jaw jerk, dysarthric speech and pseudobulbar affect). Patients with clinical or EMG signs of LMN involvement or with history of spastic para/tetraparesis in family such as hereditary spastic paraplegia are excluded. It has a low incidence rate with peak in the sixth decade in both genders, Median survival time is the longest among ALS phenotype (more than 10 years) [4].

Phenotype	No of cases (%)	Age at onset (years) (mean (SD))	Age at onset (years) (median (IQR))‡	Diagnostic delay (months) (mean (SD))	Diagnostic delay (months) (median (IQR))‡	Cases with FTD (%)
Classic	404 (30.3)	62.8 (11.3)	64.6 (56.1–70.6)	10.9 (9.6)	8 (5–13)	16 (4.0)
Bulbar	456 (34.2)	68.8 (9.7)	69.9 (62.9–75.0)	9.8 (7.0)	8 (5–12)	41 (9.0)
Flail arm	74 (5.5)	62.6 (11.8)	63.3 (54.8–72.2)	12.8 (11.0)	9 (5–15)	1 (1.4)
Flail leg	173 (13.0)	65.0 (9.6)	65.6 (58.5–71.2)	13.1 (10.1)	11 (7–17)	7 (4.1)
Pyramidal	120 (9.1)	58.3 (13.5)	60.1 (49.2–68.3)	15.9 (13.4)	12 (6–22)	3 (2.5)
Respiratory	14 (1.1)	62.2 (8.6)	62.0 (58.3–65.3)	6.4 (4.3)	5 (3–9)	–
PLMN	38 (2.9)	56.2 (11.3)	55.2 (45.7–61.3)	15.5 (12.4)	14 (10–19)	–
PUMN	53 (4.0)	58.9 (10.9)	56.5 (48.3–62.6)	15.9 (14.3)	15 (10–19)	2 (3.8%)
Overall ALS	**1332**	**64.3 (11.3)**	**65.3 (59.7–71.8)**	**10.8 (10.4)**	**9 (5–14)**	**70 (5.4%)**
		p=0.0001*		p=0.0001*		p=0.0001†

*ANOVA.
†χ^2 test.
‡Q1–Q3.
ALS, amyotrophic lateral sclerosis; FTD, frontotemporal dementia; PLMN, pure lower motor neuron phenotype; PUMN, pure upper motor neuron phenotype.

Table 2. Mean age at onset, mean time delay from onset to diagnosis and frequency of frontotemporal dementia [4].

Phenotype	Overall, incidence rate (95% CI)	Men, incidence rate (95% CI)	Women, incidence rate (95% CI)	Men to women incidence rate ratio
Classic	0.94 (0.85 to 1.04)	1.17 (1.03 to 1.32)	0.71 (0.61 to 0.83)	1.65:1
Bulbar	1.05 (0.96 to 1.15)	1.04 (0.91 to 1.19)	1.06 (0.94 to 1.20)	0.98:1
Flail arm	0.17 (0.13 to 0.21)	0.28 (0.21 to 0.36)	0.07 (0.04 to 0.12)	4.00:1
Flail leg	0.40 (0.34 to 0.47)	0.40 (0.32 to 0.50)	0.39 (0.31 to 0.48)	1.03:1
Pyramidal	0.28 (0.23 to 0.34)	0.28 (0.21 to 0.36)	0.27 (0.21 to 0.35)	1.04:1
Respiratory	0.03 (0.02 to 0.05)	0.06 (0.03 to 0.10)	0.01 (0 to 0.03)	6.00:1
PLMN	0.08 (0.06 to 0.11)	0.11 (0.07 to 0.17)	0.05 (0.03 to 0.08)	2.04:1
PUMN	0.12 (0.09 to 0.16)	0.12 (0.08 to 0.18)	0.12 (0.08 to 0.17)	0.98:1
Overall ALS	**3.07 (2.89 to 3.25)**	**3.46 (3.23 to 3.71)**	**2.68 (2.44 to 2.90)**	**1.29:1**

ALS, amyotrophic lateral sclerosis; PLMN, pure lower motor neuron phenotype; PUMN, pure upper motor neuron phenotype.

Table 3. Amyotrophic lateral sclerosis phenotypes. Overall and men versus women mean annual crude incidence raters (/100000 population), 95% CIs and gender incidence rate ratios [4].

http://dx.doi.org/10.5772/56547

In this chapter we would deep investigate the correlation between genetic and clinical features in the ALS population that we better know, the Italian one. However, heterogeneity between and among families implies that other environmental and genetic influences contribute to not only the rate of evolution and which signs predominate but also whether the disease will appear at all during life. Considerable work lies ahead in determining the genetic and environmental factors that most contribute to ALS. Altogether one determinant of ALS phenotype is the underlying causative mutation.

We will focus this book section on the correlation between genotype and phenotype in Italian ALS disease population. This chapter will be organized in different paragraphs about the genes mostly mutated in Italian ALS patients, *SOD1, FUS, TARDBP, ANG, C9orf72* and *OPTN* genes (Table 2), and each paragraphs will be subdivided in two parts about genotype and phenotype. Moreover we will try to define and understand particular connection between phenotype and genotype in Italian population and in our experience in Pavia to characterize the Italian ALS population in relation to the genetic aspects.

Obviously in literature different mutations are known for every genes and many other ones will be discovered in future.

In this chapter we cannot deepen the importance of every mutation in relation to the phenotypic characteristic of ALS patients.

For this reason in this book section we will develop speech on more frequent alterations and on which we have met during our daily activity in Pavia or in our collaborations with other groups.

2. Cu/Zn Superoxide Dismutase (SOD1 gene)

Superoxide dismutase [Cu-Zn] also known as superoxide dismutase 1 or SOD1 is a soluble protein acting as a 32 kDa homodimeric enzyme. SOD1 is one of three human superoxide dismutases.

Its main function is the conversion, naturally occurring, but harmful, superoxide radicals to molecular oxygen and hydrogen peroxide.

SOD1 binds copper and zinc ions and is one of three superoxide dismutases responsible for destroying free superoxide radicals in the body. The encoded isozyme is a soluble cytoplasmic and mitochondrial inter-membrane space protein, acting as a homodimer to convert naturally occurring, but harmful, superoxide radicals to molecular oxygen and hydrogen peroxide

2.1. Genotype

The human *SOD1* gene (Entrez Gene ID 6647) is located on chromosome 21q22.11, and it codes for the monomeric SOD1 polypeptide (153 amino acids, molecular weight 16 kDa).

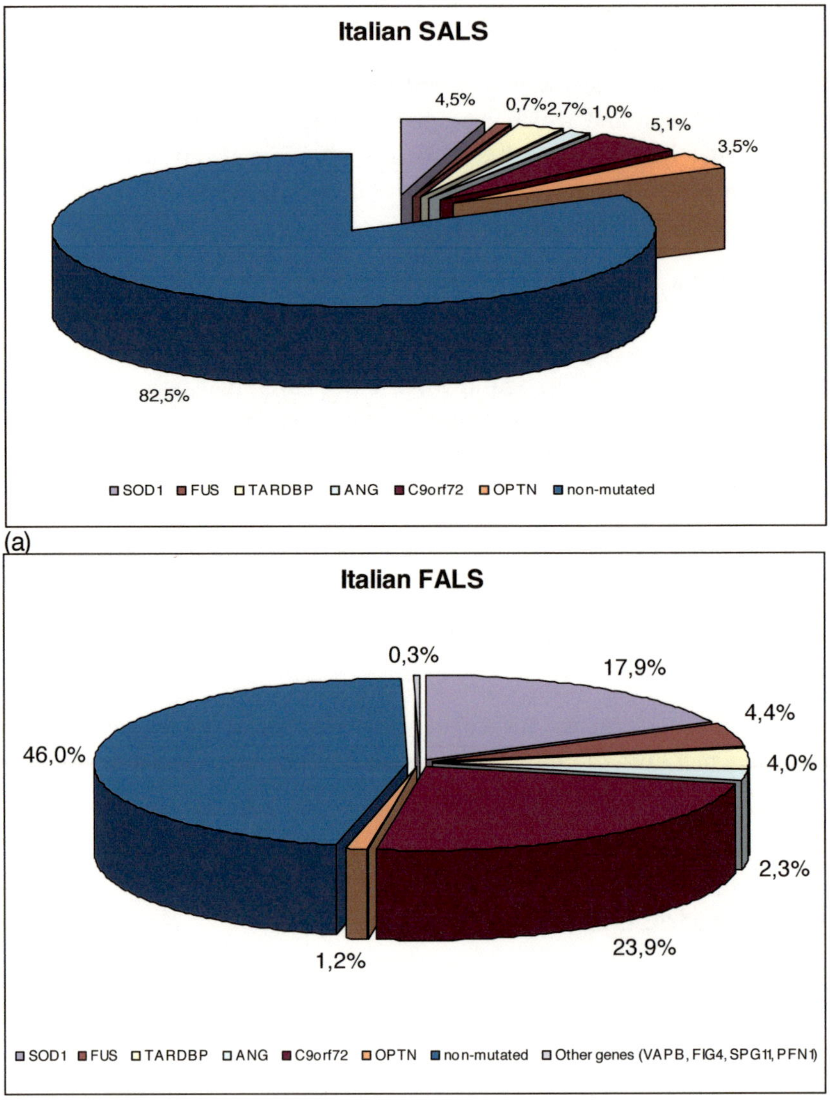

(b)

Figure 1. Summarize the percentage of mutations in Italian ALS patients, (a) SALS, (b) FALS [2, 9, 10, 11, 12, 13, 14].

In 1991, Siddique and collaborators [15] identified a linkage between familial ALS and the SOD1 locus on chromosome 21q22 and demonstrated genetic locus heterogeneity in FALS studying 23 ALS families.

In 1993, Rosen and collaborators [16] have reported tight genetic linkage between ALS and *SOD1* gene, establishing *SOD1* as the first causative gene for ALS. More than 150 *SOD1* mutations have been reported in 68 of the 153 codons, spread over all five exons (ALS Online Genetic Database, ALSOD: http://alsod.iop.kcl.ac.uk/).

http://dx.doi.org/10.5772/56547

The vast majority of which are missense substitutions distributed throughout the five exons of the gene. Also frame-shift deletions and insertions, all clustered in exons 4 and 5, which lead to a premature truncation of the protein have been described (Figure 2).

Collectively, SOD1 mutations are found in ~20% of all FALS patients, and in ~3% of SALS cases [17].

In Italian ALS population, different screening have been performed [2, 18] and both confirmed that the percentage of mutation in SOD1 gene in Italian SALS was 4.5%.

About FALS the percentage of SOD1-mutated FALS patients was 14.7% [18]. In the most recent screening of 480 SALS patients in 48 FALS has been found that the percentage of mutations was totally 2.1% [19].

Novel mutations are continuous discovered, the last one in Italian patient has been described in January 2012 [20].

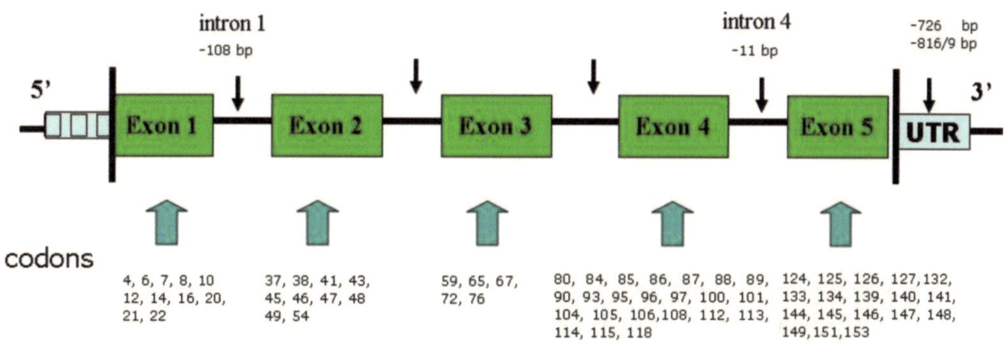

Figure 2. Distribution of *SOD1* mutations detected in sporadic ALS patients.

2.2. Phenotype

Patients with SOD1 mutations, FALS and SALS, show a phenotypic heterogeneity even within the same mutation although some sporadic missense mutations carry a consistently worse or better prognosis. A lot of mutations have been described during the time, we have focused in this paragraph on the most interesting in the Italian population for eventually presence of correlation between genotype and phenotype, both for FALS and SALS.

Patients with FALS and G41S mutations have similar clinical phenotype with early upper and lower motor neuron involvement in one or both lower limbs, rapidly spreading to upper limbs, appearance of bulbar signs within 1 years and death a few months later [21].

In 2010 Battistini et al. [22] described a family with 9 members ALS affected, in which there was evidence of a missense mutation in exon 4 (L106F) in SOD1 gene. In this family there was autosomal dominant inheritance. The clinical presentation was characterized by relatively early age of onset, spinal onset with proximal distribution weakness, bulbar involvement and a rapid disease course about two years.

Another mutation, L106P, has been found in a patient who presented similar clinical pattern with spinal onset with weakness mainly in proximal areas; however in this patient, 30 months after disease onset, weakness remained restricted to the upper limbs without pyramidal signs and it was consistent with brachial amyotrophic diplegia, a relatively slowly progressive variant of motor neuron disease [23].

Corrado et al. [2] suggested that the nonsense mutation in exon 5 was present in SALS patients with severe and rapid clinical course, analogous to what found for most SOD1 mutations leading to a truncated protein. Conversely, N65S and A95T are both associated to a slowly progressive course of the disease, similarly to other mutations (H46R, D76V, H13T, L144P, G93V, I151T, D90A, A89T) detected in patients with a disease duration >10 years. In addition N65S seems to be strictly correlated to a prevalent involvement of the lower motor neurons and only at the spinal cord.

In 2011 in their article, Del Grande et al. [3] showed a similar phenotype in three unrelated patients with sporadic SOD1 mutation D11Y: slow progression, initial distal limbs muscles involvement and predominant lower motor neurons signs. The topographic distribution in distal muscles was a constant feature over many years, with only late impairment of proximal or bulbar muscles (respiratory muscles involvement after 7-10 years). All three patients had slight pyramidal signs (hyperactive reflexes, Babinski sign without increase of muscular tone).

In 2011 Luigetti et al. [24] described a strange case report of a sporadic patient with SOD1 G93D mutation disclosing a rapid progression of the disease. The beginning of symptoms was weakness in upper limbs, without involvement of lower limbs or bulbar functions. Over a 2-year-follow up the patient showed a rapidly progressive course with involvement of lower limbs, bulbar and respiratory muscles and the patient died after 30 months since the onset.

This case is in contrast with literature data [25-27]: other patients with SOD1 mutation (FALS) presented a slowly progressive diseas with a long-lasting paucisymptomatic phase. The authors discovered a novel heterozygous ANG missense mutation (c. 433 C>T, p.R145C), so they hypothesised a role in pathogenesis and clinical phenotype [24].

Penco et al. [28] described a family with same mutation of SOD1, in which there was wide variability of disease expression among family members. The ANG IVS1+27 variant in the heterozygous state was found in the proband that disclosed an aggressive clinical course. Though this variant occurred in noncoding region and no prediction of splicing alteration was made, the authors speculated that this variant contributed to the clinical phenotype.

These findings support a possible pathogenetic role of ANG mutation with influence on clinical manifestations in patient with SOD1 mutation.

Often bulbar onset is associated with older age of disease presentation without significant difference of distribution between FALS and SALS [21].

These data are confirmed by international literature [29-32].

3. TAR DNA-Binding Protein 43 (TARDBP gene)

TAR DNA-binding protein 43 is homologous to the heterogeneous nuclear ribonucleoproteins (hnRNPs) [33], which are involved in RNA processing, and its abnormal cellular distribution is one of the key feature of ALS and frontotemporal lobar degeneration (FTLD) [34].

The protein is highly conserved, widely expressed and predominantly localized to the nucleus with a very small amount being present in the cytoplasm [34-35].

3.1. Genotype

The human *TARDBP* gene (Entrez Gene ID 23435) is located on chromosome 1p36.22, and it codes for a protein of 414 amino acids.

Mutations in *TARDBP* gene associated with ALS disease have been discovered fro the first time in 2008 [34, 36].

The proposed mutational frequency is ~5% for FALS and 0.5-2% for SALS. To date, more than 30 different TARDBP mutations have been described, all of which are missense substitutions. With a single exception, all of them are clustered in the C-terminal glycine-rich region encoded by exon 6. The most common mutation is A382T.

Mutations in *TARDBP* gene associated with ALS disease have been discovered fro the first time in 2009 and in the same year a Italian screening has been performed [9]. The Italian results showed a higher frequency of *TARDBP* mutations in SALS Italian patients compared to individuals of mainly Northern European origin (2.7% vs. 1%).

The frequency of mutations in *TARDBP* gene in Italian patients (4.4%) are similar to other population studies (about 3 to 4% of FALS cases) [37, 38].

Most *TARDBP* mutations are missense changes in exon 6, encoding for Gly-rich C-terminal region that allows to bind single-stranded DNA, RNA and proteins [39, 40] (Figure 3).

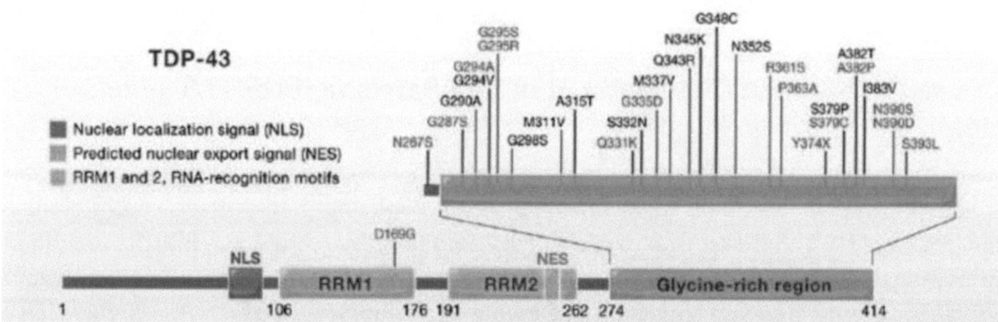

Figure 3. Distribution of TDP-43 mutations detected in sporadic ALS patients [41].

3.2. Phenotype

Many individuals who present with a pure ALS phenotype also develop pathological features of FTD and vice versa. Recently TDP-43 is identified as the major protein of inclusions in FTD and ALS brain tissues, suggesting that both degenerative diseases belong to a clinio-pathological spectrum of overlapping central nervous system disorders. Dominant mutations in the gene encoding the deposited protein account for at least some cases of these diseases.

Corrado et al. [9] described 12 different missense mutations in TARDBP, all located in exon 6, in 18 patients with ALS, both FALS and SALS. Patients don't share a homogeneous clinical phenotype: the average age at onset is 53,2 +/- 14,5 years, the site of onset is mainly spinal (88%), disease duration varies from 17 to 87 months. But in contrast to what is expected from the similarity of TDP-43 pathological deposits in ALS and FTD, none of patients tested worldwide with FTD carried TARDBP mutations. On the contrary, a TARDBP mutation (p.G294V) is discovered in patients with ALS and dementia of Alzheimer type. He developed dementia 3 years before the onset of MND. It is possible that the concurrence of the two diseases is only by chance.

Piaceri et al. [42] described clinical heterogeneity in patients with ALS and mutations in TARDBP. Age at onset is between 49 and 62 years, site of onset is both spinal and bulbar with different involvement of upper or lower motor neuron, disease duration varies from 9 to 85 years. Nobody has FTD. One patient has p.ALA382Thr mutation in exon 6.

In literature also [9, 36] this mutation is associated with some differences in phenotype, that are in site of onset (bulbar-spinal in France and spinal in Italy), disease duration (28-73 months in France, 17-60 months in Italy) and age at onset (50 years in France, 32-69 years in Italy). Italian and French patients shared a common haplotype with allele D1S2667 and D1S489, so there was a common founder for the mutation.

Literature datas [43] suggested that in TARDBP patients site of onset is in the upper limbs, with both upper and lower motor neuron signs but with disease progression lower signs became predominant. Age at onset is mean of 54 years, disease duration mean of 58 months. Some patients presented cognitive impairment that met criteria for FTD.

4. Fused in Sarcoma, Translocated in LipoSarcoma (FUS/TLS gene)

Fused in Sarcoma, Translocated in LipoSarcoma (FUS/TLS) is a heterogeneous ribonucleoprotein (hnRNP) that is involved, as TARDBP, in RNA splicing, transportation and stabilization [38, 44]. FUS/TLS (fused in sarcoma/translocated in liposarcoma) was initially identified by investigators as a component of fusion proteins found in a variety of cancers such as myxoid liposarcoma, acute myeloid leukemia, and Ewing's tumour. More recently, researchers have found several mutations of FUS/TLS in ALS and FTLD (frontotemporal lobar degeneration) patients that causes cytoplasmic mislocalization of FUS/TLS.

4.1. Genotype

The human *FUS/TLS* gene (Entrez Gene ID 2521) is located on chromosome 16p11.2, and it codes for a protein of 525 amino acids.

Mutations in *FUS/TLS* gene in ALS patients have been discovered for the first time in 2009 [37, 45], as *TARDBP*.

Following the original reports [37, 45], several other groups identified additional variants in ALS cohorts of different ethnicities, proposing an overall mutational frequency of ~4% in FALS and ~1% in SALS [46, 47, 48].

To date more than 30 different mutations have been described, the vast majority of which are missense substitutions and the rest are frameshift or nonsense mutations (Figure 3).

In the next year a Italian screening has been performed [10]. The results of the Italian screening are in accord with the interanation screening. The Italian data showed that the percentage of *FUS* missense mutations is 0.7% of Italian SALS cases, 4.4% in FALS.

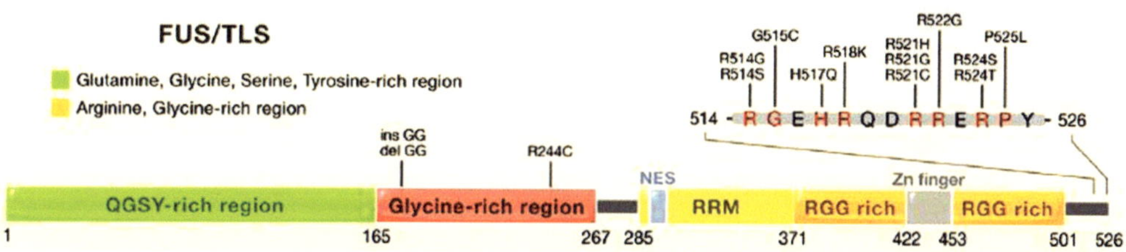

Figure 4. Distribution of FUS mutations detected in sporadic ALS patients [41].

4.2. Phenotype

In 2010 Corrado et al. [10] identified 9 SALS or FALS patients carrying FUS missense mutations. Site of onset was both in upper and lower limbs, age at onset was lower (median 50 years). One of these patients with sporadic ALS and FUS mutation presented, at the age of 34, bilateral scapular girdle muscle weakness with unusual neck flexor/extensor muscle weakness with cramps and fasciculations, no weakness in the lower limbs has been demonstrated. Another patient with FALS and FUS mutation, at the age of 54, slowly developed weakness of the neck flexor/extensor muscles and bilateral scapular girdle and proximal upper limb muscle weakness, with subsequent impairment of the pelvic girdle, no bulbar involvement has been shown but slight proximal weakness in the lower limbs; one year after onset, the symptoms extended to the bulbar region. So these two patients developed an unusual proximal symmetrical upper limbs onset and axial involvement.

Ticozzi N et al. in 2009 [49] described two patients with FALS and mutation of FUS that presented the same clinical phenotype.

In 2011 Lai SL et al. [50] described 4 Italian patients with sporadic ALS and FUS mutations (p.Y66Y, p.G507D, p.R521C, p.R521H). All of these cases initially manifested limb weakness and symptoms onset was before 50 years of age in more cases.

In 2009 Chiò et al. [51] described a patient with mutation in FUS and a very young age at onset (<30 years) with a bulbar presentation and a short duration.

In literature [37, 45] confirmed this correlations between genotype and phenotype in FUS mutations in ALS both FALS and SALS patients.

Millecamps S et al. [43] suggested that FUS patients had a shorter lifespan, more rapid disease, younger onset than other mutations.

5. Angiogenin (ANG)

Angiogenin is a angiogenic ribonuclease whose activity is related to its ability in regulating ribosomal RNA (rRNA) transcription. ANG induces angiogenesis by activating vessel endothelial and smooth muscle cells and triggering a number of biological processes, including cell migration, invasion, proliferation, and formation of tubular structures [52].

5.1. Genotype

The human *ANG* gene (Entrez Gene ID 283) is located on chromosome 14q11.1-q11.2, and it codes for a protein of 147 amino acids.

ANG, encoding a 14 kDa angiogenic ribonuclease, is the first loss-of-function gene identified in ALS. Since original discovery of *ANG* as an ALS candidate gene, a total of 15 missense mutations in the coding region of ANG have been identified in 37 of the 4,193 ALS patients. Among them, 10 have been characterized in detail and shown to be loss-of-function mutations. ANG gene has been found mutated in 2.3% of FALS and 1% of SALS patients [53].

The percentage of *ANG* gene mutations has been confirmed in the Italian ALS population [11].

5.2. Phenotype

Gellera et al. [11] identified 9 patients with new ANG mutation, 6 SALS and 3 FALS. Two patients presented bulbar onset, while 7 patients spinal onset. Patients with P-4S mutation presented signs of LMN involvement in both legs at age of 55 years and subsequently a rapidly progressive course with signs of UMN and LMN involvement. Two patients had G20G mutation but two different clinical course: first patient had slowly progressive lower limb onset MND at age 62 with prevalence of LMN signs and 3 years later manifested cognitive dysfunction of frontal lobe type, second patient presented distal weakness of upper limb at age 21 with a slowly progressive course characterized by prevalence of LMN signs. SALS Patient with V113I mutation developed spasticity of the right arm and atrophy of the right hand muscles at age 51, one year later the same symptoms appeared in the controlateral upper limb with prevalence of UMN signs. Patient with H114R mutation started with bulbar signs at age of 68.

Patients with previously described I46V mutation presented distal weakness of lower limbs, predominance of LMN signs, slow course of disease (only in one case more rapid with bulbar involvement). Age at onset was between 50-60 years.

So there was a wide phenotypic variability in these patients, for both district of onset and involvemenent of UMN/LMN.

Greenway et al. [53] reported that bulbar onset was more frequent in patients with ANG mutations.

6. Chromosome 9 open reading frame 72 (C9orf72)

Chromosome 9 open reading frame 72 is a protein localized on plasma membrane and cytoskeleton. There are two isoforms of C9orf72 that are produced as a result of alternative splicing events and the molecular weight of *C9orf72* isoforms is 54/25 kDa. Normally, it is nuclear protein, even if the mutated form has been described in the cytoplasm [54].

6.1. Genotype

The human *C9orf72* gene (Entrez Gene ID 203228) is located on chromosome 9p21.2, and it codes for a protein of 481 amino acids.

Recently, a hexanucleotide repeat expansion within the *C9orf72* gene was identified as the cause of chromosome 9p21-linked ALS-FTD [54, 55].

About the Italian population, a screening *C9orf72* in a large cohort of 259 familial ALS, 1275 sporadic ALS, and 862 control individuals has been performed [12]. It has been found RE in 23.9% familial ALS, 5.1% sporadic ALS, and 0.2% controls. Two cases carried the RE together with mutations in other ALS-associated genes.

Genotype data revealed that 95% of RE carriers shared a restricted 10-single nucleotide polymorphism haplotype within the previously reported 20-single nucleotide polymorphism risk haplotype, detectable in only 27% of nonexpanded ALS cases and in 28% of controls, suggesting a common founder with cohorts of North European ancestry. Although *C9orf72* RE segregates with disease, the identification of RE both in controls and in patients carrying additional pathogenic mutations suggests that penetrance and phenotypic expression of *C9orf72* RE may depend on additional genetic risk factors.

6.2. Phenotype

Ratti et al. [12] observed that the phenotype of RE carriers was characterized in higher proportion by bulbar-onset compared with nonexpanded patients, while in individuals with spinal onset expanded patients displayed an early involvement of the upper limbs less frequently than other patients, with predominance of upper motor neuron signs. RE carriers had a shorter survival compared with noncarriers. There was a correlation between more frequent bulbar onset in expanded patients and shorter survival time. The concurrence of FTD was significantly higher in expanded cases compared with wild type individuals and also ALS-FTD patients with RE manifested cognitive behaviour before the onset of motor symptoms. In most cases the phenotype was compatible with a behavioural variant of FTD and frequently dominated by psychiatric symptoms, such as visual hallucination, paranoid behaviour with persecutory delusions, aggressive behaviour and/or suicidal thoughts.

Reports in literature were in according [56-59].

Extrapyramidal and cerebellar signs were also observed in two patients, while a patients presented continuous lingual myclonus at disease onset. These cases suggested that clinical phenotype associated with RE in C9orf72 may be broader than originally thought, possibly involving extramotoneuronal structures such as the basal ganglia, cerebellum, brainstem nuclei.

Sabatelli et al. and Chiò et al. [60, 61, 62] studied clinical phenotype of patients with repeat expansion in large population and also two Sardinian families with neurodegenerative diseases (FTD-ALS) in which mutations in different genes (TARDBP p.A382T mutation and repeat expansion GGGGCC C9orf72) co-existed as pathogenetic causes, giving varied phenotypes.

7. Optineurin

Optineurin is an inhibitor protein that play an important role in the maintenance of the Golgi complex, in membrane trafficking and in exocytosis. Alternative splicing results in multiple transcript variants encoding the same protein., three different isoforms are known.

7.1. Genotype

The human *OPTN* gene (Entrez Gene ID 10133) is located on chromosome 10p13, and it codes for a protein of 577 amino acids. In 2010 *OPTN* mutations have been described, for the first time, in ALS patients [63]. In the first paper about OPTN mutation three type of mutation have been found, two point mutation and one deletion. In 2011, a screening in the Caucasian population in SALS and FALS patients showed that *OPTN* mutations causing ALS are rare, especially in mainly Caucasian ALS subjects [64]. About Italian population, Del Bo and collaborators screened 274 ALS patients, 161 FALS and 113 SALS and the results showed six novel variants in both FALS and SALS patients, all occurring in an heterozygous state [13]. This data support the involvement of *OPTN* in ALS, especially in FALS patients, due to the 1.2% cases found mutated [13].

7.2. Phenotype

Del Bo et al. [13] suggested that ALS patients carrying OPTN mutations showed a prevalent lower-limb onset, with large variable age of onset (from 24 to 71 years of age) and progression (very aggressive forms with survival time < 1 year and very slow disease course over 10 years) with no differencies between SALS and FALS patients. Many patients were characterized by a prevalence of upper motor neuron signs.

8. Conclusions

Amyotrophic Lateral Sclerosis is a multifactorial and multigenic disease with still unknown aetiology and pathogenesis. We know many causative mutations in particular genes, both in familial and sporadic patients, and different clinical presentation of ALS. Genetic factors may play a role in determining the range of ALS phenotypes although in this moment no genes have been demonstrated to have a definite effect on phenotype (Chiò et al., 2011) [4]. Heterogeneity between and among families and patients with same mutation suggests that environmental and other influences contribute to not only the rate of evolution and which signs predominate but also whether the disease will appear at all during life.

In this chapter we have identified cases in which connection between phenotype and genotype is possible and relevant.

We started from the ALS patients part of the recruitment of our Institute to define the possible clinical features that may be related to specific genes alteration.

For ALS patients with mutations in some genes, such as *SOD1*, there are an important clinical phenotypic heterogeneity at onset and during evolution of disease, different time of survival and velocity of progression with rapidly or slowly involvement of bulbar functions.

TARDBP is involved both in pathogenesis of frontotemporal dementia and ALS, but it's not sure that all patients with ALS will develop FTD and they don't demonstrated an homogenous clinical pattern.

In particular we will focus attention on connection between FUS mutations, and clinical presentation with upper limbs onset, developed weakness of the neck flexor/extensor muscles and bilateral scapular girdle and proximal muscle. In many cases this phenotype is correlated with rapidly bulbar evolution and frontotemporal behaviour alterations, with negative prognosis in short time. This focus is in particular due to the presence of FUS mutated patients in our cohort and the "poverty" of the literature about FUS and clinical features.

Another interesting suggestion is that sometimes mutated patients (i.e. SOD1) can have particular clinical course modulated by other causative or associated modified genes (ANG). It is an important issue that maybe indicates a central role of genotype in developing phenotype.

For other genes it's difficult discovering association between genotype and phenotype for rarity of manifestation compared with more frequent mutations.

In conclusion, at this time, in front of a patient with ALS, a neurologist should has some "milestones" considering clinical phenotype:

- if patient's history suggests a familial form, it is important to perform a screening of four principal genes (SOD1, TARDBP, FUS, C9ORF) because they cover more than 50% of FALS;
- if onset of disease is in early age, the probability of a mutation is high and four principal genes are still first candidates in SALS;
- if patient presents frontotemporal characters or premature respiratory involvement, TARDBP, FUS, C9ORF are essential in screening;
- if clinical phenotype is characterized by proximal muscles involvement in upper and/or lower limbs, FUS has to be suspected.

Our idea is that a specific mutation can cause a particular clinical onset, involvement and evolution of ALS, with a pathogenetic mechanism still unknown.

On the other side, now we have some ideas for type of disease correlated with particular mutations (i.e. FUS and TARDBP give a early onset, short duration of disease for early bulbar involvement) but it's impossible predict exactly what kind of phenotype can be developed by patient.

Different genes are involved in ALS disease, the importance of a good clinical characterization may help in choosing the genetic approach. We hypothesized that in the future, the symptoms observation may became more specific to indicate which gene is the most probably mutated. This idea may proceed in the same time of a better collaboration between clinicians and biologist to create a direct link from bed to bench.

This approach may be relevant for diagnostic use, so starting from neurological exam, that remains the essential element, and we can formulate diagnostic hypothesis that it can be surely confirmed by genetic test.

Acknowledgement

We are grateful to the patients and their families. We thank other members of General Neurology Department and Laboratory of Experimental Neurobiology for continuous working activity.

Author details

L. Diamanti[1,2], S. Gagliardi[3], C. Cereda[3] and M. Ceroni[1,2]

1 General Neurology Department, IRCCS, National Neurological Institute "C. Mondino", Pavia, Italy

2 Department of Public Health, Neuroscience, Experimental and Forensic Medicine, University of Pavia, Pavia, Italy

3 Laboratory of Experimental Neurobiology, IRCCS, National Neurological Institute "C. Mondino", Pavia, Italy

References

[1] Ropper AH, Samuels MA. Adams & Victor's, Principles of Neurology, 9th edition, 2009; chapter 39, p. 1059.

[2] Corrado L, D'Alfonso S, Bergamaschi L, Testa L, Leone M, Nasuelli N, Momigliano-Richiardi P, Mazzini L. SOD1 gene mutations in Italian patients with sporadic ALS. Neuromuscolar disorders 2006; 16: 800-804.

[3] Del Grande A, Conte A, Lattante S, Luigetti M, Marangi G, Zollino M, Madia F, Bisogni G, Sabatelli M. D11Y SOD1 mutation and benign ALS: a consitent genotype-phenotype correlation. Journal of neurological science 2011; 309: 31-33.

[4] Chiò A, Calvo A, Moglia C, Mazzini L, Mora G; PARALS study group. Phenotypic heterogeneity of amyotrophic lateral sclerosis: a population based study. J Neurol Neurosurg Psychiatry 2011; 82:740-6.

[5] Brooks BR, El Escorial World Federation of Neurology criteria for diagnosis of amyotrophic lateral sclerosis: Subcommittee on Motor Neuron Diseases/Amyotrophic Lateral Sclerosis of the World Federation of Neurology Research Group on Neuromuscular Diseases and the El Escorial Clinical Limits of Amyotrophic Lateral Sclerosis workshop contributors. J Neurol Sci 1994; 124: 96-107.

[6] Brooks BR, Miller RG, Swash M, Munsat TL, World Federation of Neurology Research Group on Motor Neuron Diseases. El Escorial revisited: revised criteria for the diagnosis of Amyotrophic Lateral Sclerosis. Amyotroph Lateral Scler Other Motor Neuron Disord 2000; 1: 293-9.

[7] Neary D, Snowden JS, Gustafson L, Passant U, Stuss D, Black S, freedman M, Kertesz A, Robert PH, Albert M, Boone K, Miller BL, Cummings J, Benson DF. Frontotemporal lobar degeneration: a consensus on clinical diagnostic criteria. Neurology 1998; 51: 1546-54.

[8] The Lund and Manchester Group. Clinical and neuropathological criteria for frontotemporal dementia. J Neurol Neurosurg Psychiatry 1994; 57: 416-18.

[9] Corrado L, Ratti A, Gellera C, Buratti E, Castellotti B, Carlomagno Y, Ticozzi N, Mazzini L, Testa L, Taroni F, Baralle FE, Silani V, D'Alfonso S. High frequency of TARDBP gene mutations in Italian patients with amyotrophic lateral sclerosis. Hum Mutat 2009 ; 30: 688-94.

[10] Corrado L, Del Bo R, Castellotti B, Ratti A, Cereda C, Penco S, Sorarù G, Carlomagno Y, Ghezzi S, Pensato V, Colombrita C, Gagliardi S, Cozzi L, Orsetti V, Mancuso M, Siciliano G, Mazzini L, Comi GP, Gellera C, Ceroni M, D'Alfonso S, Silani V. Mutations of FUS gene in sporadic amyotrophic lateral sclerosis. J Med Genet. 2010; 47:190-4.

[11] Gellera C, Colombrita C, Ticozzi N, Castellotti B, Bragato C, Ratti A, Taroni F, Silani V. Identification of new ANG gene mutations in a large cohort of Italian patients with amyotrophic lateral sclerosis. Neurogenetics 2008; 9: 33-40.

[12] Ratti A, Corrado L, Castelletti B, Del Bo R, Fogh I, Cereda C, Tiloca C, D'Ascenzo C, Bagarotti A, Pensato V, Ranieri M, Gagliardi S, Calini D, Mazzini L, Taroni F, Corti S, Ceroni M, Oggioni GD, Lin K, Powell JF, Sorarù G, Ticozzi N, Comi GP, D'Alfonso S, Gellera C, Silani V and the SLAGEN Consortium. C9ORF72 repeat expansion in a large Italian ALS cohort: evidence of a founder effect. Neurobiology of aging 2012; 33: 2528.e7-e14.

[13] Del Bo R, Tiloca C, Pensato V, Corrado L, Ratti A, Ticozzi N, Corti S, Castellotti B, Mazzini L, Sorarù G, Cereda C, D'Alfonso S, Gellera C, Comi GP, Silani V; SLAGEN Consortium. Novel optineurin mutations in patients with familial and sporadic amyotrophic lateral sclerosis. J Neurol Neurosurg Psychiatry 2011; 82:1239-43.

[14] Nishimura AL, Mitne-Neto M, Silva HC, Richieri-Costa A, Middleton S, Cascio D, Kok F, Oliveira JR, Gillingwater T, Webb J, Skehel P, Zatz M. A mutation in the vesicle-trafficking protein VAPB causes late-onset spinal muscular atrophy and amyotrophic lateral sclerosis. Am J Hum Genet 2004; 75: 822-31.

[15] Siddique T, Figlewicz DA, Pericak-Vance MA, Haines JL, Rouleau G, Jeffers AJ, Sapp P, Hung WY, Bebout J, McKenna-Yasek D, et al. Linkage of a gene causing familial amyotrophic lateral sclerosis to chromosome 21 and evidence of genetic-locus heterogeneity. N Engl J Med 1991; 324:1381-4.

[16] Rosen DR, Siddique T, Patterson D, Figlewicz DA, Sapp P, Hentati A, Donaldson D, Goto J, O'Regan JP, Deng HX, Rahmani Z, Krizus A, McKenna Yasek D, Cayabyab A, Gaston SM, Berger R, Tanzi RE, Halperin JJ, Herzfeltd B, Van den Bergh R, Hung W-Y, Bird T, Deng G, Mulder DW, Smyth C, Laing NG, Soriano E, Pericak-Vance MA, Haines J, Rouleau GA, Gusella JS, Horvitz HR, Brown RH Jr. Mutations in Cu/Zn superoxide dismutase gene are associated with familial amyotrophic lateral sclerosis. Nature 1993; 362: 59-62.

[17] Andersen PM, Sims KB, Xin WW, Kiely R, O'Neill G, Ravits J, Pioro E, Harati Y, Brower RD, Levine JS, Heinicke HU, Seltzer W, Boss M, Brown RH Jr. Sixteen novel mutations in the Cu/Zn superoxide dismutase gene in amyotrophic lateral sclerosis: a decade of discoveries, defects and disputes. Amyotroph. Lateral Scler Other Motor Neuron Disord 2003; 4: 62-73.

[18] Gellera C. Genetics of ALS in Italian families. Amyotrophic Lateral Scler Other Motor Neuron Disord 2001; 2: S43-46.

[19] Lattante S, Conte A, Zollino M, Luigetti M, Del Grande A, Marangi G, Romano A, Marcaccio A, Meleo E, Bisogni G, Rossini PM, Sabatelli M. Contribution of major amyotrophic lateral sclerosis genes to the etiology of sporadic disease. Neurology 2012; 79:66-72.

[20] Origone P, Caponnetto C, Mantero V, Cichero E, Fossa P, Geroldi A, Verdiani S, Bellone E, Mancardi G, Mandich P. Fast course ALS presenting with vocal cord paralysis: clinical features, bioinformatic and modelling analysis of the novel SOD1 Gly147Ser mutation. Amyotroph Lateral Scler 2012; 13: 144-8.

[21] Battistini S, Giannini F, Greco G, Bibbò G, Ferrera L, Marini V, Causarano R, Casula M, Lando G, Patrosso MC, Caponnetto C, Origone P, Marocchi A, Del Corona A, Siciliano G, Carrera P, Mascia V, Giagheddu M, Carcassi C, Orrù S, Garrè C, Penco S. SOD1 mutations in amyotrophic lateral sclerosis. Results from a multicenter Italian study. J Neurol 2005; 252: 782-8.

[22] Battistini S, Ricci C, Lotti EM, Benigni M, Gagliardi S, Zucco R, Bondavalli M, Marcello N, Ceroni M, Cereda C. Severe familial ALS with a novel exon 4 mutation (L106F) in the SOD1 gene. Journal of the neurological sciences 2010; 293: 112-115.

[23] Valentino P, Conforti FL, Pirritano D, Nisticò R, Mazzei R, Patitucci A, Sprovieri T, Gabriele AL, Muglia M, Clodomiro A, Gambardella A, Zappia M, Quattrone A. Brachial amyotrophic diplegia associated with a novel SOD1 mutation (L106P). Neurology 2005; 64:1477-8.

[24] Luigetti M, Lattante S, Zollino M, Conte A, Marangi G, Del Grande A, Sabatelli M. SOD1 G93D sporadic ALS patient with rapid progression and concomitant novel ANG variant. Neurobiology of aging 2011; 32: 1924e15-18.

[25] Luigetti M, Madia F, Conte A, Marangi G, Zollino M, Del Grande A, Dileone M, Tonali PA, Sabatelli M. SOD1 G93D mutation presenting as paucisymptomatic amyotrophic lateral sclerosis. Amyotroph Lateral Scler 2009;10:479-82.

[26] Luigetti M, Conte A, Madia F, Marangi G, Zollino M, Mancuso I, Dileone M, Del Grande A, Di Lazzaro V, Tonali PA, Sabatelli M. Heterozygous SOD1 D90A mutation presenting as slowly progressive predominant upper motor neuron amyotrophic lateral sclerosis. Neurol Sci 2009; 30: 517-20.

[27] Restagno G, Lombardo F, Sbaiz L, Mari L, Gellera C, Alimenti D, Calvo A, Tarenzi L, Chiò A. The rare G93D mutation causes a slowly progressing lower motor neuron disease. Amyotr Lat Scler 2008; 9: 35-39.

[28] Penco S, Lunetta C, Mosca L, Maestri E, Avemaria F, Tarlarini C, Patrosso MC, Marocchi A, Corbo M. Phenotypic heterogeneity in a SOD1 G93D Italian ALS family; an example of human model to study a complex disease. J Mol Neurosci 2011; 44: 25-30.

[29] Andersen PM, Nilsson P, Keranen ML, Forsgren L, Hagglund J, Karlsborg M, Ronnevi LO, Gredal O, Marklund SL. Phenotypic heterogeneity in motor neuron disease patients with CuZn-SOD mutations in Scandinavia. Brain 1997; 120: 1723-1737.

[30] Andersen PM. Amyotrophic lateral sclerosis associated with mutations in the CuZn SOD gene. Curr Neurol Neurosci Rep 2006; 6: 37-46.

[31] Rosen DR, Bowling A, Patterson D, Usdin TB, Sapp P, Mezey E et al. A frequent ala4val SOD1 mutations is associated with a rapidly progressive familial amyotrophic lateral sclerosis. Hum Mol Genet 1994; 4: 981-7.

[32] Georgoulopoulou E, Gellera C, Bragato C, Sola P, Chiari A, Bernabei C, Mandrioli J. A novel SOD1 mutation in a young ALS patient with a very slowly progressive clinical corse. Muscle nerve 2010; 42: 596-7.

[33] Colombrita C, Onesto E, Tiloca C, Ticozzi N, Silani V, Ratti A. RNA-binding proteins and RNA metabolism: a new scenario in the pathogenesis of Amyotrophic lateral sclerosis. Arch Ital Biol 2011; 149:83-99.

[34] Sreedharan J, Blair IP, Tripathi VB, Hu X, Vance C, Rogelj B, Ackerley S, Durnall JC, Williams KL, Buratti E, Baralle F, de Belleroche J, Mitchell JD, Leigh PN, Al-Chalabi A, Miller CC, Nicholson G, Shaw CE. TDP-43 mutations in familial and sporadic amyotrophic lateral sclerosis. Science 2008; 319:1668-72.

[35] Minvielle-Sebastia L, Beyer K, Krecic AM, Hector RE, Swanson MS, Keller W.Winton MJ, Van Deerlin VM, Kwong LK, Yuan W, Wood EM, Yu CE, Schellenberg GD, Rademakers R, Caselli R, Karydas A, Trojanowski JQ, Miller BL, Lee VM. A90V TDP-43 variant results in the aberrant localization of TDP-43 in vitro. FEBS Lett 2008; 582: 2252-6.

[36] Kabashi E, Valdmanis PN, Dion P, Spiegelman D, McConkey BJ, Vande Velde C, Bouchard JP, Lacomblez L, Pochigaeva K, Salachas F, Pradat PF, Camu W, Meininger V, Dupre N, Rouleau GA. TARDBP mutations in individuals with sporadic and familial amyotrophic lateral sclerosis. Nat Genet 2008; 40: 572-574.

[37] Kwiatkowski TJ Jr, Bosco DA, Leclerc AL, Tamrazian E, Vanderburg CR, Russ C, Davis A, Gilchrist J, Kasarskis EJ, Munsat T, Valdmanis P, Rouleau GA, Hosler BA, Cortelli P, de Jong PJ, Yoshinaga Y, Haines JL, Pericak-Vance MA, Yan J, Ticozzi N, Siddique T, McKenna-Yasek D, Sapp PC, Horvitz HR, Landers JE, Brown RH Jr. Mutations in the FUS/TLS gene on chromosome 16 cause familial amyotrophic lateral sclerosis. Science 2009; 323:1205-8.

[38] Kamada M, Maruyama H, Tanaka E, Morino H, Wate R, Ito H, Kusaka H, Kawano Y, Miki T, Nodera H, Izumi Y, Kaji R, Kawakami H. Screening for TARDBP mutations in Japanese familial amyotrophic lateral sclerosis. J Neurol Sci 2009; 284: 69-71.

[39] Ayala YM, Zago P, D'Ambrogio A, Xu YF, Petrucelli L, Buratti E, Baralle FE. Structural determinants of the cellular localization and shuttling of TDP-43. J Cell Sc 2008; 121: 3778-85.

[40] Wang HY, Wang IF, Bose J, Shen CK. Structural diversity and functional implications of the eukaryotic TDP gene family. Genomics 2004; 83:130-9.

[41] Liscic RM, Breljak D. Molecular basis of amyotrophic lateral sclerosis. Prog Neuropsychopharmacol Biol Psychiatry 2011; 35:370-2.

[42] Piaceri I, Del Mastio M, Tedde A, Bagnoli S, Latorraca S, Massaro F, Paganini M, Corrado A, Sorbi S, Nacmias B. Clinical heterogeneity in Italian patients with amyotrophic lateral sclerosis. Clin Genet 2012; 82: 83-87.

[43] Millecamps S, Salachas F, Cazeneuve c, Gordon P, Bricka B, Camuzat A, Guillot-Noel L, Russaouen O, Bruneteau G, Pradat PF, Le Forestier N, Vandenberghe N, Danel-Brunaud V, Guy N, Thauvin-Robinet C, Lacomblez L, Couratier P, Hannequin D, Seilhean D, Le Ber I, Corcia P, Camu W, Brice A, Rouleau G, leGuern E, Meininger V. SOD1, ANG, VAPB, TARDBP and FUS mutations in familial ALS : genotype-phenotype correlations. J Med Genet 2010; 47 : 554-560.

[44] Lagier-Tourenne C, Polymenidou M, Cleveland DW. TDP-43 and FUS/TLS: emerging roles in RNA processing and neurodegeneration. Hum Mol Genet 2010; 19:R46-64.

[45] Vance C, Rogelj B, Hortobagyi T, De Vos KJ, Nishimura AL, Sreedharan J, Hu X, Smith B, Ruddy D, Wright P, Ganesalingham J, Williams KL, Tripathi V, Al-Saraj S, Al Chalabi A, Leigh PN, Blair IP, Nicholson G, de Belleroche J, Gallo JM, Miller CC, Shaw CE. Mutations in FUS, an RNA processing protein, cause familial amyotrophic lateral sclerosis type 6 Science 2009; 323: 1208-1211.

[46] Belzil VV, Valdmanis PN, Dion PA, Daoud H, Kabashi E, Noreau A, Gauthier J, Hince P, Desjarlais A, Bouchard JP, Lacomblez L, Salachas F, Pradat PF, Camu W, Meininger V, Dupre N, Rouleau GA Mutations in FUS cause familial amyotrophic lateral sclerosis and sporadic amyotrophic lateral sclerosis in French and French Canadian populations. Neurology 2009; 73: 1176-1179.

[47] Blair IP, Williams KL, Warraich ST, Durnall JC, Thoeng AD, Manavis J, Blumbergs PC, Vucic S, Kiernan MC, Nicholson GA FUS mutations in amyotrophic lateral sclerosis: clinical, pathological, neurophysiological and genetic analysis. J Neurol Neurosurg Psychiatry 2009; 81: 639-45.

[48] Waibel S, Neumann M, Rabe M, Meyer T, Ludolph AC. Novel missense and truncating mutations in FUS/TLS in familial ALS. Neurology 2010; 75: 815- 817.

[49] Ticozzi N, Silani V, LeClerc LA, Keagle P, Gellera C, Ratti A, Taroni F, Kwiatkowski TJ Jr, McKenna-Yasek DM, Sapp PC, Brown RH Jr, Landers JE. Analysis of FUS gene mutation in familial amyotrophic lateral sclerosis within an Italian cohort. Neurology 2009; 73: 1171-3.

[50] Lai SL, Abramzon Y, Schymick JC, Stephan DA, Dunckley T, Dillman A, Cookson M, Calvo A, Battistini S, Giannini F, Caponnetto C, Mancardi GL, Spataro R, Monsurro MR, Tedeschi G, Marinou K, Sabatelli M, Conte A, Mandrioli J, Sola P, Salvi F, Bartolomei I, Lombardo F, the ITALSGEN Consortium, Mora G, Restagno G, Chiò A, Traynor BJ. FUS mutations in sporadic ALS. Neurobiology of aging 2011; 32: 550e1-e4.

[51] Chiò A, Restagno G, Brunetti M, Ossola I, Calvo A, Mora G, Sabatelli M, Monsurrò MR, Battistini S, Mandrioli J, Salvi F, Spataro R, Schymick J, Traynor BJ, LaBella V.

ITALSGEN Consortium. Two Italian kindreds with familial amyotrophic lateral sclerosis due to FUS mutations. Neurobiol aging 2009; 30: 1272-75.

[52] Russo N, Shapiro R, Acharya KR, Riordan JF, Vallee BL. Role of glutamine-117 in the ribonucleolytic activity of human angiogenin. Proc Natl Acad Sci USA 1994; 91: 2920–2924.

[53] Greenway MJ, Andersen PM, Russ C, Ennis S, Cashman S, Donaghy C, Patterson V, Swingler R, Kieran D, Prehn J, Morrison KE, Green A, Acharya KR, Brown RH Jr, Hardiman O. ANG mutations segregate with familial and 'sporadic' amyotrophic lateral sclerosis. Nat Genet 2006; 38: 411-3.

[54] DeJesus-Hernandez M, Mackenzie IR, Boeve BF, Boxer AL, Baker M, Rutherford NJ, Nicholson AM, Finch NA, Flynn H, Adamson J, Kouri N, Wojtas A, Sengdy P, Hsiung GY, Karydas A, Seeley WW, Josephs KA, Coppola G, Geschwind DH, Wszolek ZK, Feldman H, Knopman DS, Petersen RC, Miller BL, Dickson DW, Boylan KB, Graff-Radford NR, Rademakers R. Expanded GGGGCC hexanucleotide repeat in noncoding region of C9ORF72 causes chromosome 9p-linked FTD and ALS. Neuron 2011; 72: 1-12.

[55] Renton AE, Majounie E, Waite A, Simón-Sánchez J, Rollinson S, Gibbs JR, Schymick JC, Laaksovirta H, van Swieten JC, Myllykangas L, Kalimo H, Paetau A, Abramzon Y, Remes AM, Kaganovich A, Scholz SW, Duckworth J, Ding J, Harmer DW, Hernandez DG, Johnson JO, Mok K, Ryten M, Trabzuni D, Guerreiro RJ, Orrell RW, Neal J, Murray A, Pearson J, Jansen IE, Sondervan D, Seelaar H, Blake D, Young K, Halliwell N, Callister JB, Toulson G, Richardson A, Gerhard A, Snowden J, Mann D, Neary D, Nalls MA, Peuralinna T, Jansson L, Isoviita VM, Kaivorinne AL, Hölttä-Vuori M, Ikonen E, Sulkava R, Benatar M, Wuu J, Chiò A, Restagno G, Borghero G, Sabatelli M; ITALSGEN Consortium, Heckerman D, Rogaeva E, Zinman L, Rothstein JD, Sendtner M, Drepper C, Eichler EE, Alkan C, Abdullaev Z, Pack SD, Dutra A, Pak E, Hardy J, Singleton A, Williams NM, Heutink P, Pickering-Brown S, Morris HR, Tienari PJ, Traynor BJ. A hexanucleotide repeat expansion in C9ORF72 is the cause of chromosome 9p21-linked ALS-FTD. Neuron 2011; 72: 257-68.

[56] Byrne S, Elamin M, Bede P, Shatunov A, Walsh C, Corr B, Heverin M, Jordan N, Kenna K, Lynch C, McLaughlin RL, Iyer PM, O'Brien C, Phukan J, Wynne B, Bokde AL, Bradley DG, Pender N, Al-Chalabi A, Hardiman O. Cognitive and clinical characteristics of patients with ALS carrying a C9ORF72 RE; a population-based cohort study. Lancet Neurol 2012; 11: 232-240.

[57] Gijselinck I, Van Langenhove T, Van der Zee J, Sleegers K, Philtjens S, Kleinberger G, Janssens J, Bettens K, Van Cauwenberghe C, Pereson S, Engelborghe S, Sieben A, De Jonghe P, Vandenberghe R, Santens P, De Bleecker J, Maes G, Baumer V, Dillen L, Joris G, Cuijt I, Corsmit E, Elinck E, Van Dongen J, Vermeulen S, Van den Broeck M, Vaerenberg C, Mattheijssens M, Peeters K, Robberecht W, Cras P, Martin JJ, De Deyn PP, Cruts M, Van Broeckhoven C. A C9ORF72 promoter RE in a Flanders-Belgian co-

hort with disorders of the frontotemporal lobar degeneration-amyotrophic lateral sclerosis spectrum: a gene identification study. Lancet Neurol 2012; 11: 54-65.

[58] Simón-Sánchez J, Dopper EG, Cohn-Hokke PE, Hukema RK, Nicolaou N, Seelaar H, de Graaf JR, de Koning I, van Schoor NM, Deeg DJ, Smits M, Raaphorst J, van den Berg LH, Schelhaas HJ, De Die-Smulders CE, Majoor-Krakauer D, Rozemuller AJ, Willemsen R, Pijnenburg YA, Heutink P, van Swieten JC. The clinical and pathological phenotype of C9ORF72 hexanucleotide repeat expansions. Brain 2012; 135: 723-35.

[59] Snowden JS, Rollinson S, Thompson JC, Harris JM, Stopford CL, Richardson AM, Jones M, Gerhard A, Davidson YS, Robinson A, Gibbons L, Hu Q, DuPlessis D, Neary D, Mann DM, Pickering-Brown SM. Distinct clinical and pathological characteristics of frontotemporal dementia associated with C9ORF72 mutations. Brain 2012; 135:693-708.

[60] Chiò A, Restagno G, Brunetti M, Ossola I, Calvo A, Canosa A, Moglia C, Floris G, Tacconi P, Marrosu F, Marrosu MG, Murru MR, Majounie E, Renton AE, Abramzon Y, Pugliatti M, Sotgiu MA, Traynor BJ, Borghero G; SARDINIALS Consortium. ALS/FTD phenotype in two Sardinian families carrying both C9ORF72 and TARDBP mutations. J Neurol Neurosurg Psychiatry 2012; 83:730-3.

[61] Chiò A, Borghero G, Restagno G, Mora G, Drepper C, Traynor BJ, Sendtner M, Brunetti M, Ossola I, Calvo A, Pugliatti M, Sotgiu MA, Murru MR, Marrosu MG, Marrosu F, Marinou K, Mandrioli J, Sola P, Caponnetto C, Mancardi G, Mandich P, La Bella V, Spataro R, Conte A, Monsurrò MR, Tedeschi G, Pisano F, Bartolomei I, Salvi F, Lauria Pinter G, Simone I, Logroscino G, Gambardella A, Quattrone A, Lunetta C, Volanti P, Zollino M, Penco S, Battistini S; ITALSGEN consortium, Renton AE, Majounie E, Abramzon Y, Conforti FL, Giannini F, Corbo M, Sabatelli M. Clinical characteristics of patients with familial amyotrophic lateral sclerosis carrying the pathogenic GGGGCC hexanucleotide repeat expansion of C9ORF72. Brain 2012; 135: 784-93.

[62] Sabatelli M, Conforti FL, Zollino M, Mora G, Monsurrò MR, Volanti P, Marinou K, Salvi F, Corbo M, Giannini F, Battistini S, Penco S, Lunetta C, Quattrone A, Gambardella A, Logroscino G, Simone I, Bartolomei I, Pisano F, Tedeschi G, Conte A, Spataro R, La Bella V, Caponnetto C, Mancardi G, Mandich P, Sola P, Mandrioli J, Renton AE, Majounie E, Abramzon Y, Marrosu F, Marrosu MG, Murru MR, Sotgiu MA, Pugliatti M, Rodolico C; ITALSGEN Consortium, Moglia C, Calvo A, Ossola I, Brunetti M, Traynor BJ, Borghero G, Restagno G, Chiò A. C9ORF72 hexanucleotide repeat expansions in the Italian sporadic ALS population. Neurobiol Aging 2012; 33:1848.e15-20.

[63] Maruyama H, Morino H, Ito H, Izumi Y, Kato H, Watanabe Y, Kinoshita Y, Kamada M, Nodera H, Suzuki H, Komure O, Matsuura S, Kobatake K, Morimoto N, Abe K, Suzuki N, Aoki M, Kawata A, Hirai T, Kato T, Ogasawara K, Hirano A, Takumi T,

Kusaka H, Hagiwara K, Kaji R, Kawakami H. Mutations of optineurin in amyotrophic lateral sclerosis. Nature 2010; 465:223-6.

[64] Sugihara K, Maruyama H, Kamada M, Morino H, Kawakami H. Screening for OPTN mutations in amyotrophic lateral sclerosis in a mainly Caucasian population. Neurobiol Aging 2011; 32: 1923.e9-10.

Chapter 4

The Neuroinflammation in the Physiopathology of Amyotrophic Lateral Sclerosis

Melissa Bowerman, Thierry Vincent,
Frédérique Scamps, William Camu and Cédric Raoul

Additional information is available at the end of the chapter

http://dx.doi.org/10.5772/56489

1. Introduction

Neuroinflammation is an inflammatory response that takes place within the central nervous system (CNS) during a neurodegenerative process or following a neuronal injury. The main effectors of neuroinflammation, which are astrocytes, microglia and immune cells can confer in a context- and time-dependent manner both neuroprotective and neurotoxic effects. It has now become evident that neuroinflammation is a prominent pathological hallmark of several neurodegenerative diseases such as Alzheimer's disease, Parkinson's disease and Amyotrophic Lateral Sclerosis (ALS)(reviewed in [1, 2]). Indeed, reactive astrocytes and microglia as well as infiltrating T lymphocytes have been identified in ALS experimental models and patients. In the present chapter, we will describe the neuroinflammatory phenotype that characterizes ALS and discuss how the aberrant astrocytes, microglia and immune cells may actively participate in the neurodegenerative process. Further, we will examine the therapeutic potential of targeting neuroinflammation in both pre-clinical disease models and ALS patients.

2. The contribution of astrocytes in the neuroinflammatory response

2.1. Activation profile of astrocytes in human and animal models of ALS

Under normal and healthy conditions, astrocytes, which are the most abundant cell type within the CNS, are typically found in a resting state. Activation of astrocytes follows an acute or chronic injury, where the cells adopt a different morphology, become proliferative, express the intermediate filament glial fibrillary acidic protein (GFAP) release pro-inflammatory cytokines and growth factors as well as produce nitric oxide (NO)(reviewed in [3]). The phenomenon of astrocytosis has been well characterized in both ALS patients and animal models. Analysis of human ALS brains reveals the presence of reactive astrocytes within the subcortical white matter in a widespread fashion [4]. Importantly, the same brain regions from patients with non-ALS neurological disorders display a distinct histopathology, suggesting that the ALS astrocytosis is not simply an indirect result of the ongoing neurodegenerative process [4]. Similarly, the cortical gray matter tissue and the primary motor area from both sporadic and familial ALS patients are characterized by the omnipresence of reactive astrocytes [5, 6]. Studies performed on spinal cords from ALS patients show the occurrence of astrocytosis in both the ventral and dorsal horn region of the spinal cord [7, 8]. In addition to the above-mentioned post-mortem observations, in vivo brain imaging of ALS patients using deuterium-substituted [^{11}C](L)-deprenyl positron emission tomography has allowed the visualization of astrocytosis in live patients [9]. Hence, a thorough analysis of the CNS of ALS patients has uncovered and highlighted astrocytosis as a *bona fide* feature of ALS pathology, whether sporadic or inherited. While human ALS tissue represents most accurately the hallmarks that typify the disease, the caveat is that it limits our knowledge of the cellular events that occur prior to disease onset.

The generation of both mouse and rat models of ALS has helped elucidate more precisely the contributory role of astrocytosis during the neurodegenerative process. Analysis of different *superoxide dismutase 1* (*SOD1*) mutant mouse models identifies astrocytic alterations such as reactive morphological changes, proliferation as well as the presence of SOD1- and ubiquitin-positive inclusions, as occurring prior or close-to axonal degeneration and neuronal loss [10-13]. Furthermore, the process of astrocytosis significantly intensifies as the disease progresses [10, 11]. Three-dimensional reconstruction of *SOD1*^{G93A} spinal cord sections shows that astrocytic processes actually target and envelop pathological vacuoles within the degenerating neurons [11]. Similarly to the murine models, the transgenic *SOD1*^{G93A} rats also display signs of astrocytosis prior to significant motoneuron loss. As the disease progresses, there is an increase of astrocytic hypertrophy and proliferation as well as an accumulation of ubiquitin and tau-positive aggregates [14, 15]. Thus, while the human data provided the first insights into astrocytosis as a pathological hallmark of ALS, the observation in pre-clinical models of astrocytic inflammation prior to neurodegeneration strengthened the proposed contributory role of astrocytes in ALS pathogenesis.

2.2. A role for astrocytes in ALS pathogenesis

Once the astrocytic histopathology was thoroughly characterized in both human and animal ALS models, a comprehensive assessment of its functional influence on motoneuron loss thus ensued. One of the first indications of astrocyte-dependent neurodegeneration in ALS comes from the generation of chimeric mice, composed of both normal cells and SOD1 mutant-expressing cells [16]. This study demonstrates that mutant SOD1-positive motoneurons surrounded by wildtype non-neuronal cells have a better survival rate than those enclosed by mutant SOD1-positive non-neuronal cells [16]. A complementary approach consisting in deleting the human mutant SOD1 specifically within astrocytes of the *SOD1*^{G37R} mice suggests that mutant astrocytes contribute to progression, but not onset of the disease [17]. However, knocking down the mutant SOD1 in astrocytes of the *SOD1*^{G85R} mouse model results in increased survival by delaying disease onset as well as the early stage of the disease [18]. Despite minor differences between the targeted disease stages in both models, the key finding is that mutant SOD1-expressing astrocytes regulate the disease progression of murine ALS.

Another approach used to address the astrocytic-induced motoneuron loss in ALS is the *in vitro* co-culture of both cell types. Indeed, when cultured alone, primary *SOD1*^{G93A} astrocytes express high levels of pro-inflammatory effectors such as tumor necrosis factor alpha (TNFα), interferon gamma (IFNγ), interleukins (IL)-1 beta (IL-1β) and -18 (IL-18), 5-lipoxygenase (5-LOX), leukotriene B4, cyclooxygenase (COX-2) and prostaglandin E_2 (PGE_2), thus displaying an inflammatory phenotype with potential neurotoxic effects [19]. Consequently, primary wildtype and mutant motoneurons or motoneurons derived from murine or human embryonic stem cells show decreased survival when cultured in the presence of astrocytes expressing different mutated forms of SOD1 [20-24]. While the above-mentioned *in vivo* and *in vitro* studies suggest a contributory role for astrocytes in ALS pathogenesis, the targeted ablation of GFAP-expressing proliferating astrocytes in *SOD1*^{G93A} mice has no effect on the onset or the progression of the neurodegenerative process [25]. Recently, a subtype of astrocytes from spinal cord cultures of *SOD1*^{G93A} rats that displayed an aberrant phenotype has been isolated (termed Aba cells). Aba cells, that highly express S100β and connexin-43, but weakly express GFAP, are distinguished by their increased proliferative abilities and the absence of replicative senescence. Specifically, they are localized in proximity of motoneurons *in vivo*, increase drastically upon disease onset and demonstrate a greater neurotoxicity compared to non-Aba astrocytes isolated from *SOD1*^{G93A} rats [26]. Combined, these studies suggest that different subpopulations of astrocytes with different functional features and different cellular origin coexist during the pathological processes.

An additional important feature of the astrocytic contribution in ALS relates to the observation that the expression of SOD1^{G85R} solely in astrocytes does not give rise to motoneuron loss despite the fact that astrocytosis occurs prominently [27]. Likewise, the specific expression of SOD1^{G37R} in spinal cord motoneurons or the accumulation of SOD1^{G93A} in postnatal motoneurons does not impact motor function, neurodegeneration or disease onset and progression [28, 29]. Together, these observations therefore point to the critical communication that takes place between astrocytes and motoneurons, which might in turn lead to the initiation of neuronal death pathways.

2.3. Misregulation of neuronal transmission by astrocytes

The glutamate hypothesis proposes that a glutamate imbalance, leading to a calcium (Ca^{2+})-mediated excitotoxic insult, represents a major mechanism of motoneuron injury [30]. Astrocytes actively participate in modulating neuronal excitability and neurotransmission by controlling the extracellular levels of ions and neurotransmitters. The astroglial glutamate transporter excitatory amino-acid transporter 2 (EAAT2) in humans or glutamate transporter 1 (GLT-1) in rodents is the primary means of maintaining low extracellular glutamate levels. EAAT2/GLT-1 rapidly removes glutamate from the extracellular milieu and thereby prevents excitotoxic injury to neurons that occurs by overstimulation of the post-synaptic N-methyl-D-aspartic acid (NMDA) and α-amino-3-hydroxy-5-methyl-4-isoxazolepropionic acid (AMPA)/kainate ionotropic glutamate receptors [31, 32]. Decreased expression of EAAT2/GLT-1, which leads to elevated levels of extracellular glutamate, has been found in a vast majority of sporadic and familial ALS patients as well as ALS mice and rats [10, 33-35], suggesting the participation of astrocytes in glutamate-induced excitotoxicity.

In addition to the relationship between glutamate excitotoxicity and glutamate transporter loss, other glutamatergic pathways have been implicated in motoneuron degeneration. Functional AMPA receptors consist of various combinations of four subunits (designated glutamate receptor (GluR)1-4) and are involved in fast excitatory synaptic transmission in the CNS [36]. The GluR2 subunit is functionally dominant and renders AMPA receptors impermeable to Ca^{2+}, preventing Ca^{2+} influx-induced toxicity. Thus, high levels of GluR2 in neuronal tissues might confer neuroprotection against glutamate-induced excitotoxicity. Within normal human spinal motoneurons, there is a low relative abundance of the GluR2 subunit mRNA compared to other GluR subunits and to other neuronal tissues, which may make them unduly susceptible to Ca^{2+}-mediated toxic events following glutamate receptor activation [37]. However, work from another group does not observe any significant quantitative changes in GluR2 mRNA within spinal cord motoneurons, suggesting that a selective decrease of the GluR2 subunit might not be the only mechanism mediating the AMPA receptor-dependent neurotoxicity in ALS [38]. Indeed, it has been demonstrated that RNA editing of GluR2 mRNA at the glutamine/arginine (Q/R) site is decreased in autopsy-obtained spinal motoneurons from patients with sporadic ALS [39], a molecular event that confers Ca^{2+} permeability to the GluR2 receptor [40]. Therefore, reductions in both GluR2 expression and GluR2 Q/R site editing may contribute to increased Ca^{2+} influx and neurotoxicity through AMPA receptors in ALS.

The molecular basis for lower GluR2 abundance in motoneurons compared to other CNS neurons has been investigated using two different rat strains that show differential vulnerability to AMPA-mediated excitotoxicity [41]. It has thus been demonstrated that astrocytes derived from the ventral spinal cord, but not those derived from the dorsal spinal cord, cerebellum, or the cortex, have the ability to regulate GluR2 expression in motoneurons. Interestingly, expression of mutant SOD1 abolishes their GluR2-regulating capacity. Although, the astrocytic factor responsible for GluR2 regulation in motoneurons remains to be identified, the regulation of motoneuron electrical activity through neuronal GluR2 expression and the uptake of glutamate by the glial transporter EAAT2/GLT-1 are major mechanisms by which astrocytes may mediate excitotoxic neurodegeneration in ALS.

2.4. Additional mechanisms of astrocytic neurotoxicity

While the astrocytic influence on neuronal excitability is seldom disputed, various reports suggest that they may also participate in the neurodegenerative process via the release of neurotoxic factors. Typically, the activation and/or reaction of astrocytes that characterize neuroinflammation occurs following a CNS injury, including chronic neurodegenerative diseases (reviewed in [42]). In experiments where the spinal cords of neonatal rats were injected with cerebrospinal fluid (CSF) from ALS patients, there is an increased GFAP immunoreactivity within the grey and white matter [43], suggesting that the astrocytosis in ALS might in fact be a responsive phenomenon. Conversely, many research groups have identified specific factors that are abnormally regulated in ALS astrocytes that could potentially trigger the motoneuron loss that typifies the disease.

2.4.1. The interferon response

Type I, II and III IFNs are an important family of immunomodulatory cytokines (reviewed in [44]). Elevated levels of IFNγ, a potent pro-inflammatory mediator, are found in the CSF of ALS patients, in the serum as the disease progresses and in spinal cord of sporadic ALS patients [45-47]. Further, the analysis of spinal cord sections from ALS patients shows that IFNγ is detected in ventral horn neurons, glial cells and plausibly immune cells [47]. In addition, the IFNγ-inducible protein, IP-30 and the interferon-stimulated gene 15 (ISG15) are significantly upregulated in human ALS spinal cord [48, 49]. In spinal cord extracts and serum of ALS mice, elevated levels of IFNγ mRNA and protein are also documented [24, 50, 51]. The expression of IFNγ is found within motoneurons and astrocytes of $SOD1^{G93A}$ and $SOD1^{G85R}$ spinal cords at both disease onset and symptomatic stages [24]. Similarly, a gene expression array analysis of pre-symptomatic $SOD1^{G93A}$ spinal cord reveals an induction of several genes regulated by type I IFNα, IFNβ and type II IFNγ, with specifically an increased expression of ISG15 in spinal cord astrocytes. Further, the phosphorylation of signal transducer and activator of transcription (STAT) 1 and 2, downstream effectors of IFNs [52], and STAT4, an inducer of IFNγ, is also elevated in $SOD1^{G93A}$ spinal cords [51]. Functionally, the genetic deletion of *Ifnα/β receptor 1* in $SOD1^{G93A}$ mice significantly prolongs life expectancy [49]. Importantly, astrocytic IFNγ triggers a motoneuron-selective death pathway via the activation of lymphotoxin beta receptor (LT-βR) by LIGHT. LIGHT is also upregulated in sporadic ALS spinal cords and the genetic ablation of *Light* in $SOD1^{G93A}$ mice delays disease progression [24]. Combined, these observations in rodent and human models of the disease suggest that the neuroinflammatory role of IFNs may contribute to the neurodegenerative process in ALS.

2.4.2. The contribution of nerve growth factor

The low affinity p75 neurotrophin receptor ($p75^{NTR}$) has a well-described role in mediating neuronal death signaling (reviewed in [53]). In symptomatic $SOD1^{G93A}$ mice and in ALS patients, $p75^{NTR}$ is overexpressed within spinal motoneurons [54]. Correspondingly, the immunoreactivity of nerve growth factor (NGF), a $p75^{NTR}$ ligand [55], is increased in spinal cord astrocytes of symptomatic $SOD1^{G93A}$ mice and in primary $SOD1^{G93A}$ astrocyte cultures [56, 57]. Further, the excessive expression of fibroblast growth factor 1 (FGF-1) by $SOD1^{G93A}$ motoneurons stimulates the nuclear accumulation of FGF receptor 1 (FGFR1) in astrocytes, consequently triggering astrocytic NGF production [58]. Importantly, primary $SOD1^{G93A}$ motoneuron cultures are hypersensitive to the NGF-$p75^{NTR}$ apoptotic signaling [59]. Thus, the astrocyte-dependent activation of the neurotoxic NGF-$p75^{NTR}$ pathway might participate to the neurodegeneration that typifies ALS.

2.4.3. *Cyclooxygenase-2*

COX-2 is a pro-inflammatory enzyme that converts arachidonic acid into prostanoids such as PGE_2, a potent inflammatory mediator (reviewed in [60]). In the anterior horn region of the spinal cord of *SOD1*^{G93A} mice, at both the early and end stage of the disease, COX-2 immunoreactivity is elevated in astrocytes [61]. Similarly, spinal cord astrocytes from sporadic ALS patients also display increased COX-2 expression [61, 62]. The expression of COX-2 can be modulated by the binding of CD40, a member of the TNF family (reviewed in [63]), with its ligand CD40L [64]. Interestingly, spinal cord astrocytes of symptomatic *SOD1*^{G39A} mice show an upregulation of CD40, concomitant with COX-2 astrocytic expression. Moreover, the activation of COX-2 in astrocytes upon CD40 stimulation leads to motoneuron death *in vitro* [65], suggesting that an astrocytic CD40-COX-2 pathway could also participate in ALS pathogenesis. The contribution of the CD40/CD40L pathway has recently been proposed in ALS mice, though its role in astrocytic neurotoxicity role has not been established [66]. Finally, another facet of the COX-2 pathway relates to the ability of PGE_2 to promote glutamate release from astrocytes, emphasizing further the complex multimodality of neuroinflammatory signals [67].

2.4.4. *The Wnt/β-catenin signaling pathway*

The canonical Wnt/β-catenin transduction pathway, which comprises multiple Wnt genes, regulates many biological functions (reviewed in [68]), including neuronal survival, as demonstrated by its involvement in other neurodegenerative disease such as Alzheimer's disease and Parkinson's disease [69, 70]. In the ventral region of symptomatic *SOD1*^{G93A} spinal cords, there is an increase in the number of Wnt3a- and β-catenin-positive astrocytes [71]. An upregulation of Wnt2 and Wnt7 within astrocytes of symptomatic *SOD1*^{G93A} spinal cords is also reported [72]. Among its biological functions, the Wnt/β-catenin pathway mediates the activity of cyclin D1 [73], a nuclear transcription factor important for cell cycle regulation (reviewed in [74]). The upregulation of cyclin D1 in *SOD1*^{G93A} astrocytes suggests that the increased activation of the Wnt/β-catenin/cyclin D1 may plausibly direct astrocytosis [71]. Interestingly, a study performed in colorectal cancer cell lines uncovers the possible regulation of COX-2 by the Wnt/β-catenin pathway [75]. Thus, an astrocytic increased activation of Wnt and β-catenin may not only impact cyclin D1 expression but potentially that of COX-2, for which a possible role in ALS neurodegeneration has been described above.

2.4.5. *Monoamine oxidase-B*

Monoamine oxidase-B (MAO-B) is an outer mitochondrial membrane-bound enzyme that catalyzes the oxidative deamination of biogenic amines, thus producing reactive oxygen species (ROS). MAO-B is primarily found in the CNS where it localizes mainly in astrocytes and radial glial [76]. The spinal cord lumbar region from symptomatic ALS patients displays more MAO-B, due to the general astrocyte proliferation and to a cell-intrinsic increased expression [77]. Using ^{3}H-L deprenyl *in vitro* autoradiography, a more in-depth follow-up study in the *post-mortem* ALS CNS reveals an increased expression in the corticospinal tract, the ventral white matter and in the vicinity of motoneurons. Further, reactive astrocytes

http://dx.doi.org/10.5772/56489

displayed a higher content of MAO-B compared to microglial cells [8, 78]. Finally, an epidemiological analysis has uncovered that the MAO-B allelic phenotype influences the age of ALS onset [79]. Excessive astrocytic MAO-B expression, which results in elevations of extracellular ROS levels, may have damaging effects on neighboring motoneurons. Additional mechanisms could also involve mitochondrial dysfunction by the selective inhibition of respiratory complex I, which further leads to increased production of superoxide as well as microglial activation [80].

2.4.6. *Mitochondrial dysfunctions*

While there is a vast amount of research on the mitochondrial dysfunction in ALS motoneurons (reviewed in [81]), not much is known about the impact of toxic genetic mutations on the mitochondria of astrocytes. There is evidence however, that ALS astrocytes do in fact display pathological mitochondrial dysfunction that subsequently leads to oxidative damage, sustaining their reactive status. Indeed, primary astrocytes isolated from the cerebral cortex of neonatal rats and overexpressing *SOD1*^{G93A} display a decreased mitochondrial respiration rate, an increased superoxide formation and a decreased membrane potential [82]. In co-culture experiments, modulating the mitochondrial defects of SOD1^{G93A}-expressing astrocytes via small chemical compounds improves astrocytic-dependent motoneuron survival. Conversely, induction of mitochondrial damage to wildtype astrocytes increases motoneuron death [82]. Thus, organelle dysfunction within ALS astrocytes may be an important contributor to the neurodegenerative process. In addition, a positive amplification system could take place during the degenerative process, since the inflammatory mediator NO, mainly produced by the inducible form of nitric oxide synthase (iNOS) in reactive astrocytes, can in turn induce mitochondrial dysfunction in astrocytes [83].

2.4.7. *Activation of microglial cells*

A fundamental role for astrocytes in the neuroinflammation process is the recruitment of microglia [84], the resident macrophages of the CNS (reviewed in [85]). In *SOD1*^{G37R} mice where the mutant *SOD1* gene is specifically deleted in astrocytes, the delay in the progression of the later stages of disease is accompanied with an inhibition of microglial activation and microglia-dependent detrimental NO production [17]. Thus, astrocytosis in ALS may promote neuroinflammation events through microglial recruitment, which in turn may participate directly or indirectly to the motoneuron loss in ALS. Several pro-inflammatory contributors including TNFα, IFNγ, IL-1β and NO, which are aberrantly produced by mutant astrocytes can indeed enhance the activation of microglia. The specific role of microglia in the neuroinflammatory aspects of ALS will therefore be discussed below.

Figure 1 illustrates the potential non-cell-autonomous mechanisms implicating reactive astrocytes in the selective death of motoneurons in ALS.

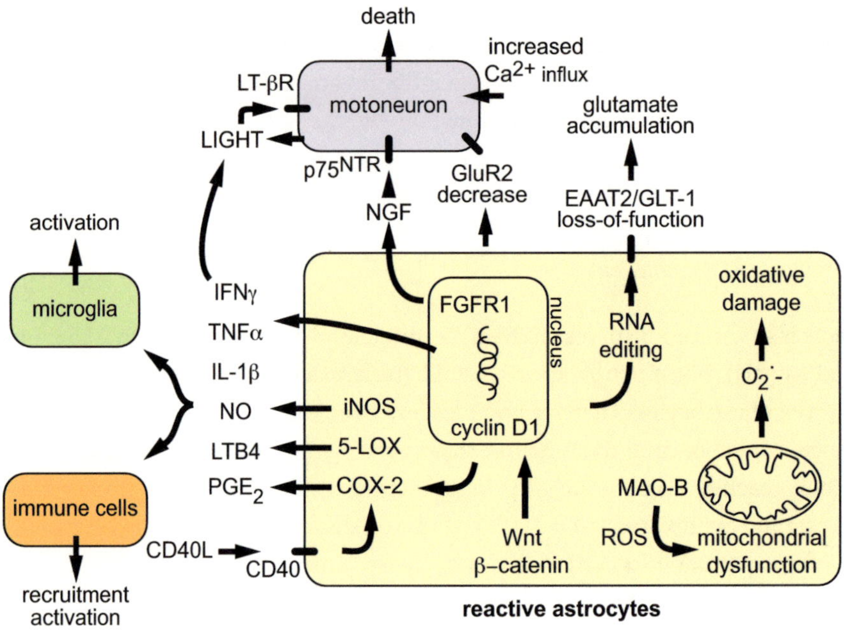

Figure 1. Proposed mechanisms for astrocytic-mediated neuroinflammation and toxicity towards motoneurons. Reactive astrocytes contribute to the degenerative process by influencing the activity of microglial and immune cells as well as by releasing soluble factors that are toxic to motoneurons (as described in section 2).

3. A role for microglia in neuroinflammation

3.1. Activation profile in human and animal models of ALS

Microglia are often termed the immune cells of the CNS as they constantly monitor the neuronal environment in a resting state and become activated upon acute or chronic neuronal damage, eliciting a strong pro-inflammatory response (reviewed in [86]). In ALS patients, reactive microglia are observed in the motor cortex, the motor nuclei of the brainstem, the ventral horn of the spinal cord, along the entire corticospinal tract and within the CSF [87-89]. Given the relationship between astrocytes and microglia [17, 84] and the importance of astrocytosis in ALS, it has been hypothesized that microgliosis may also participate in ALS pathogenesis.

To better understand at which developmental point of the disease reactive microglia appear, microgliosis has been characterized in rodent ALS models at various stages of the disease. Microgliosis occurs in pre-symptomatic and symptomatic *SOD1*^{G93A} spinal cords as well as within various CNS compartments [90-93]. Similarly, *SOD1*^{G37R} mice display microgliosis at both onset and early-stage of the disease [94]. An in-depth characterization of microgliosis in

http://dx.doi.org/10.5772/56489

SOD1^{G93A} mice via *in vivo* imaging by two-photon laser-scanning microscopy shows that microglia are highly reactive in pre-symptomatic stages while they lose their ability to respond to injury and to monitor the environment as the disease progresses [95]. Indeed, comparison of microglia populations during disease progression reveals that microglia isolated from either neonatal or early onset *SOD1*^{G93A} mice display an alternatively activated M2 phenotype and enhance motoneuron survival while microglia isolated from either adult or endstage *SOD1*^{G93A} mice have a classically activated M1 phenotype and induce motoneuron death [96, 97]. In the pre-symptomatic and symptomatic *SOD1*^{G93A} rat model, microglia aggregates are detected in both the spinal cord and brainstem [98, 99]. Interestingly, the microglia in endstage *SOD1*^{G93A} rats display a degenerative and apoptotic phenotype [98]. Further, in the lumbar spinal cord of pre-symptomatic *SOD1*^{H46R} rats, the microglia express the proliferating marker Ki67 and the phagocytic markers ED1 and major histocompatibility complex (MHC) class II [100, 101]. The thorough investigation of microglial events in rodents therefore suggests that microgliosis not only typifies ALS but that the function of microglia changes during disease progression, thus exerting differential effects on the degenerating motoneurons.

3.2. A role for microglia in ALS pathogenesis

Experimental endeavors have been undertaken to better understand the precise contribution of microglia in the neurodegenerative process. A key finding in support of the proposed direct contribution of microglia to ALS pathogenesis is in ALS mice where the mutant SOD1 (G37R or G85R) is specifically deleted from macrophages and microglial lineages [94, 102]. This results in a delay in the progression but not onset of the disease and a significant extension in lifespan. The importance of microgliosis in ALS pathology was also ascertained in *SOD1*^{G93A} mice bred with *PU.1*$^{-/-}$ mice that lack CNS microglia at birth [103, 104]. While the bone marrow transplantation of *SOD1*^{G93A} microglia into *PU.1*$^{-/-}$ mice did not induce neurodegeneration, the bone marrow transplantation of wildtype microglia into *SOD1*^{G93A};*PU.1*$^{-/-}$ mice improved survival compared to the bone marrow transplantation of *SOD1*^{G93A} microglia [103]. Further, administration of extracellular murine SOD1^{G93A} to primary cultures of microglia activates these cells and renders them neurotoxic [105]. However, phenotypical analysis of microglia in different regions of *SOD1*^{G93A} spinal cord suggests that both neuroprotective and neurotoxic population of microglial cells may coexist during the disease [106]. In fact, the depletion of proliferative microglia does not prevent motoneuron degeneration [107]. Together, these studies suggest that microglia participate, through a complex balance between neuroprotective and neurotoxic signals, in the course of the disease.

3.3. Proposed mechanisms of microglial-derived neurotoxicity

While the injection of motoneuron-directed or ALS patient-derived immunoglobulin G into the spinal cord of mice initiates the recruitment of reactive microglia [108], a study looking at cerebral cortex of ALS patients shows that the phagocytosis of degenerating neurons is mediated by perivascular macrophages and not microglia [109]. This finding already suggested that reactive microglia might play a more complex function in ALS than simply eliminating dying motoneurons. Indeed, various misregulated pathways within ALS microglia have been identified that may influence motoneuron survival.

3.3.1. Endoplasmic reticulum stress

When a cell starts to excessively accumulate misfolded or unfolded proteins, the over-activated endoplasmic reticulum (ER) stress induces apoptosis (reviewed in [110]). Importantly, ER stress is an established characteristic of ALS pathogenesis (reviewed in [111]). In spinal cord microglia of both sporadic ALS patients and symptomatic $SOD1^{G93A}$ mice, there is an increased expression of C/EBP homologous protein (CHOP) [112], a member of the apoptotic ER stress pathway (reviewed in [113]). It remains unclear however if the aberrant levels of CHOP reflect an upstream defect in protein folding or if they directly participate in microglial neurotoxicity. It is noteworthy that the exposure of microglial cells to IFNγ induces iNOS expression, and the subsequent increased NO production can cause an ER stress response involving CHOP [114]. Interestingly, the analysis of selectively vulnerable motoneurons from low-expression $SOD1^{G93A}$, high-expression $SOD1^{G93A}$ and $SOD1^{G85R}$ mice shows the initiation of a specific ER stress response accompanied by microglial activation [115]. Thus, the interaction between ALS motoneurons and microglia may be important in the modulation of the neurodegenerative process.

3.3.2. CD14-toll-like receptor signaling

Once the ligand-dependent CD14 lipopolysaccharide (LPS) receptor located at the microglial surface [116] is activated, it initiates a pro-inflammatory signaling cascade dependent on Toll-like receptors (TLRs), specifically TLR2 and TLR4 [117, 118]. Interestingly, the neurotoxic activation of microglia by extracellular $SOD1^{G93A}$ is mediated by the CD14-TLR pathway [105, 119]. Indeed, immortalized microglia cells expressing mutant SOD1 display an increased TLR2 stimulation and subsequent release of pro-inflammatory cytokines, including TNFα and IL-1β. Importantly, an analysis of spinal cord microglia from sporadic ALS patients shows an enhanced TLR2 immunoreactivity [120]. Recently, it has been shown that the endocytosis of extracellular mutant SOD1 by microglia is required for the activation of caspase-1, which is required for the maturation of IL-1β [121]. This can be paralleled with the finding that the microgliosis caused by fibrillar amyloid beta (Aβ), the main component of the aggregates that are a pathological signature of Alzheimer's disease, also requires CD14, TLR2 and TLR4 [122]. All together, these studies suggest that microglia may participate in motoneuron loss following the specific activation of the CD14-TLR pathway by secreted SOD1 mutant, therefore propagating pro-inflammatory stimuli.

3.3.3. Purinergic signaling

The release of extracellular nucleoside di- and tri-phosphates by degenerating neurons can elicit the activation of microglia through the ionotropic P2X and metabotropic P2Y purinergic receptors. A general alarm signal for microglia is ATP, which can subsequently elicit a pro-inflammatory response, chemotaxis and phagocytosis (reviewed in [123, 124]). Embryonic immortalized microglia and neonatal primary microglial cultures isolated from mutant *SOD1* mice display an upregulation of $P2X_4$, $P2X_7$ and $P2Y_6$ receptors [125]. Notably, the immunoreactivity of P2X is increased within spinal cord microglia of ALS patients [126]. Activation of $P2X_7$ in *SOD1^{G93A}* microglial cells produces significantly higher levels of TNFα, which has a neurotoxic effect on motoneuron cultures [127], and of COX-2, compared to non-mutant microglia [125]. In addition, a reduced ATP hydrolysis activity, possibly implicating the ecto-NTPDase CD39, is observed in mutant SOD1 microglia, suggesting that a potentiation of a purinergic-mediated inflammation can participate to the neuroinflammatory state of microglial cells. Since ATP induces an astrocytic neurotoxic phenotype through $P2X_7$ [128], it is thus feasible to hypothesize that increased extracellular ATP in ALS, whether exacerbated by motoneurons and/or microglia contributes to the pathogenic microgliosis.

3.4. The potential influence of microglia on neuronal excitability

To our knowledge, there is presently no direct assessment of the influence of microglia on motoneuron electrophysiology. However, studies on peripheral nerve injury or spinal cord injury show that microglia activation has prominent effects on neuronal inhibitory control. Importantly, loss of inhibitory control is a contributing mechanism to the motoneuron hyperexcitability that typifies ALS pathogenesis in humans [129].

Loss of neuronal inhibitory control occurs by several means including decrease in gamma-aminobutyric acid (GABA)ergic interneurons [130] combined with changes in the expression of the $GABA_A$ receptor mRNA subunit [131]. $GABA_A$ and glycine receptors are chloride (Cl^-) channels and the expression of cation-chloride co-transporter contributes to inhibitory effects of these Cl^- currents [132]. Indeed, the entry of Cl^- following the opening of $GABA_A$ and glycine receptor-gated Cl^- channels inhibits neuron excitability by hyperpolarizing membrane potential. Under physiological condition, low $[Cl^-]_i$ is maintained by the potassium (K^+)-chloride co-transporter KCC2 that extrudes Cl^- from mature neurons [133]. Stimulation of spinal microglia following peripheral nerve injury induces a decrease in KCC2 expression among dorsal horn nociceptive neurons [134]. KCC2 decrease is induced by the brain-derived neurotrophic factor (BDNF) and this is consistent with the previous observation that BDNF can be produced by non-neuronal cells involved in immune responses, including T and B lymphocytes, monocytes and microglia [135, 136]. BDNF produces a depolarizing shift in the anion reversal potential of dorsal horn lamina I neurons due to an increase in $[Cl^-]_i$. This shift prompts an inversion of inhibitory GABA currents that contributes to neuropathic pain following nerve injury [135]. Decrease in KCC2 expression is thus responsible for the excitatory effects of GABA on neurons. Microglia activation and BDNF secretion are mediated through ATP activation of microglial P2X receptors. As described earlier, P2X receptors might be involved in ALS pathology since a higher density of $P2X_7$-immunoreactive microglial cells/macrophages are found in affected regions of spinal cords from ALS patients [126]. Levels of BDNF have been found to be increased in microglial cells isolated from ALS mice at the onset of disease and KCC2 is decreased in vulnerable motoneurons in *SOD1^{G93A}* mice [96, 137]. Additionally, BDNF might play a role in the microglia's influence on motoneuron electric activity as suggested by work on spasticity. Spasticity is characterized by a velocity-dependent increase in muscle tone resulting from hyperexcitable stretch reflexes, spasms and hypersensitivity to normally innocuous sensory stimulations. Spasticity develops following spinal cord injury and is also regarded as an ALS clinical symptom [138]. The main mechanisms hypothesized to be responsible for spasticity are increased motoneuron excitability and increased synaptic inputs in response to muscle stretch due to reduced inhibitory mechanisms. Recently, it has been demonstrated that, following spinal cord injury, increased levels of BDNF mediated spasticity, due to post-transcriptional down regulation of KCC2 [139]. Together, these studies suggest that reactive microglia in ALS may exert an aberrant effect on the electrical activity of motoneurons and highlight the importance of furthering our understanding of this functional interaction.

Lastly, a hypothetical scenario relates to the defect in astrocytic glutamate transporter and the neurotoxic accumulation of the excitatory amino acid that we have mentioned above. It has been demonstrated that TNFα promotes the release of glutamate by activated microglia through the cystine/glutamate exchanger (Xc)[140]. Though the implication of the Xc system in ALS has not yet been investigated, it is intriguing that the Aβ peptide induces a neurotoxic phenotype in microglia through the Xc-mediated release of glutamate Therefore, system Xc represents a potential mechanism of microglia-mediated excitotoxicity that warrants further study [141].

The potential non-cell-autonomous mechanisms involving microglial cells in the selective degeneration of motoneurons in ALS are illustrated in Figure 2.

4. Involvement of neuroimmunity in motoneuron degeneration

4.1. Pathological phenotype of the immune system in ALS

In addition to astrocytes and microglia, immune cells may also play synergistic and critical roles in ALS neuroinflammation and disease progression. Presence of a systemic immune activation is suggested by abnormalities observed in the blood and CSF of ALS patients such as increased numbers of circulating lymphocytes (CD4+ helper T cells, CD8+ cytotoxic T lymphocytes (CTL) and natural killer (NK) cells), increased expression of MHC class II molecules on monocytes as well as higher levels of inflammatory chemokines and cytokines (regulated on activation normal T cell expressed and secreted (RANTES), monocyte chemotactic protein (MCP-1), IL-12, IL-15, IL-17 and IL-23)[142-146]. Further, *post-mortem* studies of brain and spinal cord from ALS patients show that the activation and proliferation of microglia is associated with an infiltration of activated macrophages, mast cells and T lymphocytes which are found in close proximity to degenerating tissues [147-149]. An in-depth autopsy of six ALS patients reveals an enrichment of T-cell receptor Vβ2 positive T cells in the spinal cord and CSF, suggesting an antigen-driven T cell selection [150]. Finally, ALS patients with a more rapidly progressing pathology show decreased numbers of regulatory T lymphocytes (Tregs), suggesting that the numbers of Tregs are inversely correlated with disease progression [144, 151]. Tregs secrete anti-inflammatory cytokines such as IL-4, IL-10 and transforming growth factor beta (TGF-β) as well as the neurotrophic growth factors glial-derived neurotrophic factor (GDNF) and BDNF. Tregs are also able to dampen a Th1 pro-inflammatory response and

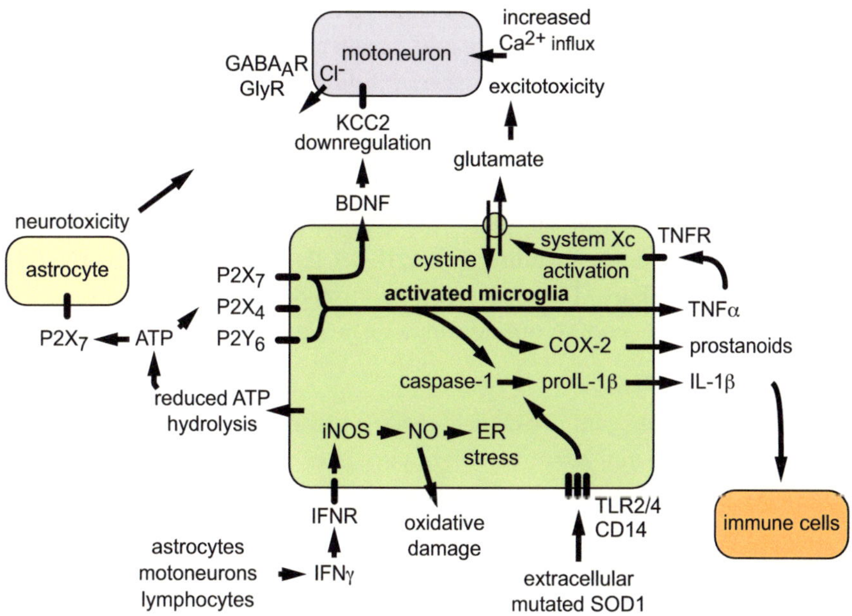

Figure 2. Proposed mechanisms by which microglial activation and inflammation contribute to the neurodegenerative process in ALS. Microglia can influence astrocytes and immune cells as well as directly impact motoneuron viability via several mechanisms.

attenuate toxic microglial responses. Contribution of the innate immune system is also suggested by the presence of immunoglobulins and complement deposition as well as a significant increase of NK cells in the blood of ALS patients [87, 144, 152]. While these investigations of ALS samples and tissues do not assess the contributory role of the immune system to the disease pathogenesis, they do highlight its active presence.

In support of what is observed in humans, ALS rodent models also display a particular immunological phenotype. Indeed, *SOD1*^{G93A} mice demonstrate that the inflammatory cell subtypes are phenotypicaly and functionally different depending upon the disease stage [96]. During the initial stages, infiltrating CD4+ T cells are almost mainly Th2 (IL-4+) while as the disease progresses there is a skew toward Th1 (IFNγ+) cells and CD8+ T cells (both IL-17A positive and negative)[106, 153]. Alteration in inflammatory cell subtypes is associated with, and maybe driven by, differences in Tregs. Interestingly, early symptomatic *SOD1*^{G93A} mice have increased numbers of Tregs and a decreased proliferation of effectors T lymphocytes (Teffs), whereas decreased numbers of Tregs and increased proliferation of Teffs is found in end-stage animals [151, 154]. The innate immune system is also affected in ALS rodents, displayed by the substantial increase of NK and NKT in the spinal cord of *SOD1*^{G93A} mice [155, 156].

Whether neuroinflammation is a cause or a consequence of motoneuron death is still debated. It is interesting to note that inflammation is not limited to the CNS but systemic with increased levels of plasma LPS associated with increased numbers of activated circulating monocytes and T lymphocytes that correlate with disease evolution [142, 157]. A thymic dysfunction is also observed in parallel to the neurodegenerative process in mutant SOD1 mice and ALS patient [158]. In the CNS of ALS patients, TAR DNA-binding protein 43 (TDP-43) increased and interacts with nuclear factor kappa B (NF-κB) in glial and neuronal cells. LPS-activation of NF-κB in microglial cells expressing the TDP-43 mutant is associated with the production of pro-inflammatory cytokines, including TNFα, IL-1β, IL-6 and IFNγ [159]. The central role of inflammation and NF-κB in ALS was recently confirmed by the description in familial ALS of mutations in the gene encoding optineurin, a negative regulator of TNF-induced NF-κB activation [160].

Altogether, the information from pre-clinical models and ALS patients suggest that systemic immune activation (innate and adaptive) might play a key role in ALS pathogenesis and may represent an interesting target for the development of novel treatments. However, a better understanding of the specific roles played by the different subtypes of immune cells is of utmost necessity. Indeed, accumulative evidence suggests that inflammatory cells mediate both protective and deleterious effects on motoneuron survival and that these functions vary during disease progression.

4.2. The protective function of the immune response in ALS

Protective immunity, a homeostatic phenomenon important in the repair of damaged tissues, results from both the clearance of debris and the effects of cytokines and growth factors delivered by inflammatory T-cells to the site of injury [161, 162]. The neuroprotective ability of immune cells is also evident in ALS. Indeed, when *SOD1*^{G93A} mice are bred with mice lacking functional T cells or CD4+ T cells, microglia skew towards an M1 inflammatory phenotype and disease progression accelerates, suggesting that CD4+ T cells provide neuroprotection by suppressing the cytotoxic activation of microglia. Accordingly, reconstitution of T cells following bone marrow transplantation of *SOD1*^{G93A} mice lacking functional T and B cells prolonged their survival and suppressed the activation of M1 microglia [163]. Further analysis shows that the increased numbers of CD4+/CD25+/Foxp3+ Tregs during early symptomatic stages secrete IL-4, thus promoting the M2 protective microglia while inhibiting the neurotoxic Th1 response and IFNγ secretion. As described above, these neuroprotective Tregs are decreased as the disease progression accelerates. Co-culture experiments show that Tregs suppress the expression of cytotoxic factors Nox2 and iNOS from *SOD1*^{G93A} microglia through IL-4. Tregs also inhibit the proliferation of *SOD1*^{G93A} Teffs via the combined secretion of IL-4, IL-10 and TGF-β[154]. The neuroprotective properties of Tregs are also reinforced by their ability to secrete GDNF and BDNF, thus attenuating toxic microglial responses [164]. Importantly, the passive transfer of endogenous Tregs into *SOD1*^{G93A} mice lengthens disease duration and prolongs survival, suggesting that Tregs is likely the neuroprotective subpopulation among CD4+ T lymphocytes. Therefore, a subtype of immune cells appear to have a beneficial role in ALS and targeting the Tregs/M2 signaling pathway may be an attractive therapeutic strategy for this neurodegenerative disease.

4.3. The neurotoxic function of the immune response in ALS

T lymphocytes could mediate motoneuron damage either directly through cell-cell contact, secretion of cytokines or indirectly through activation of microglia and macrophages [165]. As mentioned above, the effect of the immune system varies during disease progression from a protective role at early stages to a neurotoxic activity when disease accelerates [151]. Neuroprotective activity has been associated with a Tregs/M2 response and expression of trophic and anti-inflammatory factors such as BDNF, GDNF and IL-4 whereas neurotoxic effects are associated with an M1/Th1/CTL pro-inflammatory immune response [106]. Accordingly, mutated SOD1 Teffs proliferate to a greater extend and produce more IFNγ (Th1-driven) during the rapidly progressing phase than Teffs isolated during slowly progressing phase [154]. Different death pathways can be induced by Th1/CTL lymphocytes and promote motoneuron loss in ALS. For instance, activation of Fas (CD95) has been demonstrated to trigger a motoneuron-restricted death pathway. Motoneurons expressing ALS-linked SOD1 mutants showed an increased susceptibility to Fas-mediated death through activation of an amplification loop [166-168]. Accordingly, mutant *SOD1* mice with homozygous FasL mutation present a reduced loss of motoneurons and a prolonged life expectancy [169]. Likewise, the RNA interference-mediated silencing of Fas following intrathecal delivery of Fas-specific small interfering RNA improves motor function and survival in ALS mice [170]. While it remains unclear if T lymphocytes contribute to Fas-induced motoneuron degeneration, these studies suggest the possibility of their direct participation in the degenerative process.

T lymphocytes could also amplify the neuroinflammation in ALS via glial cells. Upon activation, microglia cells increase membrane expression of MHC class II molecules, becoming efficient antigen presenting cells able to actively drive T cell activation and differentiation. In turn, cytokines secreted by T cells modulate microglia phenotype and function. For instance, TNFα and IFNγ, two major pro-inflammatory cytokines produced by Th1 lymphocytes induce and activate M1 microglial cells and cause neurotoxicity toward motoneurons. Experimental studies in ALS mice demonstrated that inflammatory cell subtypes were phenotypicaly and functionally different depending upon the disease stage [96]. At initial stages, microglia exhibits anti-inflammatory M2 phenotype (Ym1+, CD163+) and infiltrating T cells are almost exclusively CD4+ while end-stage disease is associated with a skew of microglia toward a pro-inflammatory M1 phenotype (Nox2+) and T lymphocytes are mainly Th1 cells [106].

The neurotoxic effect of NK cells is suggested by the neuroprotective effect of the immunomodulation of NK cells, which increases lifespan of ALS mice and is accompanied by a reduced astrocytosis. While the pathological modalities of NK cells in ALS remain elusive, several hypothetical mechanisms can be raised. Indeed, activated NK (and to a lesser extent CD8+ T cells) inhibit neurite outgrowth of cerebellar neurons in a cell contact-dependent manner *in vitro* [171]. In sensory neurons, IL-2-activated NK cells have a killing activity that requires cellular contact and perforin [172]. Further, the production of IFNγ by activated NK cells might directly trigger motoneuron death through the LIGHT/LT-βR pathway or potentiate a cytotoxic Th1/CTL response via the combined action of other NK-related cytokines such as IL-17 or IL-22 [173]. Of note, NK cells also produce IL-4 upon activation, which as described earlier, mediates a neuroprotective effect. Therefore, NK cells represent an appealing branch of the immunopathology that could be considered as a therapeutic target for ALS.

In addition to the adaptive immune system, several studies suggest that humoral immunity and immunoglobulins could also contribute to the disease. Autoantibodies to voltage-gated Ca^{2+} or K^{+} channels have been described in ALS patients, which induce specific motoneuron alterations both *in vitro* and *in vivo* after passive transfer in mice [174-178]. Accordingly, C5a and other complement activation products released after activation of the classical complement pathway by antibodies are elevated in the CSF and spinal cord of ALS mice and patients and specific inhibition of C5a receptor ameliorates disease in *SOD1*^{G93A} mice [179, 180]. Additionally, abnormal levels of anti-Fas antibodies, able to induce neuronal apoptosis *in vitro*, have been detected in the serum of patients with ALS [181, 182]. Thus, both the innate and adaptive immune system appear to have deleterious consequences on the survival and maintenance of motoneurons in ALS.

Figure 3 illustrates the potential mechanisms implicating different populations of immune cells in ALS pathogenesis.

5. Pre-clinical therapies targeting neuroinflammation

5.1. Pharmacological targeting of the neuroinflammatory response

In light of the salient evidence supporting the contribution of neuroinflammation in ALS, several drug- or cell-based therapeutic approaches have been evaluated in ALS mice for their ability to modulate the pathologic process. Those that have shown a positive effect on astrocytosis and microgliosis are described below and have been categorized based on their desired functional target.

In order to mitigate the detrimental effects of the overactive $p75^{NTR}$ pathway in ALS, an antagonist that mimics the short NGF β loop region that binds the $p75^{NTR}$ has been utilized [183]. Unfortunately, the intraperitoneal (i.p.) delivery of the $p75^{NTR}$ antagonist from asymptomatic stage up until the endpoint of the disease does not improve the phenotype or survival of *SOD1*^{G93A} mice [183]. However, antisense peptide nucleic acid-based silencing of $p75^{NTR}$ following early systemic i.p. administration delays by about 10% both onset and progression of the disease [184]. Although, alternative route of administration or development of more efficient molecules should be assessed, $p75^{NTR}$ represents a therapeutic target that needs to be further explored.

COX-2 appears as an appealing therapeutic target for ALS as it promotes both pro-inflammatory events and astrocytic glutamate release [60, 67]. Celecoxib, a COX-2 inhibitor, fed to *SOD1*^{G93A} mice from asymptomatic to end-stage results in a delayed onset and an increased lifespan of approximately 25%. Celecoxib treatment prevents loss of spinal motoneurons and

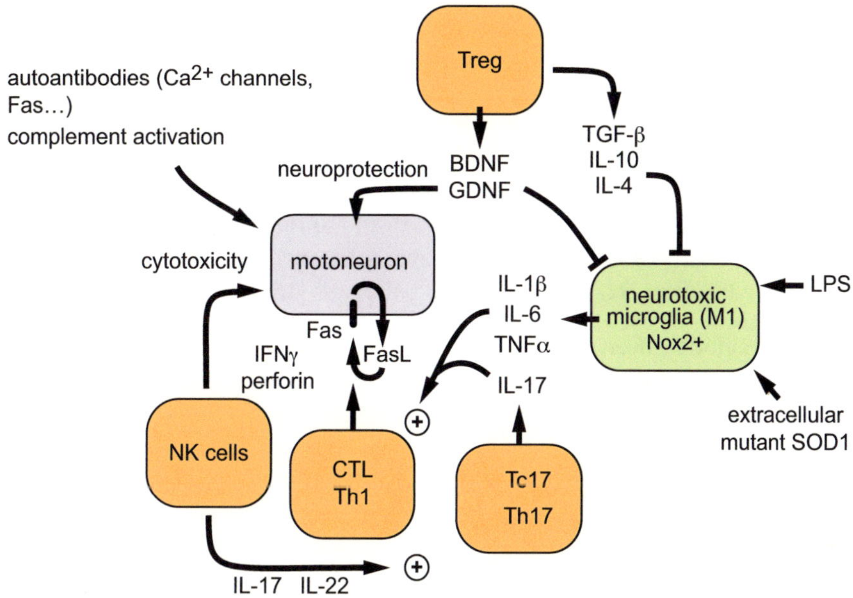

Figure 3. Potential Mechanisms by which peripheral and central immunity might contribute to the neurodegenerative process in ALS. Both neuroprotective and neurotoxic functions can be proposed for the involvement of lymphocytes in ALS pathogenesis (as described in section 3).

reduces astrocytosis [185]. Importantly, celecoxib-treated *SOD1*^{G93A} spinal cords display reduced levels of PGE2, a potent pro-inflammatory mediator as well as a signal for glutamate release from astrocytes [67].

Lenalidomide, an immunomodulatory drug with pleiotropic properties derived from thalidomide, has been evaluated in mutant SOD1 mice due to its inhibitory effect on TNFα production by monocytes [186]. A lenalidomide-diet given to *SOD1*^{G93A} mice retards disease onset, ameliorates motoneuron survival and extends survival by 18%. A significant decrease in IL-1α and TNFα as well as an increase in IL-1 receptor antagonist (IL-1RA) and TGF-β1 is observed in the spinal cord of Lenalidomide-treated mice [187]. In a similar study, the lifespan of ALS mice treated with lenalidomide at onset of symptoms is increased by 12%. Concomitantly, there is an improved survival of motoneurons, decreased levels of the pro-inflammatory cytokines TNFα and Fas associated Factor as well as an increased expression of the anti-inflammatory cytokines TGF-β3 and IL-1RA [188].

Epigallocathecin gallate (EGCG) is a green tea polyphenol that can prevent microglial neurotoxicity through the modulation of TNFα mRNA transcription and release as well as iNOS production [189]. The daily oral administration of EGCG to *SOD1*^{G93A} mice daily from asymptomatic to endstage delays disease onset and lifespan by approximately 10 and 14%, respectively. EGCG also moderately mitigates motoneuron loss and reduces microglia activation [190].

Pioglitazone is a drug that was initially developed to treat type II diabetes patients that also exerts ant-inflammatory and neuroprotective activities (reviewed in [191]). For these reasons, it has been hypothesized that it may improve ALS pathology. Indeed, pioglitazone-fed $SOD1^{G93A}$ mice have a delayed onset of 10% and a prolonged lifespan of about 8% [192]. Pioglitazone significantly reduces microgliosis and astrocytosis in $SOD1^{G93A}$ mice as well as alters the expression profile of spinal cord lysates from pro-inflammatory to anti-inflammatory [192, 193]. Further analysis of spinal cords reveals that pioglitazone may act through the inhibition of the p38 kinase, NF-κB and STAT3 pathways [167, 193, 194].

Olesoxime has previously been selected as a neuroprotective agent via a motoneuron survival-based screen [195]. Interestingly, $SOD1^{G93A}$ mice fed an olesoxime diet from asymptomatic stage to end-stage survive 10% longer than non-treated mice and also demonstrate a reduction in both astrocytosis and microgliosis [195, 196].

Dicatechol nordihydroguaiaretic acid (NDGA) is a selective inhibitor of 5-LOX that presents TNFα antagonizing activity in microglial cells. $SOD1^{G93A}$ mice on an NDGA-diet from pre-symptomatic stage to end-point have a 32% increase in median lifespan as well as a reduced motoneuron loss and astrocytosis [197].

Minocycline is a member of the tetracycline molecules that can enter the CNS and mediates inflammation and microgliosis (reviewed in [198]). Asymptomatic $SOD1^{G93A}$ mice that received daily minocycline by i.p. injection have a delayed disease onset, a 16% increase in lifespan as well as a preservation of spinal motoneurons [199]. Similarly, minocycline-fed late pre-symptomatic $SOD1^{G37R}$ mice display a 6% longer survival, an increased number of spinal cord motoneurons and a reduced microgliosis [200]. However, a minocycline diet in symptomatic $SOD1^{G93A}$ has no effect on survival while amplifying both astrocytosis and microgliosis [201]. These results strikingly illustrate the time-dependent dynamics of the neuroinflammation response, highlighting not only the requirement to target the most pertinent therapeutic molecular and cellular effectors but to also do so at the proper stage of the disease.

5.2. Advances and possible applications of protein therapy

In addition to chemical compounds, the therapeutic delivery of proteins has also been assessed as a potential modulator of neuroinflammation in ALS. Indeed, the granulocyte-colony stimulating factor (G-CSF), a hematopoietic growth factor, has been delivered to $SOD1^{G93A}$ mice by osmotic pump starting at asymptomatic stage for a continuance of 8 weeks [202]. G-CSF-recipient ALS mice display a delay in disease onset as well as an increased motoneuron survival. The time to clinical endstage is increased by 10% in $SOD1^{G93A}$ mice receiving G-CSF. Importantly, while G-CSF was initially used for its neuroprotective effects and its ability to readily cross the blood-brain barrier [203, 204], further characterization of treated $SOD1^{G93A}$ mice shows a reduced spinal cord astrocytosis and microgliosis as well as an increased availability of migratory healing monocytes, suggesting that G-CSF may be beneficial in ALS via its modulation of neuroinflammation [205].

http://dx.doi.org/10.5772/56489

Another potential protein therapy is the administration of the activated protein C (APC), a plasma protease with anti-coagulant, neuroprotective and anti-inflammatory functions (reviewed in [206]). A daily i.p. injection of APC to symptomatic *SOD1^G93A^* mice until death slows disease progression, leading to a 25% increase in lifespan [207]. Further, APC appears to exert its beneficial effects via a downregulation of mutant SOD1 expression in both motoneurons and microglia, thus resulting in delayed neuroinflammatory events [207].

Anakinra (Kineret), a recombinant form of human IL-1RA, that inhibits the pro-inflammatory activity of both IL-1α and IL-1β, is approved by the U.S food and drug administration for rheumatoid arthritis [208]. When administrated by i.p. daily to asymptomatic stage to *SOD1^G93A^* mice, it ameliorates motor function and prolongs lifespan by approximately 4% [121].

The CD40 costimulatory pathway, which plays an important role in B and T cell activation [209], has been proposed to contribute to ALS pathogenesis. The weekly delivery of a blocking anti-CD40L antibody by i.p. injection starting at an asymptomatic stage delays onset and prolongs survival by approximately 7%. Consistently, anti-CD40L delivery reduces significantly the percentage of peripheral CD8+ T cells as well as GFAP+ astrocytes and Mac2+ microglia in the spinal cord [66], suggesting that the CD40 pathway, an integral component of neuroimmunity, is a potential therapeutic target in ALS.

5.3. Cell therapy perspectives

While drugs and protein therapy target the misregulated pathways within astrocytes and microglia, the aim of cell therapy is to replace these aberrantly functional cells by healthy ones or use implanted cells as a therapeutic platform to deliver neurotrophic support, thus hopefully alleviating neuroinflammation in ALS.

5.3.1. Glial precursor cells

Glial cell therapy has indeed been evaluated by isolating human neural progenitor cells (hNPCs) and genetically modifying them to express GDNF [210, 211]. Prior to direct injection in the spinal cord of *SOD1^G93A^* rats, hNPCs were pre-differentiated into astrocytes [210]. Despite the fact that the hNPC injection did not increase the lifespan of *SOD1^G93A^* rats, they do localize within both the grey and white matter of the spinal cord and survive until the death of the animal. Further investigation of this method reveals that hNPCs preserve dying motoneuron cell bodies in *SOD1^G93A^* rats without improving their innervations at the neuromuscular junction [212]. In *SOD1^G93A^* mice, GDNF-expressing hNPCs also migrate to the spinal cord where a subset of them differentiates into astrocytes, again without improving survival or neurodegeneration [213]. However, the lack of beneficial outcome is most likely due to the regional specificity of GDNF's biological activity, as intramuscular but not intraspinal delivery of GDNF exerts its neuroprotective effect [214, 215]. Another astrocyte precursor with potential benefits is the glial-restricted progenitors (GRPs), isolated from the spinal cord of embryonic rats [216]. The transplantation of GRPs in the ventral horn of *SOD1^G93A^* rats shows that these cells differentiate into astrocytes and can survive and migrate along the spinal cord [217]. Importantly, GRP-recipient ALS rats survive longer as well as show a slower cervical neurodegeneration and a reduced spinal cord microgliosis. In *SOD1*^{G93A} mice however, while the GRPs efficiently differentiate into astrocytes, survive, and locate to both grey and white matter of the spinal cord, they do not influence lifespan and do not prevent motoneuron loss [218].

Human umbilical cord blood cells (hUCBCs) also have the potential to differentiate into glial cells (reviewed in [219]). Pre-symptomatic *SOD1*^{G93A} mice received either native hUCBCs or cells engineered to overexpress vascular endothelial growth factor (VEGF) and/or FGF [220]. Two weeks following the orbital injection, analysis of the spinal cords reveals the presence of the transplanted hUCBCs with the non-modified cells preferentially differentiating into microglia while the cells expressing the growth factors became astrocytes [220]. Importantly, the administration of hUCBCs to pre-symptomatic and symptomatic *SOD1*^{G93A} mice via intravenous injections delays disease progression, increases lifespan by approximately 8%, prevents motoneuron loss and reduces both astrocytosis and microgliosis [221].

5.3.2. Mesenchymal stem cells

Mesenchymal stem cells (MSCs) are multipotent stem cells that can differentiate in a broad variety of cells and instigate a reparative environment. MSCs have been therapeutically assessed in light of their immunosuppressive capacities, limiting inflammatory responses in their surroundings [222]. MSCs isolated from rat muscle injected into the CSF of *SOD1*^{G93A} rats subsequently localize to the spinal cord and adopt astrocytic characteristics [223]. The injected ALS rats display motor deficits at the same age than vehicle-injected animals. However, the MSC-injected *SOD1*^{G93A} rats show an increased survival of approximately 11%, an increased number of motoneurons as well as a reduced neuroinflammation [223]. Similarly, the intravenous injection of MSCs after the onset of disease in *SOD1*^{G93A} mice increases lifespan by 13% and reduces both astrocytosis and microgliosis [224]. Alternatively, a combination of intraspinal and intravenous transplantation of MSCs has been evaluated in *SOD1*^{G93A} rats at disease onset and leads to a 6% increased in survival [225]. Similarly, the intracisternal delivery at asymptomatic stage of human MSCs derived from ALS patients also prolongs survival ALS mice by about 6% [226]. Further, intramuscular administration of MSCs genetically engineered to produce GDNF in asymptomatic *SOD1*^{G93A} rats does not influence the time of disease onset but prolongs survival of implanted ALS rats. However, the beneficial effect of MSCs transplantation was not correlated with decreased astrocytosis or microgliosis [227]. Although this pre-clinical evidence proposes MSC-based therapy as a potential means to intervene in the course of disease, the neuroprotective mechanisms involved remain elusive, especially regarding the immunosuppressive abilities of MSCs.

6. Clinical aspects

As discussed in the present book and chapter, the molecular pathways and cellular effectors responsible for ALS are numerous and their precise contributions to disease pathogenesis are still debated. While this has made translational therapy a challenge, it has shifted the devel-

http://dx.doi.org/10.5772/56489

opment of neuronal-specific therapies toward those targeting more general phenomena characterizing ALS, including neuroinflammation.

The pattern of neurodegeneration in ALS has been described as overall linear, albeit with some variations [228, 229]. One of the biggest discrepancies between individuals is the evolution of the disease, which ranges from death in less than 6 months to a limited handicap after more than 10 years following the initial diagnosis. Either rapid or slow, the topography of neurodegenerative events is rather reproducible, usually spreading from one limb to the opposite one and then to another level. Thus, from the moment a patient presents himself at the clinic with symptoms, there is a progressive extension and diffusion of the pathological process. This spreading of neurodegeneration over time may result from the infiltration and migration of non-neuronal cells or by the exchange of molecules from one cell to another. This hypothesis, based on pre-clinical and clinical observations, highlights the importance of developing therapies that modulate immunity and/or neuroinflammation.

As described in section 2.3, the excitotoxic theory suggests that glutamate accumulates within the intercellular space and induce a pathological synaptic excitotoxic transmission, leading to motoneuron death [230]. This hypothesis motivated a series of clinical trials with riluzole, a potent glutamate antagonist, culminating in the demonstration that riluzole is efficient in slowing down disease progression [231]. To date, only riluzole is marketed as a *bona fide* treatment for ALS. While riluzole is thought to reduce glutamate release in neurons via the inhibition of voltage-gated sodium channels [232], riluzole may also have some important anti-inflammatory functions. Indeed, riluzole significantly decreases IL-1β, TNFα and iNOS levels as well as increases IL-10 levels in LPS-activated microglial cells [233]. Another neuroprotective mechanism mediated by riluzole may include the production of BDNF and GDNF by astrocytes, as demonstrated in cultures [234]. In experimental autoimmune encephalomyelitis (EAE), a commonly used murine model of multiple sclerosis, riluzole administration significantly ameliorates motor functions. Importantly, the decrease in the clinical severity of riluzole-treated EAE mice is associated with a diminished inflammatory response and a marked reduction in lymphocytes infiltrating the spinal cord [235]. Together, these results suggest a more complex mode of action for riluzole where a modulation of inflammation should be acknowledged as one of its therapeutic activity.

Other immunomodulatory agents have also been tested in ALS clinical trials, but their therapeutic benefits have not been as promising as those demonstrated by riluzole [236]. Indeed, immunosuppressants such as cyclosporine or cyclophosphamide as well as the more aggressive total lymphoid irradiation were not successful. The intravenous immunoglobulin G (IVIg) treatment has been proposed to suppress inflammatory responses by inducing an IFNγ-refractory state in macrophages [237]. Interestingly, an open-label pilot study of IVIg administration in ALS patients led to a transient clinical improvement in subjects with bulbar-ALS but not in patients with lower signs, suggesting that immunomodulation may have therapeutic potential [238]. Nevertheless, the combined administration of cyclophosphamide and IVIg in another cohort of 7 patients with upper and lower signs did not lead to clinical improvement [239]. These studies highlight the importance of a better identification of targets as well as a more efficient and specific design of therapies by specifically taking into account the clinical heterogeneity of the disease.

Among the drugs mentioned that have been evaluated in pre-clinical models, celecoxib and pioglitazone were both assessed in a randomized, double-blind, placebo-controlled trial, but gave disappointing results as there were no effects on motor function and survival rate [240, 241]. When minocycline was tested in a randomized placebo-controlled phase III trial, it not only did not show any benefits, it in fact displayed serious harmful effect in patients [242]. Thalidomide, an analogue of lenalidomide, which showed therapeutic potential in SOD1 mutant mice, was used in a single arm, open label phase II study. Unfortunately, similar to minocycline, thalidomide led to undesirable side effects, without any positive effects [243]. A pilot trial (double-blind, placebo-controlled, randomized) where G-CSF was administered to ALS patients for over 25 days does however show encouraging results on the prevention of degeneration of several white matter tracts [244]. This study supports a larger scale trial in which the immunomodulatory aspect of G-CSF should be further explored.

The translational therapy of neuroinflammatory and immunomodulatory effectors has thus shown both exciting and disappointing outcomes. There are many factors that could help explain the discrepancy between pre-clinical and clinical evaluations of potential therapies. Firstly, most drugs are typically assessed in the mutant SOD1 animal models. This poses an important caveat, as not only there exists an obvious difference between humans and animals, but SOD1 models also represent hereditary ALS, which account for only 4% of ALS cases. Thus, a drug may show a positive influence on an inherited disease model without having any effect on sporadic cases. There is therefore the risk of wrongly eliminating or pushing forward an ALS treatment due to the lack of diverse familial and sporadic pre-clinical models. Secondly, the exact timing of a specific treatment could also impact its efficiency. Indeed, as described in the present chapters, neuroinflammation consists of dynamic mechanisms, combining over time and space, different cell types with opposing neuroprotective and neurotoxic functions. Thus, depending on the desired target, the therapeutic window of various drugs may differ one from another. Thirdly, while establishing a dosage regimen (concentration of drug and treatment length) is amenable in pre-clinical models, determining the exact dose and duration of a therapy in human patients is somewhat more complex. Further, it remains unclear if the treatment of ALS patients should take place daily for several months or periodically in pulses. It thus becomes imperative to develop new analytical methods to adequately extract from pre-clinical studies the equivalent doses for humans as well as the optimal treatment protocol. Finally, in light of the high heterogeneity of ALS forms, it is possible that not all patients will respond equally to a particular therapy. Therefore, all of these parameters, including additional ones not mentioned herein, have to be thoroughly considered and analyzed to ensure that we do not wrongly disregard or promote a drug.

When dealing with neuroinflammation in ALS, the therapeutic intervention is of a different kind than the previous major clinical trials. It is not compulsorily a matter of influencing the disease process, that is the motoneuron death itself, but a matter of stopping a potential amplification and/or diffusion phenomenon. In animal models, this strategy has given interesting results but there still remains a lot of work before a successful therapy targeting neuroinflammation is translated into humans.

7. Future directions

In the present chapter, we have described the cellular and molecular events characterizing the neuroinflammation in ALS. We have also highlighted the beneficial potential of various therapeutic approaches specifically targeting these neuroinflammatory effectors. While the reports discussed herein support a role for astrocytes, microglia and immune cells in ALS, it remains unclear how they influence disease onset, progression or both. Hence, a thorough investigation of the neuroinflammatory pathways that impact neurodegeneration will ultimately enhance our understanding of how and when to therapeutically modulate this pathological process. Further, it is important to remember that the astrocytosis and microgliosis that typify ALS stem from the chronicity of this neurodegenerative disorder and thus, there is an active communication with the neurotoxic environment that is composed of neurons, glial cells and immune cells. Therefore, it is with caution that we should proceed with defining a causal or consequential role for neuroinflammation in ALS, but instead, our focus should be on identifying its exact pathological contribution.

List of abbreviations

5-LOX, 5-lipoxygenase; Aβ, amyloid beta; ALS, amyotrophic lateral sclerosis; AMPA, α-amino-3-hydroxy-5-methyl-4-isoxazolepropionic acid; APC, activated protein C; BDNF, brain-derived neurotrophic factor; CHOP, C/EBP homologous protein; CNS, central nervous system; COX-2, cyclooxygenase; CSF, cerebrospinal fluid; CTL, cytotoxic T lymphocytes; EAE, experimental autoimmune encephalomyelitis; EGCG, Epigallocathecin Gallate; excitatory amino-acid transporter 2; FDA, food and drug administration; FGF, fibroblast growth factor; G-CSF, granulocyte-colony stimulating factor; GABA, gamma-aminobutyric acid; GDNF, glial-derived neurotrophic factor; GFAP, glial fibrillary acidic protein; GLT-1, glutamate transporter 1; GRP, glial-restricted progenitor; glutamate receptor, GluR; IL-1RA, IL-1 receptor antagonist, IFN, interferon; IL, interleukin; i.p., intraperitoneal; ISG15, interferon-stimulated gene 15; IVIg, Intravenous immunoglobulin G; KCC, potassium (K^+)-chloride co-transporter; LPS, lipopolysaccharide; LT-βR, lymphotoxin beta receptor; MAO-B, monoamine oxidase-B; MHC, major histocompatibility complex; MSC, mesenchymal stem cell; NDGA, dicatechol nordihydroguaiaretic acid; NF-κB, nuclear factor kappa B; NK, natural killer; NMDA, N-methyl-D-aspartic acid; NPC, neural progenitor cell; NO, nitric oxide; NTF, neurotrophic factor; $p75^{NTR}$, p75 neurotrophin receptor; PGE_2 prostaglandin E_2; ROS, reactive oxygen species; SOD1, superoxide dismutase 1; STAT, signal transducer and activator of transcription; TDP-43, TAR DNA-binding protein 43; Teff, effectors T lymphocyte; TGF-β, transforming growth factor beta; TLR, Toll-like receptor; TNF, tumor necrosis factor; Treg, regulatory T lymphocyte; UCBC, umbilical cord blood cell; VEGF, vascular endothelial growth factor.

Acknowledgements

Our work is supported by grants from the Institut National de la Santé et de la Recherche Médicale (Inserm), Association Française contre les Myopathies (AFM), Association Française pour la Recherche sur la SLA (ARS), Direction de l'Hospitalisation et de l'Organisation des soins (DHOS) and the Thierry Latran foundation. M.B is a recipient of a long-term EMBO Marie Curie Fellowship. We apologize to authors whose work could not have been cited due to space limitations.

Author details

Melissa Bowerman[1], Thierry Vincent[1,2], Frédérique Scamps[1], William Camu[1,3] and Cédric Raoul[1*]

*Address all correspondence to: cedric.raoul@inserm.fr

1 The Neuroscience Institute of Montpellier, INM, Inserm UMR1051, Saint Eloi Hospital, Montpellier, France

2 Department of Immunology, Saint Eloi Hospital, Montpellier, France

3 Department of Neurology, ALS Reference Center, Gui-de-Chauliac Hospital, Montpellier, France

References

[1] Czlonkowska A, Kurkowska-Jastrzebska I. Inflammation and gliosis in neurological diseases--clinical implications. J Neuroimmunol. 2011 Feb;231(1-2):78-85.

[2] Philips T, Robberecht W. Neuroinflammation in amyotrophic lateral sclerosis: role of glial activation in motor neuron disease. Lancet Neurol. 2011 Mar;10(3):253-63.

[3] Liu W, Tang Y, Feng J. Cross talk between activation of microglia and astrocytes in pathological conditions in the central nervous system. Life Sci. 2011 Aug 1;89(5-6): 141-6.

[4] Kushner PD, Stephenson DT, Wright S. Reactive astrogliosis is widespread in the subcortical white matter of amyotrophic lateral sclerosis brain. J Neuropathol Exp Neurol. 1991 May;50(3):263-77.

[5] Nagy D, Kato T, Kushner PD. Reactive astrocytes are widespread in the cortical gray matter of amyotrophic lateral sclerosis. J Neurosci Res. 1994 Jun 15;38(3):336-47.

[6] Murayama S, Inoue K, Kawakami H, Bouldin TW, Suzuki K. A unique pattern of astrocytosis in the primary motor area in amyotrophic lateral sclerosis. Acta neuropathologica. 1991;82(6):456-61.

[7] Schiffer D, Cordera S, Cavalla P, Migheli A. Reactive astrogliosis of the spinal cord in amyotrophic lateral sclerosis. J Neurol Sci. 1996 Aug;139 Suppl:27-33.

[8] Jossan SS, Ekblom J, Aquilonius SM, Oreland L. Monoamine oxidase-B in motor cortex and spinal cord in amyotrophic lateral sclerosis studied by quantitative autoradiography. J Neural Transm Suppl. 1994;41:243-8.

[9] Johansson A, Engler H, Blomquist G, Scott B, Wall A, Aquilonius SM, et al. Evidence for astrocytosis in ALS demonstrated by [11C](L)-deprenyl-D2 PET. J Neurol Sci. 2007 Apr 15;255(1-2):17-22.

[10] Bruijn LI, Becher MW, Lee MK, Anderson KL, Jenkins NA, Copeland NG, et al. ALS-linked SOD1 mutant G85R mediates damage to astrocytes and promotes rapidly progressive disease with SOD1-containing inclusions. Neuron. 1997 Feb;18(2):327-38.

[11] Levine JB, Kong J, Nadler M, Xu Z. Astrocytes interact intimately with degenerating motor neurons in mouse amyotrophic lateral sclerosis (ALS). Glia. 1999 Dec;28(3): 215-24.

[12] Acevedo-Arozena A, Kalmar B, Essa S, Ricketts T, Joyce P, Kent R, et al. A comprehensive assessment of the SOD1G93A low-copy transgenic mouse, which models human amyotrophic lateral sclerosis. Dis Model Mech. 2011 Sep-Oct;4(5):686-700.

[13] Morrison BM, Janssen WG, Gordon JW, Morrison JH. Time course of neuropathology in the spinal cord of G86R superoxide dismutase transgenic mice. J Comp Neurol. 1998 Feb 2;391(1):64-77.

[14] Rafalowska J, Fidzianska A, Dziewulska D, Gadamski R, Ogonowska W, Grieb P. Progression of morphological changes within CNS in a transgenic rat model of familial amyotrophic lateral sclerosis. Folia Neuropathol. 2006;44(3):162-74.

[15] Gadamski R, Chrapusta SJ, Wojda R, Grieb P. Morphological changes and selective loss of motoneurons in the lumbar part of the spinal cord in a rat model of familial amyotrophic lateral sclerosis (fALS). Folia Neuropathol. 2006;44(3):154-61.

[16] Clement AM, Nguyen MD, Roberts EA, Garcia ML, Boillee S, Rule M, et al. Wild-type nonneuronal cells extend survival of SOD1 mutant motor neurons in ALS mice. Science. 2003 Oct 3;302(5642):113-7.

[17] Yamanaka K, Chun SJ, Boillee S, Fujimori-Tonou N, Yamashita H, Gutmann DH, et al. Astrocytes as determinants of disease progression in inherited amyotrophic lateral sclerosis. Nat Neurosci. 2008 Mar;11(3):251-3.

[18] Wang L, Gutmann DH, Roos RP. Astrocyte loss of mutant SOD1 delays ALS disease onset and progression in G85R transgenic mice. Hum Mol Genet. 2011 Jan 15;20(2): 286-93.

[19] Hensley K, Mhatre M, Mou S, Pye QN, Stewart C, West M, et al. On the relation of oxidative stress to neuroinflammation: lessons learned from the G93A-SOD1 mouse model of amyotrophic lateral sclerosis. Antioxidants & redox signaling. 2006 Nov-Dec;8(11-12):2075-87.

[20] Di Giorgio FP, Carrasco MA, Siao MC, Maniatis T, Eggan K. Non-cell autonomous effect of glia on motor neurons in an embryonic stem cell-based ALS model. Nat Neurosci. 2007 May;10(5):608-14.

[21] Nagai M, Re DB, Nagata T, Chalazonitis A, Jessell TM, Wichterle H, et al. Astrocytes expressing ALS-linked mutated SOD1 release factors selectively toxic to motor neurons. Nat Neurosci. 2007 May;10(5):615-22.

[22] Di Giorgio FP, Boulting GL, Bobrowicz S, Eggan KC. Human embryonic stem cell-derived motor neurons are sensitive to the toxic effect of glial cells carrying an ALS-causing mutation. Cell stem cell. 2008 Dec 4;3(6):637-48.

[23] Marchetto MC, Muotri AR, Mu Y, Smith AM, Cezar GG, Gage FH. Non-cell-autonomous effect of human SOD1 G37R astrocytes on motor neurons derived from human embryonic stem cells. Cell stem cell. 2008 Dec 4;3(6):649-57.

[24] Aebischer J, Cassina P, Otsmane B, Moumen A, Seilhean D, Meininger V, et al. IFN-gamma triggers a LIGHT-dependent selective death of motoneurons contributing to the non-cell-autonomous effects of mutant SOD1. Cell death and differentiation. 2011 May;18(5):754-68.

[25] Lepore AC, Dejea C, Carmen J, Rauck B, Kerr DA, Sofroniew MV, et al. Selective ablation of proliferating astrocytes does not affect disease outcome in either acute or chronic models of motor neuron degeneration. Exp Neurol. 2008 Jun;211(2):423-32.

[26] Diaz-Amarilla P, Olivera-Bravo S, Trias E, Cragnolini A, Martinez-Palma L, Cassina P, et al. Phenotypically aberrant astrocytes that promote motoneuron damage in a model of inherited amyotrophic lateral sclerosis. Proc Natl Acad Sci U S A. 2011 Nov 1;108(44):18126-31.

[27] Gong YH, Parsadanian AS, Andreeva A, Snider WD, Elliott JL. Restricted expression of G86R Cu/Zn superoxide dismutase in astrocytes results in astrocytosis but does not cause motoneuron degeneration. J Neurosci. 2000 Jan 15;20(2):660-5.

[28] Pramatarova A, Laganiere J, Roussel J, Brisebois K, Rouleau GA. Neuron-specific expression of mutant superoxide dismutase 1 in transgenic mice does not lead to motor impairment. J Neurosci. 2001 May 15;21(10):3369-74.

[29] Lino MM, Schneider C, Caroni P. Accumulation of SOD1 mutants in postnatal motoneurons does not cause motoneuron pathology or motoneuron disease. J Neurosci. 2002 Jun 15;22(12):4825-32.

[30] Van Den Bosch L, Van Damme P, Bogaert E, Robberecht W. The role of excitotoxicity in the pathogenesis of amyotrophic lateral sclerosis. Biochim Biophys Acta. 2006 Nov-Dec;1762(11-12):1068-82.

[31] Arundine M, Tymianski M. Molecular mechanisms of calcium-dependent neurodegeneration in excitotoxicity. Cell Calcium. 2003 Oct-Nov;34(4-5):325-37.

[32] Lee A, Pow DV. Astrocytes: Glutamate transport and alternate splicing of transporters. The international journal of biochemistry & cell biology. 2010 Dec;42(12):1901-6.

[33] Rothstein JD. Excitotoxic mechanisms in the pathogenesis of amyotrophic lateral sclerosis. Adv Neurol. 1995;68:7-20; discussion 1-7.

[34] Lin CL, Bristol LA, Jin L, Dykes-Hoberg M, Crawford T, Clawson L, et al. Aberrant RNA processing in a neurodegenerative disease: the cause for absent EAAT2, a glutamate transporter, in amyotrophic lateral sclerosis. Neuron. 1998 Mar;20(3):589-602.

[35] Howland DS, Liu J, She Y, Goad B, Maragakis NJ, Kim B, et al. Focal loss of the glutamate transporter EAAT2 in a transgenic rat model of SOD1 mutant-mediated amyotrophic lateral sclerosis (ALS). Proc Natl Acad Sci U S A. 2002 Feb 5;99(3):1604-9.

[36] Hollmann M, Heinemann S. Cloned glutamate receptors. Annu Rev Neurosci. 1994;17:31-108.

[37] Heath PR, Shaw PJ. Update on the glutamatergic neurotransmitter system and the role of excitotoxicity in amyotrophic lateral sclerosis. Muscle Nerve. 2002 Oct;26(4): 438-58.

[38] Kawahara Y, Kwak S, Sun H, Ito K, Hashida H, Aizawa H, et al. Human spinal motoneurons express low relative abundance of GluR2 mRNA: an implication for excitotoxicity in ALS. J Neurochem. 2003 May;85(3):680-9.

[39] Kwak S, Hideyama T, Yamashita T, Aizawa H. AMPA receptor-mediated neuronal death in sporadic ALS. Neuropathology. 2010 Apr;30(2):182-8.

[40] Burnashev N, Monyer H, Seeburg PH, Sakmann B. Divalent ion permeability of AMPA receptor channels is dominated by the edited form of a single subunit. Neuron. 1992 Jan;8(1):189-98.

[41] Van Damme P, Bogaert E, Dewil M, Hersmus N, Kiraly D, Scheveneels W, et al. Astrocytes regulate GluR2 expression in motor neurons and their vulnerability to excitotoxicity. Proc Natl Acad Sci U S A. 2007 Sep 11;104(37):14825-30.

[42] Streit WJ, Mrak RE, Griffin WS. Microglia and neuroinflammation: a pathological perspective. J Neuroinflammation. 2004 Jul 30;1(1):14.

[43] Shahani N, Nalini A, Gourie-Devi M, Raju TR. Reactive astrogliosis in neonatal rat spinal cord after exposure to cerebrospinal fluid from patients with amyotrophic lateral sclerosis. Exp Neurol. 1998 Jan;149(1):295-8.

[44] Borden EC, Sen GC, Uze G, Silverman RH, Ransohoff RM, Foster GR, et al. Interferons at age 50: past, current and future impact on biomedicine. Nat Rev Drug Discov. 2007 Dec;6(12):975-90.

[45] Babu GN, Kumar A, Chandra R, Puri SK, Kalita J, Misra UK. Elevated inflammatory markers in a group of amyotrophic lateral sclerosis patients from northern India. Neurochemical research. 2008 Jun;33(6):1145-9.

[46] Tateishi T, Yamasaki R, Tanaka M, Matsushita T, Kikuchi H, Isobe N, et al. CSF chemokine alterations related to the clinical course of amyotrophic lateral sclerosis. J Neuroimmunol. 2010 May;222(1-2):76-81.

[47] Aebischer J, Moumen A, Sazdovitch V, Seilhean D, Meininger V, Raoul C. Elevated levels of IFNgamma and LIGHT in the spinal cord of patients with sporadic amyotrophic lateral sclerosis. Eur J Neurol. 2012 May;19(5):752-9, e45-6.

[48] Dangond F, Hwang D, Camelo S, Pasinelli P, Frosch MP, Stephanopoulos G, et al. Molecular signature of late-stage human ALS revealed by expression profiling of postmortem spinal cord gray matter. Physiol Genomics. 2004 Jan 15;16(2):229-39.

[49] Wang R, Yang B, Zhang D. Activation of interferon signaling pathways in spinal cord astrocytes from an ALS mouse model. Glia. 2011 Jun;59(6):946-58.

[50] Hensley K, Fedynyshyn J, Ferrell S, Floyd RA, Gordon B, Grammas P, et al. Message and protein-level elevation of tumor necrosis factor alpha (TNF alpha) and TNF alpha-modulating cytokines in spinal cords of the G93A-SOD1 mouse model for amyotrophic lateral sclerosis. Neurobiol Dis. 2003 Oct;14(1):74-80.

[51] Takeuchi S, Fujiwara N, Ido A, Oono M, Takeuchi Y, Tateno M, et al. Induction of protective immunity by vaccination with wild-type apo superoxide dismutase 1 in mutant SOD1 transgenic mice. J Neuropathol Exp Neurol. 2010 Oct;69(10):1044-56.

[52] Darnell JE, Jr., Kerr IM, Stark GR. Jak-STAT pathways and transcriptional activation in response to IFNs and other extracellular signaling proteins. Science. 1994 Jun 3;264(5164):1415-21.

[53] Underwood CK, Coulson EJ. The p75 neurotrophin receptor. The international journal of biochemistry & cell biology. 2008;40(9):1664-8.

[54] Lowry KS, Murray SS, McLean CA, Talman P, Mathers S, Lopes EC, et al. A potential role for the p75 low-affinity neurotrophin receptor in spinal motor neuron degeneration in murine and human amyotrophic lateral sclerosis. Amyotroph Lateral Scler Other Motor Neuron Disord. 2001 Sep;2(3):127-34.

[55] Radeke MJ, Misko TP, Hsu C, Herzenberg LA, Shooter EM. Gene transfer and molecular cloning of the rat nerve growth factor receptor. Nature. 1987 Feb 12-18;325(6105): 593-7.

[56] Pehar M, Cassina P, Vargas MR, Castellanos R, Viera L, Beckman JS, et al. Astrocytic production of nerve growth factor in motor neuron apoptosis: implications for amyotrophic lateral sclerosis. J Neurochem. 2004 Apr;89(2):464-73.

[57] Ferraiuolo L, Higginbottom A, Heath PR, Barber S, Greenald D, Kirby J, et al. Dysregulation of astrocyte-motoneuron cross-talk in mutant superoxide dismutase 1-related amyotrophic lateral sclerosis. Brain. 2011 Sep;134(Pt 9):2627-41.

[58] Cassina P, Pehar M, Vargas MR, Castellanos R, Barbeito AG, Estevez AG, et al. Astrocyte activation by fibroblast growth factor-1 and motor neuron apoptosis: implications for amyotrophic lateral sclerosis. J Neurochem. 2005 Apr;93(1):38-46.

[59] Pehar M, Vargas MR, Robinson KM, Cassina P, Diaz-Amarilla PJ, Hagen TM, et al. Mitochondrial superoxide production and nuclear factor erythroid 2-related factor 2 activation in p75 neurotrophin receptor-induced motor neuron apoptosis. J Neurosci. 2007 Jul 18;27(29):7777-85.

[60] Mancini AD, Di Battista JA. The cardinal role of the phospholipase A(2)/cyclooxygenase-2/prostaglandin E synthase/prostaglandin E(2) (PCPP) axis in inflammostasis. Inflamm Res. 2011 Dec;60(12):1083-92.

[61] Almer G, Guegan C, Teismann P, Naini A, Rosoklija G, Hays AP, et al. Increased expression of the pro-inflammatory enzyme cyclooxygenase-2 in amyotrophic lateral sclerosis. Ann Neurol. 2001 Feb;49(2):176-85.

[62] Maihofner C, Probst-Cousin S, Bergmann M, Neuhuber W, Neundorfer B, Heuss D. Expression and localization of cyclooxygenase-1 and -2 in human sporadic amyotrophic lateral sclerosis. Eur J Neurosci. 2003 Sep;18(6):1527-34.

[63] Foy TM, Aruffo A, Bajorath J, Buhlmann JE, Noelle RJ. Immune regulation by CD40 and its ligand GP39. Annu Rev Immunol. 1996;14:591-617.

[64] Garlichs CD, Geis T, Goppelt-Struebe M, Eskafi S, Schmidt A, Schulze-Koops H, et al. Induction of cyclooxygenase-2 and enhanced release of prostaglandin E(2) and I(2) in human endothelial cells by engagement of CD40. Atherosclerosis. 2002 Jul;163(1): 9-16.

[65] Okuno T, Nakatsuji Y, Kumanogoh A, Koguchi K, Moriya M, Fujimura H, et al. Induction of cyclooxygenase-2 in reactive glial cells by the CD40 pathway: relevance to amyotrophic lateral sclerosis. J Neurochem. 2004 Oct;91(2):404-12.

[66] Lincecum JM, Vieira FG, Wang MZ, Thompson K, De Zutter GS, Kidd J, et al. From transcriptome analysis to therapeutic anti-CD40L treatment in the SOD1 model of amyotrophic lateral sclerosis. Nat Genet. 2010 May;42(5):392-9.

[67] Bezzi P, Carmignoto G, Pasti L, Vesce S, Rossi D, Rizzini BL, et al. Prostaglandins stimulate calcium-dependent glutamate release in astrocytes. Nature. 1998 Jan 15;391(6664):281-5.

[68] Wang J, Sinha T, Wynshaw-Boris A. Wnt signaling in mammalian development: lessons from mouse genetics. Cold Spring Harb Perspect Biol. 2012 May;4(5).

[69] Inestrosa NC, Varela-Nallar L, Grabowski CP, Colombres M. Synaptotoxicity in Alzheimer's disease: the Wnt signaling pathway as a molecular target. IUBMB Life. 2007 Apr-May;59(4-5):316-21.

[70] Godin JD, Poizat G, Hickey MA, Maschat F, Humbert S. Mutant huntingtin-impaired degradation of beta-catenin causes neurotoxicity in Huntington's disease. EMBO J. 2010 Jul 21;29(14):2433-45.

[71] Chen Y, Guan Y, Liu H, Wu X, Yu L, Wang S, et al. Activation of the Wnt/beta-catenin signaling pathway is associated with glial proliferation in the adult spinal cord of ALS transgenic mice. Biochem Biophys Res Commun. 2012 Apr 6;420(2):397-403.

[72] Chen Y, Guan Y, Zhang Z, Liu H, Wang S, Yu L, et al. Wnt signaling pathway is involved in the pathogenesis of amyotrophic lateral sclerosis in adult transgenic mice. Neurol Res. 2012 May;34(4):390-9.

[73] Shtutman M, Zhurinsky J, Simcha I, Albanese C, D'Amico M, Pestell R, et al. The cyclin D1 gene is a target of the beta-catenin/LEF-1 pathway. Proc Natl Acad Sci U S A. 1999 May 11;96(10):5522-7.

[74] Fu M, Wang C, Li Z, Sakamaki T, Pestell RG. Minireview: Cyclin D1: normal and abnormal functions. Endocrinology. 2004 Dec;145(12):5439-47.

[75] Araki Y, Okamura S, Hussain SP, Nagashima M, He P, Shiseki M, et al. Regulation of cyclooxygenase-2 expression by the Wnt and ras pathways. Cancer Res. 2003 Feb 1;63(3):728-34.

[76] Levitt P, Pintar JE, Breakefield XO. Immunocytochemical demonstration of monoamine oxidase B in brain astrocytes and serotonergic neurons. Proc Natl Acad Sci U S A. 1982 Oct;79(20):6385-9.

[77] Ekblom J, Jossan SS, Bergstrom M, Oreland L, Walum E, Aquilonius SM. Monoamine oxidase-B in astrocytes. Glia. 1993 Jun;8(2):122-32.

[78] Ekblom J, Jossan SS, Oreland L, Walum E, Aquilonius SM. Reactive gliosis and monoamine oxidase B. J Neural Transm Suppl. 1994;41:253-8.

[79] Orru S, Mascia V, Casula M, Giuressi E, Loizedda A, Carcassi C, et al. Association of monoamine oxidase B alleles with age at onset in amyotrophic lateral sclerosis. Neuromuscul Disord. 1999 Dec;9(8):593-7.

[80] Mallajosyula JK, Kaur D, Chinta SJ, Rajagopalan S, Rane A, Nicholls DG, et al. MAO-B elevation in mouse brain astrocytes results in Parkinson's pathology. PLoS One. 2008;3(2):e1616.

[81] Kawamata H, Manfredi G. Mitochondrial dysfunction and intracellular calcium dysregulation in ALS. Mech Ageing Dev. 2010 Jul-Aug;131(7-8):517-26.

[82] Cassina P, Cassina A, Pehar M, Castellanos R, Gandelman M, de Leon A, et al. Mitochondrial dysfunction in SOD1G93A-bearing astrocytes promotes motor neuron degeneration: prevention by mitochondrial-targeted antioxidants. J Neurosci. 2008 Apr 16;28(16):4115-22.

[83] Jacobson J, Duchen MR, Hothersall J, Clark JB, Heales SJ. Induction of mitochondrial oxidative stress in astrocytes by nitric oxide precedes disruption of energy metabolism. J Neurochem. 2005 Oct;95(2):388-95.

[84] Davalos D, Grutzendler J, Yang G, Kim JV, Zuo Y, Jung S, et al. ATP mediates rapid microglial response to local brain injury in vivo. Nat Neurosci. 2005 Jun;8(6):752-8.

[85] Ransohoff RM, Perry VH. Microglial physiology: unique stimuli, specialized responses. Annu Rev Immunol. 2009;27:119-45.

[86] Hanisch UK, Kettenmann H. Microglia: active sensor and versatile effector cells in the normal and pathologic brain. Nat Neurosci. 2007 Nov;10(11):1387-94.

[87] Engelhardt JI, Appel SH. IgG reactivity in the spinal cord and motor cortex in amyotrophic lateral sclerosis. Arch Neurol. 1990 Nov;47(11):1210-6.

[88] Kawamata T, Akiyama H, Yamada T, McGeer PL. Immunologic reactions in amyotrophic lateral sclerosis brain and spinal cord tissue. Am J Pathol. 1992 Mar;140(3): 691-707.

[89] Banati RB, Gehrmann J, Kellner M, Holsboer F. Antibodies against microglia/brain macrophages in the cerebrospinal fluid of a patient with acute amyotrophic lateral sclerosis and presenile dementia. Clin Neuropathol. 1995 Jul-Aug;14(4):197-200.

[90] Gerber YN, Sabourin JC, Rabano M, Vivanco M, Perrin FE. Early functional deficit and microglial disturbances in a mouse model of amyotrophic lateral sclerosis. PLoS One. 2012;7(4):e36000.

[91] Hall ED, Oostveen JA, Gurney ME. Relationship of microglial and astrocytic activation to disease onset and progression in a transgenic model of familial ALS. Glia. 1998 Jul;23(3):249-56.

[92] Alexianu ME, Kozovska M, Appel SH. Immune reactivity in a mouse model of familial ALS correlates with disease progression. Neurology. 2001 Oct 9;57(7):1282-9.

[93] Petrik MS, Wilson JM, Grant SC, Blackband SJ, Tabata RC, Shan X, et al. Magnetic resonance microscopy and immunohistochemistry of the CNS of the mutant SOD

murine model of ALS reveals widespread neural deficits. Neuromolecular Med. 2007;9(3):216-29.

[94] Boillee S, Yamanaka K, Lobsiger CS, Copeland NG, Jenkins NA, Kassiotis G, et al. Onset and progression in inherited ALS determined by motor neurons and microglia. Science. 2006 Jun 2;312(5778):1389-92.

[95] Dibaj P, Steffens H, Zschuntzsch J, Nadrigny F, Schomburg ED, Kirchhoff F, et al. In Vivo imaging reveals distinct inflammatory activity of CNS microglia versus PNS macrophages in a mouse model for ALS. PLoS One. 2011;6(3):e17910.

[96] Liao B, Zhao W, Beers DR, Henkel JS, Appel SH. Transformation from a neuroprotective to a neurotoxic microglial phenotype in a mouse model of ALS. Exp Neurol. 2012 Jun 23.

[97] Weydt P, Yuen EC, Ransom BR, Moller T. Increased cytotoxic potential of microglia from ALS-transgenic mice. Glia. 2004 Nov 1;48(2):179-82.

[98] Fendrick SE, Xue QS, Streit WJ. Formation of multinucleated giant cells and microglial degeneration in rats expressing a mutant Cu/Zn superoxide dismutase gene. J Neuroinflammation. 2007;4:9.

[99] Graber DJ, Hickey WF, Harris BT. Progressive changes in microglia and macrophages in spinal cord and peripheral nerve in the transgenic rat model of amyotrophic lateral sclerosis. J Neuroinflammation. 2010;7:8.

[100] Sanagi T, Yuasa S, Nakamura Y, Suzuki E, Aoki M, Warita H, et al. Appearance of phagocytic microglia adjacent to motoneurons in spinal cord tissue from a presymptomatic transgenic rat model of amyotrophic lateral sclerosis. J Neurosci Res. 2010 Sep;88(12):2736-46.

[101] Bataveljic D, Stamenkovic S, Bacic G, Andjus PR. Imaging cellular markers of neuroinflammation in the brain of the rat model of amyotrophic lateral sclerosis. Acta Physiol Hung. 2011 Mar;98(1):27-31.

[102] Wang L, Sharma K, Grisotti G, Roos RP. The effect of mutant SOD1 dismutase activity on non-cell autonomous degeneration in familial amyotrophic lateral sclerosis. Neurobiol Dis. 2009 Aug;35(2):234-40.

[103] Beers DR, Henkel JS, Xiao Q, Zhao W, Wang J, Yen AA, et al. Wild-type microglia extend survival in PU.1 knockout mice with familial amyotrophic lateral sclerosis. Proc Natl Acad Sci U S A. 2006 Oct 24;103(43):16021-6.

[104] McKercher SR, Torbett BE, Anderson KL, Henkel GW, Vestal DJ, Baribault H, et al. Targeted disruption of the PU.1 gene results in multiple hematopoietic abnormalities. EMBO J. 1996 Oct 15;15(20):5647-58.

[105] Zhao W, Beers DR, Henkel JS, Zhang W, Urushitani M, Julien JP, et al. Extracellular mutant SOD1 induces microglial-mediated motoneuron injury. Glia. 2010 Jan 15;58(2):231-43.

[106] Beers DR, Zhao W, Liao B, Kano O, Wang J, Huang A, et al. Neuroinflammation modulates distinct regional and temporal clinical responses in ALS mice. Brain Behav Immun. 2011 Jul;25(5):1025-35.

[107] Gowing G, Philips T, Van Wijmeersch B, Audet JN, Dewil M, Van Den Bosch L, et al. Ablation of proliferating microglia does not affect motor neuron degeneration in amyotrophic lateral sclerosis caused by mutant superoxide dismutase. J Neurosci. 2008 Oct 8;28(41):10234-44.

[108] Obal I, Jakab JS, Siklos L, Engelhardt JI. Recruitment of activated microglia cells in the spinal cord of mice by ALS IgG. Neuroreport. 2001 Aug 8;12(11):2449-52.

[109] Troost D, Claessen N, van den Oord JJ, Swaab DF, de Jong JM. Neuronophagia in the motor cortex in amyotrophic lateral sclerosis. Neuropathol Appl Neurobiol. 1993 Oct;19(5):390-7.

[110] Breckenridge DG, Germain M, Mathai JP, Nguyen M, Shore GC. Regulation of apoptosis by endoplasmic reticulum pathways. Oncogene. 2003 Nov 24;22(53):8608-18.

[111] Lautenschlaeger J, Prell T, Grosskreutz J. Endoplasmic reticulum stress and the ER mitochondrial calcium cycle in amyotrophic lateral sclerosis. Amyotroph Lateral Scler. 2012 Feb;13(2):166-77.

[112] Ito Y, Yamada M, Tanaka H, Aida K, Tsuruma K, Shimazawa M, et al. Involvement of CHOP, an ER-stress apoptotic mediator, in both human sporadic ALS and ALS model mice. Neurobiol Dis. 2009 Dec;36(3):470-6.

[113] Oyadomari S, Mori M. Roles of CHOP/GADD153 in endoplasmic reticulum stress. Cell death and differentiation. 2004 Apr;11(4):381-9.

[114] Kawahara K, Oyadomari S, Gotoh T, Kohsaka S, Nakayama H, Mori M. Induction of CHOP and apoptosis by nitric oxide in p53-deficient microglial cells. FEBS Lett. 2001 Oct 5;506(2):135-9.

[115] Saxena S, Cabuy E, Caroni P. A role for motoneuron subtype-selective ER stress in disease manifestations of FALS mice. Nat Neurosci. 2009 May;12(5):627-36.

[116] Lacroix S, Feinstein D, Rivest S. The bacterial endotoxin lipopolysaccharide has the ability to target the brain in upregulating its membrane CD14 receptor within specific cellular populations. Brain pathology (Zurich, Switzerland). 1998 Oct;8(4):625-40.

[117] Laflamme N, Rivest S. Toll-like receptor 4: the missing link of the cerebral innate immune response triggered by circulating gram-negative bacterial cell wall components. FASEB J. 2001 Jan;15(1):155-63.

[118] Laflamme N, Soucy G, Rivest S. Circulating cell wall components derived from gram-negative, not gram-positive, bacteria cause a profound induction of the gene-encoding Toll-like receptor 2 in the CNS. J Neurochem. 2001 Nov;79(3):648-57.

[119] Liu Y, Hao W, Dawson A, Liu S, Fassbender K. Expression of amyotrophic lateral sclerosis-linked SOD1 mutant increases the neurotoxic potential of microglia via TLR2. J Biol Chem. 2009 Feb 6;284(6):3691-9.

[120] Casula M, Iyer AM, Spliet WG, Anink JJ, Steentjes K, Sta M, et al. Toll-like receptor signaling in amyotrophic lateral sclerosis spinal cord tissue. Neuroscience. 2011 Apr 14;179:233-43.

[121] Meissner F, Molawi K, Zychlinsky A. Mutant superoxide dismutase 1-induced IL-1{beta} accelerates ALS pathogenesis. Proc Natl Acad Sci U S A. 2010 Jul 20;107(29):13046-50.

[122] Reed-Geaghan EG, Savage JC, Hise AG, Landreth GE. CD14 and toll-like receptors 2 and 4 are required for fibrillar A{beta}-stimulated microglial activation. J Neurosci. 2009 Sep 23;29(38):11982-92.

[123] Inoue K. The function of microglia through purinergic receptors: neuropathic pain and cytokine release. Pharmacol Ther. 2006 Jan;109(1-2):210-26.

[124] Bours MJ, Dagnelie PC, Giuliani AL, Wesselius A, Di Virgilio F. P2 receptors and extracellular ATP: a novel homeostatic pathway in inflammation. Front Biosci (Schol Ed). 2011;3:1443-56.

[125] D'Ambrosi N, Finocchi P, Apolloni S, Cozzolino M, Ferri A, Padovano V, et al. The proinflammatory action of microglial P2 receptors is enhanced in SOD1 models for amyotrophic lateral sclerosis. J Immunol. 2009 Oct 1;183(7):4648-56.

[126] Yiangou Y, Facer P, Durrenberger P, Chessell IP, Naylor A, Bountra C, et al. COX-2, CB2 and P2X7-immunoreactivities are increased in activated microglial cells/macrophages of multiple sclerosis and amyotrophic lateral sclerosis spinal cord. BMC Neurol. 2006;6:12.

[127] Ugolini G, Raoul C, Ferri A, Haenggeli C, Yamamoto Y, Salaun D, et al. Fas/tumor necrosis factor receptor death signaling is required for axotomy-induced death of motoneurons in vivo. J Neurosci. 2003 Sep 17;23(24):8526-31.

[128] Gandelman M, Peluffo H, Beckman JS, Cassina P, Barbeito L. Extracellular ATP and the P2X7 receptor in astrocyte-mediated motor neuron death: implications for amyotrophic lateral sclerosis. J Neuroinflammation. 2010;7:33.

[129] Douaud G, Filippini N, Knight S, Talbot K, Turner MR. Integration of structural and functional magnetic resonance imaging in amyotrophic lateral sclerosis. Brain. 2011 Dec;134(Pt 12):3470-9.

[130] Maekawa S, Al-Sarraj S, Kibble M, Landau S, Parnavelas J, Cotter D, et al. Cortical selective vulnerability in motor neuron disease: a morphometric study. Brain. 2004 Jun;127(Pt 6):1237-51.

[131] Petri S, Krampfl K, Hashemi F, Grothe C, Hori A, Dengler R, et al. Distribution of GABAA receptor mRNA in the motor cortex of ALS patients. J Neuropathol Exp Neurol. 2003 Oct;62(10):1041-51.

[132] Blaesse P, Airaksinen MS, Rivera C, Kaila K. Cation-chloride cotransporters and neuronal function. Neuron. 2009 Mar 26;61(6):820-38.

[133] Rivera C, Voipio J, Payne JA, Ruusuvuori E, Lahtinen H, Lamsa K, et al. The K+/Cl- co-transporter KCC2 renders GABA hyperpolarizing during neuronal maturation. Nature. 1999 Jan 21;397(6716):251-5.

[134] Coull JA, Boudreau D, Bachand K, Prescott SA, Nault F, Sik A, et al. Trans-synaptic shift in anion gradient in spinal lamina I neurons as a mechanism of neuropathic pain. Nature. 2003 Aug 21;424(6951):938-42.

[135] Coull JA, Beggs S, Boudreau D, Boivin D, Tsuda M, Inoue K, et al. BDNF from microglia causes the shift in neuronal anion gradient underlying neuropathic pain. Nature. 2005 Dec 15;438(7070):1017-21.

[136] Kerschensteiner M, Gallmeier E, Behrens L, Leal VV, Misgeld T, Klinkert WE, et al. Activated human T cells, B cells, and monocytes produce brain-derived neurotrophic factor in vitro and in inflammatory brain lesions: a neuroprotective role of inflammation? The Journal of experimental medicine. 1999 Mar 1;189(5):865-70.

[137] Fuchs A, Ringer C, Bilkei-Gorzo A, Weihe E, Roeper J, Schutz B. Downregulation of the potassium chloride cotransporter KCC2 in vulnerable motoneurons in the SOD1-G93A mouse model of amyotrophic lateral sclerosis. J Neuropathol Exp Neurol. 2010 Oct;69(10):1057-70.

[138] Rowland LP, Shneider NA. Amyotrophic lateral sclerosis. N Engl J Med. 2001 May 31;344(22):1688-700.

[139] Boulenguez P, Liabeuf S, Bos R, Bras H, Jean-Xavier C, Brocard C, et al. Down-regulation of the potassium-chloride cotransporter KCC2 contributes to spasticity after spinal cord injury. Nat Med. 2010 Mar;16(3):302-7.

[140] Piani D, Fontana A. Involvement of the cystine transport system xc- in the macrophage-induced glutamate-dependent cytotoxicity to neurons. J Immunol. 1994 Apr 1;152(7):3578-85.

[141] Qin S, Colin C, Hinners I, Gervais A, Cheret C, Mallat M. System Xc- and apolipoprotein E expressed by microglia have opposite effects on the neurotoxicity of amyloid-beta peptide 1-40. J Neurosci. 2006 Mar 22;26(12):3345-56.

[142] Zhang R, Gascon R, Miller RG, Gelinas DF, Mass J, Hadlock K, et al. Evidence for systemic immune system alterations in sporadic amyotrophic lateral sclerosis (sALS). J Neuroimmunol. 2005 Feb;159(1-2):215-24.

[143] Rentzos M, Nikolaou C, Rombos A, Boufidou F, Zoga M, Dimitrakopoulos A, et al. RANTES levels are elevated in serum and cerebrospinal fluid in patients with amyotrophic lateral sclerosis. Amyotroph Lateral Scler. 2007 Oct;8(5):283-7.

[144] Rentzos M, Evangelopoulos E, Sereti E, Zouvelou V, Marmara S, Alexakis T, et al. Alterations of T cell subsets in ALS: a systemic immune activation? Acta Neurol Scand. 2012 Apr;125(4):260-4.

[145] McCombe PA, Henderson RD. The Role of immune and inflammatory mechanisms in ALS. Curr Mol Med. 2011 Apr 1;11(3):246-54.

[146] Rentzos M, Rombos A, Nikolaou C, Zoga M, Zouvelou V, Dimitrakopoulos A, et al. Interleukin-17 and interleukin-23 are elevated in serum and cerebrospinal fluid of patients with ALS: a reflection of Th17 cells activation? Acta Neurol Scand. 2010 Dec; 122(6):425-9.

[147] Engelhardt JI, Tajti J, Appel SH. Lymphocytic infiltrates in the spinal cord in amyotrophic lateral sclerosis. Arch Neurol. 1993 Jan;50(1):30-6.

[148] Graves MC, Fiala M, Dinglasan LA, Liu NQ, Sayre J, Chiappelli F, et al. Inflammation in amyotrophic lateral sclerosis spinal cord and brain is mediated by activated macrophages, mast cells and T cells. Amyotroph Lateral Scler Other Motor Neuron Disord. 2004 Dec;5(4):213-9.

[149] Lewis CA, Manning J, Rossi F, Krieger C. The Neuroinflammatory Response in ALS: The Roles of Microglia and T Cells. Neurol Res Int. 2012;2012:803701.

[150] Panzara MA, Gussoni E, Begovich AB, Murray RS, Zang YQ, Appel SH, et al. T cell receptor BV gene rearrangements in the spinal cords and cerebrospinal fluid of patients with amyotrophic lateral sclerosis. Neurobiol Dis. 1999 Oct;6(5):392-405.

[151] Beers DR, Henkel JS, Zhao W, Wang J, Huang A, Wen S, et al. Endogenous regulatory T lymphocytes ameliorate amyotrophic lateral sclerosis in mice and correlate with disease progression in patients with amyotrophic lateral sclerosis. Brain. 2011 May; 134(Pt 5):1293-314.

[152] Donnenfeld H, Kascsak RJ, Bartfeld H. Deposits of IgG and C3 in the spinal cord and motor cortex of ALS patients. J Neuroimmunol. 1984 Feb;6(1):51-7.

[153] Fiala M, Chattopadhay M, La Cava A, Tse E, Liu G, Lourenco E, et al. IL-17A is increased in the serum and in spinal cord CD8 and mast cells of ALS patients. J Neuroinflammation. 2010;7:76.

[154] Zhao W, Beers DR, Liao B, Henkel JS, Appel SH. Regulatory T lymphocytes from ALS mice suppress microglia and effector T lymphocytes through different cytokine-mediated mechanisms. Neurobiol Dis. 2012 Jul 17.

[155] Finkelstein A, Kunis G, Seksenyan A, Ronen A, Berkutzki T, Azoulay D, et al. Abnormal changes in NKT cells, the IGF-1 axis, and liver pathology in an animal model of ALS. PLoS One. 2011;6(8):e22374.

[156] Chiu IM, Chen A, Zheng Y, Kosaras B, Tsiftsoglou SA, Vartanian TK, et al. T lymphocytes potentiate endogenous neuroprotective inflammation in a mouse model of ALS. Proc Natl Acad Sci U S A. 2008 Nov 18;105(46):17913-8.

[157] Zhang R, Miller RG, Gascon R, Champion S, Katz J, Lancero M, et al. Circulating endotoxin and systemic immune activation in sporadic amyotrophic lateral sclerosis (sALS). J Neuroimmunol. 2009 Jan 3;206(1-2):121-4.

[158] Seksenyan A, Ron-Harel N, Azoulay D, Cahalon L, Cardon M, Rogeri P, et al. Thymic involution, a co-morbidity factor in amyotrophic lateral sclerosis. J Cell Mol Med. 2010 Oct;14(10):2470-82.

[159] Swarup V, Phaneuf D, Dupre N, Petri S, Strong M, Kriz J, et al. Deregulation of TDP-43 in amyotrophic lateral sclerosis triggers nuclear factor kappaB-mediated pathogenic pathways. The Journal of experimental medicine. 2011 Nov 21;208(12): 2429-47.

[160] Maruyama H, Morino H, Ito H, Izumi Y, Kato H, Watanabe Y, et al. Mutations of optineurin in amyotrophic lateral sclerosis. Nature. 2010 May 13;465(7295):223-6.

[161] Hohlfeld R, Kerschensteiner M, Stadelmann C, Lassmann H, Wekerle H. The neuroprotective effect of inflammation: implications for the therapy of multiple sclerosis. J Neuroimmunol. 2000 Jul 24;107(2):161-6.

[162] Schwartz M, Moalem G. Beneficial immune activity after CNS injury: prospects for vaccination. J Neuroimmunol. 2001 Feb 15;113(2):185-92.

[163] Beers DR, Henkel JS, Zhao W, Wang J, Appel SH. CD4+ T cells support glial neuroprotection, slow disease progression, and modify glial morphology in an animal model of inherited ALS. Proc Natl Acad Sci U S A. 2008 Oct 7;105(40):15558-63.

[164] Reynolds AD, Banerjee R, Liu J, Gendelman HE, Mosley RL. Neuroprotective activities of CD4+CD25+ regulatory T cells in an animal model of Parkinson's disease. J Leukoc Biol. 2007 Nov;82(5):1083-94.

[165] Holmoy T. T cells in amyotrophic lateral sclerosis. Eur J Neurol. 2008 Apr;15(4):360-6.

[166] Raoul C, Buhler E, Sadeghi C, Jacquier A, Aebischer P, Pettmann B, et al. Chronic activation in presymptomatic amyotrophic lateral sclerosis (ALS) mice of a feedback loop involving Fas, Daxx, and FasL. Proc Natl Acad Sci U S A. 2006 Apr 11;103(15): 6007-12.

[167] Raoul C, Estevez AG, Nishimune H, Cleveland DW, deLapeyriere O, Henderson CE, et al. Motoneuron death triggered by a specific pathway downstream of Fas. Potentiation by ALS-linked SOD1 mutations. Neuron. 2002 Sep 12;35(6):1067-83.

[168] Raoul C, Henderson CE, Pettmann B. Programmed cell death of embryonic motoneurons triggered through the Fas death receptor. J Cell Biol. 1999 Nov 29;147(5): 1049-62.

[169] Petri S, Kiaei M, Wille E, Calingasan NY, Flint Beal M. Loss of Fas ligand-function improves survival in G93A-transgenic ALS mice. J Neurol Sci. 2006 Dec 21;251(1-2): 44-9.

[170] Locatelli F, Corti S, Papadimitriou D, Fortunato F, Del Bo R, Donadoni C, et al. Fas small interfering RNA reduces motoneuron death in amyotrophic lateral sclerosis mice. Ann Neurol. 2007 Jul;62(1):81-92.

[171] Pool M, Rambaldi I, Darlington PJ, Wright MC, Fournier AE, Bar-Or A. Neurite outgrowth is differentially impacted by distinct immune cell subsets. Mol Cell Neurosci. 2012 Jan;49(1):68-76.

[172] Backstrom E, Chambers BJ, Kristensson K, Ljunggren HG. Direct NK cell-mediated lysis of syngenic dorsal root ganglia neurons in vitro. J Immunol. 2000 Nov 1;165(9): 4895-900.

[173] Cella M, Otero K, Colonna M. Expansion of human NK-22 cells with IL-7, IL-2, and IL-1beta reveals intrinsic functional plasticity. Proc Natl Acad Sci U S A. 2010 Jun 15;107(24):10961-6.

[174] Appel SH, Engelhardt JI, Garcia J, Stefani E. Immunoglobulins from animal models of motor neuron disease and from human amyotrophic lateral sclerosis patients passively transfer physiological abnormalities to the neuromuscular junction. Proc Natl Acad Sci U S A. 1991 Jan 15;88(2):647-51.

[175] Engelhardt JI, Siklos L, Komuves L, Smith RG, Appel SH. Antibodies to calcium channels from ALS patients passively transferred to mice selectively increase intracellular calcium and induce ultrastructural changes in motoneurons. Synapse. 1995 Jul;20(3):185-99.

[176] Demestre M, Pullen A, Orrell RW, Orth M. ALS-IgG-induced selective motor neurone apoptosis in rat mixed primary spinal cord cultures. J Neurochem. 2005 Jul; 94(1):268-75.

[177] Pagani MR, Reisin RC, Uchitel OD. Calcium signaling pathways mediating synaptic potentiation triggered by amyotrophic lateral sclerosis IgG in motor nerve terminals. J Neurosci. 2006 Mar 8;26(10):2661-72.

[178] Nwosu VK, Royer JA, Stickler DE. Voltage gated potassium channel antibodies in amyotrophic lateral sclerosis. Amyotroph Lateral Scler. 2010 Aug;11(4):392-4.

[179] Woodruff TM, Costantini KJ, Crane JW, Atkin JD, Monk PN, Taylor SM, et al. The complement factor C5a contributes to pathology in a rat model of amyotrophic lateral sclerosis. J Immunol. 2008 Dec 15;181(12):8727-34.

[180] Heurich B, El Idrissi NB, Donev RM, Petri S, Claus P, Neal J, et al. Complement upregulation and activation on motor neurons and neuromuscular junction in the SOD1 G93A mouse model of familial amyotrophic lateral sclerosis. J Neuroimmunol. 2011 Jun;235(1-2):104-9.

[181] Sengun IS, Appel SH. Serum anti-Fas antibody levels in amyotrophic lateral sclerosis. J Neuroimmunol. 2003 Sep;142(1-2):137-40.

[182] Yi FH, Lautrette C, Vermot-Desroches C, Bordessoule D, Couratier P, Wijdenes J, et al. In vitro induction of neuronal apoptosis by anti-Fas antibody-containing sera from amyotrophic lateral sclerosis patients. J Neuroimmunol. 2000 Sep 22;109(2): 211-20.

[183] Turner BJ, Murray SS, Piccenna LG, Lopes EC, Kilpatrick TJ, Cheema SS. Effect of p75 neurotrophin receptor antagonist on disease progression in transgenic amyotrophic lateral sclerosis mice. J Neurosci Res. 2004 Oct 15;78(2):193-9.

[184] Turner BJ, Cheah IK, Macfarlane KJ, Lopes EC, Petratos S, Langford SJ, et al. Antisense peptide nucleic acid-mediated knockdown of the p75 neurotrophin receptor delays motor neuron disease in mutant SOD1 transgenic mice. J Neurochem. 2003 Nov;87(3):752-63.

[185] Drachman DB, Frank K, Dykes-Hoberg M, Teismann P, Almer G, Przedborski S, et al. Cyclooxygenase 2 inhibition protects motor neurons and prolongs survival in a transgenic mouse model of ALS. Ann Neurol. 2002 Dec;52(6):771-8.

[186] Bartlett JB, Dredge K, Dalgleish AG. The evolution of thalidomide and its IMiD derivatives as anticancer agents. Nat Rev Cancer. 2004 Apr;4(4):314-22.

[187] Kiaei M, Petri S, Kipiani K, Gardian G, Choi DK, Chen J, et al. Thalidomide and lenalidomide extend survival in a transgenic mouse model of amyotrophic lateral sclerosis. J Neurosci. 2006 Mar 1;26(9):2467-73.

[188] Neymotin A, Petri S, Calingasan NY, Wille E, Schafer P, Stewart C, et al. Lenalidomide (Revlimid) administration at symptom onset is neuroprotective in a mouse model of amyotrophic lateral sclerosis. Exp Neurol. 2009 Nov;220(1):191-7.

[189] Li R, Huang YG, Fang D, Le WD. (-)-Epigallocatechin gallate inhibits lipopolysaccharide-induced microglial activation and protects against inflammation-mediated dopaminergic neuronal injury. J Neurosci Res. 2004 Dec 1;78(5):723-31.

[190] Koh SH, Lee SM, Kim HY, Lee KY, Lee YJ, Kim HT, et al. The effect of epigallocatechin gallate on suppressing disease progression of ALS model mice. Neurosci Lett. 2006 Mar 6;395(2):103-7.

[191] Kapadia R, Yi JH, Vemuganti R. Mechanisms of anti-inflammatory and neuroprotective actions of PPAR-gamma agonists. Front Biosci. 2008;13:1813-26.

[192] Schutz B, Reimann J, Dumitrescu-Ozimek L, Kappes-Horn K, Landreth GE, Schurmann B, et al. The oral antidiabetic pioglitazone protects from neurodegeneration and amyotrophic lateral sclerosis-like symptoms in superoxide dismutase-G93A transgenic mice. J Neurosci. 2005 Aug 24;25(34):7805-12.

[193] Shibata N, Kawaguchi-Niida M, Yamamoto T, Toi S, Hirano A, Kobayashi M. Effects of the PPARgamma activator pioglitazone on p38 MAP kinase and IkappaBalpha in the spinal cord of a transgenic mouse model of amyotrophic lateral sclerosis. Neuropathology. 2008 Aug;28(4):387-98.

[194] Shibata N, Yamamoto T, Hiroi A, Omi Y, Kato Y, Kobayashi M. Activation of STAT3 and inhibitory effects of pioglitazone on STAT3 activity in a mouse model of SOD1-mutated amyotrophic lateral sclerosis. Neuropathology. 2010 Aug;30(4):353-60.

[195] Bordet T, Buisson B, Michaud M, Drouot C, Galea P, Delaage P, et al. Identification and characterization of cholest-4-en-3-one, oxime (TRO19622), a novel drug candidate for amyotrophic lateral sclerosis. J Pharmacol Exp Ther. 2007 Aug;322(2):709-20.

[196] Sunyach C, Michaud M, Arnoux T, Bernard-Marissal N, Aebischer J, Latyszenok V, et al. Olesoxime delays muscle denervation, astrogliosis, microglial activation and motoneuron death in an ALS mouse model. Neuropharmacology. 2012 Jun;62(7): 2345-52.

[197] West M, Mhatre M, Ceballos A, Floyd RA, Grammas P, Gabbita SP, et al. The arachidonic acid 5-lipoxygenase inhibitor nordihydroguaiaretic acid inhibits tumor necrosis factor alpha activation of microglia and extends survival of G93A-SOD1 transgenic mice. J Neurochem. 2004 Oct;91(1):133-43.

[198] Zemke D, Majid A. The potential of minocycline for neuroprotection in human neurologic disease. Clin Neuropharmacol. 2004 Nov-Dec;27(6):293-8.

[199] Van Den Bosch L, Tilkin P, Lemmens G, Robberecht W. Minocycline delays disease onset and mortality in a transgenic model of ALS. Neuroreport. 2002 Jun 12;13(8): 1067-70.

[200] Kriz J, Nguyen M, Julien J. Minocycline slows disease progression in a mouse model of amyotrophic lateral sclerosis. Neurobiol Dis. 2002 Aug;10(3):268.

[201] Keller AF, Gravel M, Kriz J. Treatment with minocycline after disease onset alters astrocyte reactivity and increases microgliosis in SOD1 mutant mice. Exp Neurol. 2011 Mar;228(1):69-79.

[202] Pitzer C, Kruger C, Plaas C, Kirsch F, Dittgen T, Muller R, et al. Granulocyte-colony stimulating factor improves outcome in a mouse model of amyotrophic lateral sclerosis. Brain. 2008 Dec;131(Pt 12):3335-47.

[203] Schabitz WR, Kruger C, Pitzer C, Weber D, Laage R, Gassler N, et al. A neuroprotective function for the hematopoietic protein granulocyte-macrophage colony stimulating factor (GM-CSF). J Cereb Blood Flow Metab. 2008 Jan;28(1):29-43.

[204] Zhao LR, Navalitloha Y, Singhal S, Mehta J, Piao CS, Guo WP, et al. Hematopoietic growth factors pass through the blood-brain barrier in intact rats. Exp Neurol. 2007 Apr;204(2):569-73.

[205] Pollari E, Savchenko E, Jaronen M, Kanninen K, Malm T, Wojciechowski S, et al. Granulocyte colony stimulating factor attenuates inflammation in a mouse model of amyotrophic lateral sclerosis. J Neuroinflammation. 2011;8:74.

[206] Jackson C, Whitmont K, Tritton S, March L, Sambrook P, Xue M. New therapeutic applications for the anticoagulant, activated protein C. Expert Opin Biol Ther. 2008 Aug;8(8):1109-22.

[207] Zhong Z, Ilieva H, Hallagan L, Bell R, Singh I, Paquette N, et al. Activated protein C therapy slows ALS-like disease in mice by transcriptionally inhibiting SOD1 in motor neurons and microglia cells. J Clin Invest. 2009 Nov;119(11):3437-49.

[208] Mertens M, Singh JA. Anakinra for rheumatoid arthritis: a systematic review. J Rheumatol. 2009 Jun;36(6):1118-25.

[209] Munroe ME. Functional roles for T cell CD40 in infection and autoimmune disease: the role of CD40 in lymphocyte homeostasis. Semin Immunol. 2009 Oct;21(5):283-8.

[210] Klein SM, Behrstock S, McHugh J, Hoffmann K, Wallace K, Suzuki M, et al. GDNF delivery using human neural progenitor cells in a rat model of ALS. Hum Gene Ther. 2005 Apr;16(4):509-21.

[211] Blesch A, Tuszynski MH. GDNF gene delivery to injured adult CNS motor neurons promotes axonal growth, expression of the trophic neuropeptide CGRP, and cellular protection. J Comp Neurol. 2001 Aug 6;436(4):399-410.

[212] Suzuki M, McHugh J, Tork C, Shelley B, Klein SM, Aebischer P, et al. GDNF secreting human neural progenitor cells protect dying motor neurons, but not their projection to muscle, in a rat model of familial ALS. PLoS One. 2007;2(8):e689.

[213] Park S, Kim HT, Yun S, Kim IS, Lee J, Lee IS, et al. Growth factor-expressing human neural progenitor cell grafts protect motor neurons but do not ameliorate motor performance and survival in ALS mice. Exp Mol Med. 2009 Jul 31;41(7):487-500.

[214] Guillot S, Azzouz M, Deglon N, Zurn A, Aebischer P. Local GDNF expression mediated by lentiviral vector protects facial nerve motoneurons but not spinal motoneurons in SOD1(G93A) transgenic mice. Neurobiol Dis. 2004 Jun;16(1):139-49.

[215] Li W, Brakefield D, Pan Y, Hunter D, Myckatyn TM, Parsadanian A. Muscle-derived but not centrally derived transgene GDNF is neuroprotective in G93A-SOD1 mouse model of ALS. Exp Neurol. 2007 Feb;203(2):457-71.

[216] Rao MS, Noble M, Mayer-Proschel M. A tripotential glial precursor cell is present in the developing spinal cord. Proc Natl Acad Sci U S A. 1998 Mar 31;95(7):3996-4001.

[217] Lepore AC, Rauck B, Dejea C, Pardo AC, Rao MS, Rothstein JD, et al. Focal transplantation-based astrocyte replacement is neuroprotective in a model of motor neuron disease. Nat Neurosci. 2008 Nov;11(11):1294-301.

[218] Lepore AC, O'Donnell J, Kim AS, Williams T, Tuteja A, Rao MS, et al. Human glial-restricted progenitor transplantation into cervical spinal cord of the SOD1 mouse model of ALS. PLoS One. 2011;6(10):e25968.

[219] Korbling M, Robinson S, Estrov Z, Champlin R, Shpall E. Umbilical cord blood-derived cells for tissue repair. Cytotherapy. 2005;7(3):258-61.

[220] Rizvanov AA, Guseva DS, Salafutdinov, II, Kudryashova NV, Bashirov FV, Kiyasov AP, et al. Genetically modified human umbilical cord blood cells expressing vascular endothelial growth factor and fibroblast growth factor 2 differentiate into glial cells after transplantation into amyotrophic lateral sclerosis transgenic mice. Exp Biol Med (Maywood). 2011 Jan;236(1):91-8.

[221] Garbuzova-Davis S, Rodrigues MC, Mirtyl S, Turner S, Mitha S, Sodhi J, et al. Multiple intravenous administrations of human umbilical cord blood cells benefit in a mouse model of ALS. PLoS One. 2012;7(2):e31254.

[222] Uccelli A, Benvenuto F, Laroni A, Giunti D. Neuroprotective features of mesenchymal stem cells. Best Pract Res Clin Haematol. 2011 Mar;24(1):59-64.

[223] Boucherie C, Schafer S, Lavand'homme P, Maloteaux JM, Hermans E. Chimerization of astroglial population in the lumbar spinal cord after mesenchymal stem cell transplantation prolongs survival in a rat model of amyotrophic lateral sclerosis. J Neurosci Res. 2009 Jul;87(9):2034-46.

[224] Uccelli A, Milanese M, Principato MC, Morando S, Bonifacino T, Vergani L, et al. Intravenous mesenchymal stem cells improve survival and motor function in experimental amyotrophic lateral sclerosis. Mol Med. 2012;18(1):794-804.

[225] Forostyak S, Jendelova P, Kapcalova M, Arboleda D, Sykova E. Mesenchymal stromal cells prolong the lifespan in a rat model of amyotrophic lateral sclerosis. Cytotherapy. 2011 Oct;13(9):1036-46.

[226] Kim H, Kim HY, Choi MR, Hwang S, Nam KH, Kim HC, et al. Dose-dependent efficacy of ALS-human mesenchymal stem cells transplantation into cisterna magna in SOD1-G93A ALS mice. Neurosci Lett. 2010 Jan 14;468(3):190-4.

[227] Suzuki M, McHugh J, Tork C, Shelley B, Hayes A, Bellantuono I, et al. Direct muscle delivery of GDNF with human mesenchymal stem cells improves motor neuron survival and function in a rat model of familial ALS. Mol Ther. 2008 Dec;16(12):2002-10.

[228] Brooks BR, Sufit RL, DePaul R, Tan YD, Sanjak M, Robbins J. Design of clinical therapeutic trials in amyotrophic lateral sclerosis. Adv Neurol. 1991;56:521-46.

[229] Pradas J, Finison L, Andres PL, Thornell B, Hollander D, Munsat TL. The natural history of amyotrophic lateral sclerosis and the use of natural history controls in therapeutic trials. Neurology. 1993 Apr;43(4):751-5.

[230] Shaw PJ. Excitotoxicity and motor neurone disease: a review of the evidence. J Neurol Sci. 1994 Jul;124 Suppl:6-13.

[231] Lacomblez L, Bensimon G, Leigh PN, Guillet P, Meininger V. Dose-ranging study of riluzole in amyotrophic lateral sclerosis. Amyotrophic Lateral Sclerosis/Riluzole Study Group II. Lancet. 1996 May 25;347(9013):1425-31.

[232] Bellingham MC. A review of the neural mechanisms of action and clinical efficiency of riluzole in treating amyotrophic lateral sclerosis: what have we learned in the last decade? CNS Neurosci Ther. 2011 Feb;17(1):4-31.

[233] Liu BS, Ferreira R, Lively S, Schlichter LC. Microglial SK3 and SK4 Currents and Activation State are Modulated by the Neuroprotective Drug, Riluzole. J Neuroimmune Pharmacol. 2012 Apr 19.

[234] Mizuta I, Ohta M, Ohta K, Nishimura M, Mizuta E, Kuno S. Riluzole stimulates nerve growth factor, brain-derived neurotrophic factor and glial cell line-derived neurotrophic factor synthesis in cultured mouse astrocytes. Neurosci Lett. 2001 Sep 14;310(2-3):117-20.

[235] Gilgun-Sherki Y, Panet H, Melamed E, Offen D. Riluzole suppresses experimental autoimmune encephalomyelitis: implications for the treatment of multiple sclerosis. Brain Res. 2003 Nov 7;989(2):196-204.

[236] Turner MR, Parton MJ, Leigh PN. Clinical trials in ALS: an overview. Semin Neurol. 2001 Jun;21(2):167-75.

[237] Clynes R. IVIG therapy: interfering with interferon-gamma. Immunity. 2007 Jan; 26(1):4-6.

[238] Camu W, Carlander B, Cadilhac J. HIgh-dose intravenous immunoglobulin in amyotrophic lateral sclerosis with bulbar onset. In: Clifford Rose F, ed. New evidence in MND/ALS research: Smith Gordon 1991:287-9.

[239] Meucci N, Nobile-Orazio E, Scarlato G. Intravenous immunoglobulin therapy in amyotrophic lateral sclerosis. J Neurol. 1996 Feb;243(2):117-20.

[240] Cudkowicz ME, Shefner JM, Schoenfeld DA, Zhang H, Andreasson KI, Rothstein JD, et al. Trial of celecoxib in amyotrophic lateral sclerosis. Ann Neurol. 2006 Jul;60(1): 22-31.

[241] Dupuis L, Dengler R, Heneka MT, Meyer T, Zierz S, Kassubek J, et al. A randomized, double blind, placebo-controlled trial of pioglitazone in combination with riluzole in amyotrophic lateral sclerosis. PLoS One. 2012;7(6):e37885.

[242] Gordon PH, Moore DH, Miller RG, Florence JM, Verheijde JL, Doorish C, et al. Efficacy of minocycline in patients with amyotrophic lateral sclerosis: a phase III randomised trial. Lancet Neurol. 2007 Dec;6(12):1045-53.

[243] Stommel EW, Cohen JA, Fadul CE, Cogbill CH, Graber DJ, Kingman L, et al. Efficacy of thalidomide for the treatment of amyotrophic lateral sclerosis: a phase II open label clinical trial. Amyotroph Lateral Scler. 2009 Oct-Dec;10(5-6):393-404.

[244] Duning T, Schiffbauer H, Warnecke T, Mohammadi S, Floel A, Kolpatzik K, et al. G-CSF prevents the progression of structural disintegration of white matter tracts in amyotrophic lateral sclerosis: a pilot trial. PLoS One. 2011;6(3):e17770.

Chapter 5

Superoxide Dismutase and Oxidative Stress in Amyotrophic Lateral Sclerosis

María Clara Franco, Cassandra N. Dennys,
Fabian H. Rossi and Alvaro G. Estévez

Additional information is available at the end of the chapter

http://dx.doi.org/10.5772/56488

1. Introduction

Oxidative stress is defined as the imbalance between reactive species such as free radicals and oxidants and the antioxidant defenses. Free radicals are molecules with one or more unpaired electrons, while oxidants are molecules with a high potential for taking electrons from other molecules. The more recognized reactive species are the reactive oxygen species (ROS), which include oxygen and its reduction products superoxide, hydrogen peroxide and hydroxyl radical, and the reactive nitrogen species (RNS) such as the free radical nitric oxide and its by-products, including the powerful oxidant peroxynitrite and the sub-product of peroxynitrite decomposition nitrogen dioxide.

As part of the antioxidant defense system, superoxide dismutase 1 (SOD1) is an abundant and highly conserved cytosolic enzyme responsible for the disproportionation of superoxide to molecular oxygen and hydrogen peroxide (McCord and Fridovich, 1969). SOD1 is a relatively small protein of 153 amino acids that works as a tight homodimer and requires a high stability for fast catalysis (Perry et al., 2010; Trumbull and Beckman, 2009). The stability is conferred by the quaternary structure of the protein, an eight-strand beta-barrel, as well as the binding of Cu and Zn, two metal ions with catalytic roles positioned in the active site channel (Perry et al., 2010; Trumbull and Beckman, 2009). The disproportionation of superoxide is a two-step oxidation-reduction reaction that involves the cycling of the copper atom in SOD1 from Cu^{2+} to Cu^{+} and back to Cu^{+2}.

The zinc does not participate in this reaction but is essential for the structure of the active site. In addition, the formation of an intrasubunit disulfide bridge stabilizes the enzyme and plays an important role in preventing aggregation of metal-deficient SOD (Getzoff et al., 1989).

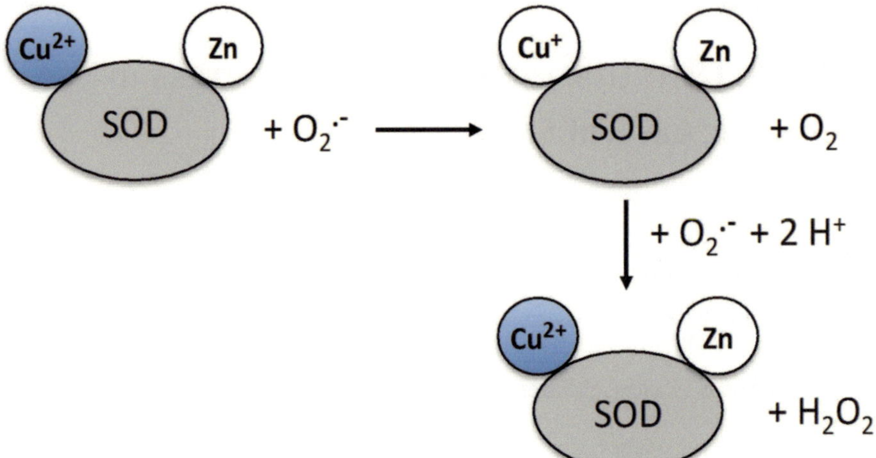

Mutations in the gene codifying for SOD1 were linked to familial ALS almost 20 years ago. Currently, over 130 point mutations on more than 70 sites on SOD1 have been described, most of these being missense single residue mutations located in critical positions that affect the stability and folding of the enzyme (Beckman et al., 2001; Perry et al., 2010; Roberts et al., 2007). The goal of this chapter is to review recent advances in our understanding of the role of oxidative stress on the gain of a toxic function associated with mutations in the gene of the copper/zinc superoxide dismutase.

2. Zn-deficient SOD1

The first proposed mechanisms linking mutations of SOD1 with ALS were based on the loss of dismutase activity (Beckman et al., 1993; Deng et al., 1993a). However, the SOD1 mutants G37R and G93A remain fully active and were linked to familial ALS (Borchelt et al., 1994; Yim et al., 1996). In addition, the mouse knockout for SOD1 developed normally and did not show signs of motor neuron deficit, although the motor neurons were more susceptible to cell death upon axonal injury (Reaume et al., 1996). This evidence indicated that a gain-of-function rather than the loss of function was responsible for motor neuron degeneration in ALS, and that the gain-of-function could be related to the redox properties of SOD1.

The discovery that mutations on the gene for an antioxidant enzyme such as SOD1 were associated with a population of familial ALS patients led to speculate on the role of oxidative stress in the pathogenesis of ALS (Beckman et al., 1993; Deng et al., 1993b; Rosen et al., 1993). From this original discovery to the present the interest on oxidative stress in ALS has been a rollercoaster. Several different groups described the presence of a variety of markers for oxidative stress in human samples and animal models of ALS, including elevated protein carbonyl and nitrotyrosine levels as well as lipid and DNA oxidation. Oxidation of proteins,

http://dx.doi.org/10.5772/56488

lipids, and DNA was also found in transgenic mice and cell culture models (Barber and Shaw, 2010). On the other hand, other groups failed to find markers of oxidative damage in animal models of ALS, casting doubt on the relevance of oxidative stress in the pathogenesis of the disease (Barber and Shaw, 2010). Currently, a role for oxidative stress in ALS is generally accepted but whether oxidative stress is responsible for the mutant SOD1 gain-of-function is still controversial.

2.1. Mutant SOD1 aggregation and Zn-deficiency

Mutant SOD1s have a tendency to aggregate when expressed in bacterial systems and transfected cells, and the presence of mutant and wild type SOD1-containing aggregates has been described in animal models of ALS (Bruijn and Cleveland, 1996; Watanabe et al., 2001). The formation of aggregates clogging the proteasome and containing other relevant proteins along with mutant SOD1 is one of the possible explanations for SOD1 toxic gain-of-function. However, in mice expressing the $SOD1^{A4V}$ mutant, the most common mutation linked to familial ALS in humans, the mutant is expressed at high levels and forms protein aggregates but does not cause disease (Gurney et al., 1994). Alternatively, other groups proposed a hypothesis in which the formation of aggregates is a protective mechanism rather than cause of toxicity. *In vitro* experiments showed that both wild type SOD1 and SOD1 with mutation of the cysteine residues involved in protein aggregation were able to stabilize the mutant SOD1 enzymes, increasing their toxicity (Clement et al., 2003; Fukada et al., 2001; Sahawneh et al., 2010; Witan et al., 2009). Additionally, it was recently described that overexpression of the deubiquitinating enzyme ataxin-3 stimulates the formation of SOD1-containing aggresomes by trimming K63-linked polyubiquitin chains. The knockdown of ataxin-3 decreases the formation of aggresomes and increases cell death induced by mutant SOD1 (Wang et al., 2012). These results suggest a toxic gain-of-function for the stabilized and soluble mutant SOD1, rather than toxicity due to aggregation. Indeed, by removing the toxic soluble mutant SOD1, the formation of aggregates has been proposed to be a protective mechanism (Trumbull and Beckman, 2009). Further support is provided by recent studies of crossbreeding showing an acceleration of the disease in mutant SOD1 transgenic mice overexpressing wild type SOD1, which was linked to the formation of disulfide bridges in the enzyme by oxidation of cysteine residues, increasing the formation of aggregates (Deng et al., 2006; Furukawa et al., 2006; Wang et al., 2009). Other investigations reproduced the acceleration of the disease in animals expressing both wild type and mutant SOD1 but failed to find a correlation between expression of wild type SOD1 and protein aggregation (Prudencio et al., 2009).

The link between the gain-of-function and the redox activity of soluble mutant SOD1 as a source of oxidative stress is based on the presence of the copper atom in the active site of the enzyme as well as the loss of zinc. The requirement for copper was challenged by genetic experiments in which the chaperone that delivers the copper metal to SOD1 was deleted. The ablation of the chaperone in the G93A, G85R, or G73R-SOD1 mutant mice decreased the activity of the enzyme but had no effect on the progression of the disease (Subramaniam et al., 2002), although it may be possible for SOD1 to acquire copper from an alternative source (Beckman et al., 2002). The transgenic expression of a SOD1 with mutations that eliminate the copper-binding site still produced disease (Prudencio et al., 2012; Wang et al., 2003). In contrast, another study showed that the mutant enzymes A4V, G85R, and G93A had a higher affinity for copper than the wild type protein, and that this aberrant copper binding was mediated by cysteine 111 (Watanabe et al., 2007), implying that the enzyme binds copper in an alternate site (Figure 1A).

Some SOD1 mutants bind copper and zinc and are fully active (Borchelt et al., 1994; Marklund et al., 1997) but many mutations affect the binding of zinc while copper remains tightly bound, thus favoring the formation of Zn-deficient SOD. In the SOD1^{G93A} mouse model of ALS, the dietary depletion of zinc accelerates the progression of the disease while moderate supplement of zinc provides protection (Ermilova et al., 2005). Indeed, a peak corresponding to one-metal SOD1 was detected *in vivo* in spinal cords from the SOD1^{G93A} rat model using the recently developed methodology of electrospray mass spectrometry. The one-metal peak was 2-fold larger in the disease-affected ventral spinal cord compare to that of the dorsal spinal cord (Rhoads et al., 2011), suggesting that Zn-deficient SOD1 may be present *in vivo* in the affected tissue.

ALS-linked mutant SOD1s have 5-50 fold less affinity for zinc than the wild type protein (Crow et al., 1997a; Lyons et al., 1996). The loss of zinc disorganizes the structure of the active site leaving the copper metal more expose and accessible to substrates other than superoxide, decreasing the normal activity of the enzyme. When replete with zinc, SOD1 mutants can generally fulfill the antioxidant activity of wild type SOD (Crow et al., 1997a). Early studies showed that mutant SOD1 has an aberrant chemistry and is reduced abnormally fast which allows the reaction with oxidants such as hydrogen peroxide and peroxynitrite (Crow et al., 1997a; Crow et al., 1997b; Lyons et al., 1996; Wiedau-Pazos et al., 1996), thus turning the antioxidant enzyme into a catalyst for oxidation. The conversion of SOD1 from antioxidant to pro-oxidant due to the loss of zinc is a simple explanation for the gain-of-function attributed to the ALS-linked SOD mutants, but is still highly controversial.

2.2. Formation of hydroxyl radical from hydrogen peroxide

In normal conditions SOD1 catalyzes the disproportionation of superoxide to hydrogen peroxide, but due to changes in mutant SOD1 conformation, the mutant enzyme can catalyze the production of hydroxyl radical from hydrogen peroxide *in vitro* (Yim et al., 1990) (Figure 1B). The G93A-SOD1 mutant has enhanced free-radical production compare to the wild type enzyme due to a more open active site, decreasing the K_m for hydrogen peroxide (Yim et al., 1996). Accordingly, an increase in the levels of hydrogen peroxide and hydroxyl radical was reported *in vivo* in the spinal cord from mice expressing the G93A mutant (Liu et al., 1999).

The aberrant chemistry of mutant SOD1 was shown to inactivate the glutamate transporter EAAT2 by oxidative reactions catalyzed by the A4V and I113T-SOD1 mutants and triggered by hydrogen peroxide (Trotti et al., 1999; Trotti et al., 1996). The function of this transporter is down regulated in human patients and animal models of ALS and its inactivation results in neuronal degeneration (Rothstein et al., 2005; Tanaka et al., 1997). Moreover, the aberrant SOD1 chemistry increases the vulnerability of a variety of cells in culture to hydrogen peroxide, with an increased susceptibility to inhibition by copper chelators. The G37R, G41D, and G85R-SOD1

http://dx.doi.org/10.5772/56488

mutants induce activation of caspase 1 and promoted apoptosis in N2a cells and tissue expressing mutant SOD1 when exposed to hydrogen peroxide. In NSC34 cells, a motor neuron model, mutant SOD1 induces cell death upon exposure of the cells to hydrogen peroxide (Pasinelli et al., 1998; Wiedau-Pazos et al., 1996). These findings suggest that the ALS phenotype may require both, the genetic background and an additional oxidative challenge.

2.3. Production of peroxynitrite

Nitric oxide alone is not toxic to normal motor neurons (Estévez et al., 1999), but when superoxide is also produced it can react with nitric oxide to form the powerful oxidant peroxynitrite, responsible for the induction of cell death. Overexpression of mutant SOD1 makes motor neurons vulnerable to exogenous and endogenous production of nitric oxide. The increased vulnerability is linked to the activation of the Fas death pathways (Raoul et al., 2002). More recently it was shown that motor neurons from mutant SOD1 transgenic animals have lower levels of a calcium-binding ER chaperone calreticulin. A decrease in the expression of this protein is necessary and sufficient to activate the Fas/NO pathways in motor neurons. Further evidence *in vivo* shows that this protein is decreased in the spinal motor neurons of $SOD1^{G93A}$ transgenic animals prior to muscle denervation (Bernard-Marissal et al., 2012). Therefore, motor neurons expressing mutant SOD1 may produce superoxide making them susceptible to the formation of peroxynitrite in the presence of nitric oxide. In the presence of reductants, Zn-deficient SOD1 is able to produce superoxide. For instance, ascorbate reduces the copper on Zn-deficient SOD1 from Cu2+ to Cu^{+}. In turn, Zn-deficient SOD1 can transfer the electrons from ascorbate to oxygen to produce superoxide slowly but significantly over a period of minutes. Indeed, Zn-deficient SOD1 is able to oxidize ascorbate 3000-fold faster than mutant or wild type Cu,Zn-SOD1 *in vitro* (Estévez et al., 1999). In the cells, ascorbate and other cellular antioxidants such as glutathione, urate, and cysteine could have a similar effect. Normally, superoxide would be removed by the dismutase activity of the remaining and fully active Cu,Zn-SOD1. However, if nitric oxide is also produced it can effectively compete with Cu,Zn-SOD1 for superoxide to produce peroxynitrite. Because nitric oxide is a small molecule able to diffuse 10-fold faster than a small size protein, the reaction of nitric oxide with superoxide occurs 10 times faster than that with SOD1 (Beckman et al., 2001; Estévez et al., 1999; Franco and Estévez, 2011; Nauser and Koppenol, 2002) (Figure 1B). Wild type Cu,Zn-SOD1 can also produce peroxynitrite by a similar mechanism but requires superoxide in the initial step to be efficiently reduced (Beckman et al., 2001).

2.4. Catalysis of tyrosine nitration

Cu,Zn-SOD1 is not only responsible for the production of peroxynitrite but it can also catalyze tyrosine nitration *in vitro* (Beckman et al., 1993; Crow et al., 1997b; Ischiropoulos et al., 1992). The mechanism for tyrosine nitration depends on the copper atom in SOD1 that reacts with peroxynitrite. The loss of zinc from Cu,Zn-SOD1 increases by 2-fold the efficiency of the enzyme to catalyze tyrosine nitration (Crow et al., 1997a) (Figure 1B). Moreover, SOD1 is not inactivated by peroxynitrite and can catalyze tyrosine nitration indefinitely. Indeed, reactivity for nitrotyrosine was found *in vivo* in the $SOD1^{G93A}$ mouse model and in patients with ALS

(Beal et al., 1997; Ferrante et al., 1997). In spite of the indirect evidence of mass spectrometry showing a peak corresponding to a one-metal SOD1 in a rat model of ALS (Rhoads et al., 2011), whether Zn-deficient SOD1 is present *in vivo* and catalyzes tyrosine nitration is still source of debate and remains to be determined.

3. Regulation of NADPH oxidase activity by mutant SOD1

Several lines of evidence support the role of oxidative stress in mutant SOD1 toxicity, but some evidence suggest that interactions other than the redox properties of the enzyme stimulate oxidative stress by different mechanisms. Mutant SOD1 can induce oxidative stress by disruption of the redox-sensitive regulation of NADPH oxidase (Nox) in microglial cells. Noxs are transmembrane proteins that catalyze the reduction of oxygen to superoxide using NADPH as an electron donor (Brown and Griendling, 2009). Superoxide is then converted to hydrogen peroxide by SOD1. Under reducing conditions, SOD1 regulates Nox2 activation by binding and stabilizing Rac1. The oxidation of Rac1 by hydrogen peroxide disrupts the complex with SOD1 and inactivates Nox2. Upon expression of certain ALS SOD1 mutants, the dissociation of Rac1 from SOD1 is impaired and Nox2 remains active (Figure 1C). In addition, the expression of Nox2 is upregulated in the $SOD1^{G93A}$ mouse model and in ALS patients. In fact, gene deletion of Nox1 or Nox2 provides the larger protection to date in animal models of ALS (Harraz et al., 2008; Marden et al., 2007).

4. Mutant SOD1 translocation to mitochondria

Mitochondria are one of the major sources of cellular ROS formed as by-products of oxidative phosphorylation. Abnormalities in the mitochondrial structure, localization and number as well as altered activity of the electron transport chain have been described in both, sporadic and familial ALS (Manfredi and Xu, 2005). The mitochondrial electron transport chain and ATP synthesis are severely impaired at disease onset in spinal cord and brain of $SOD1^{G93A}$ transgenic mice (Lin and Beal, 2006). Both, wild type and mutant SOD localize in mitochondria in the central nervous system (Higgins et al., 2002). Mutant human SOD1 was found in the mitochondrial outer membrane, intermembrane space and matrix in transgenic mice, while inactive mutant SOD1 accumulates and forms aggregates in the mitochondrial matrix in the brain (Vijayvergiya et al., 2005). Aggregates of the mutant enzyme are also selectively found in the mitochondrial outer membrane in spinal cord from mouse models of ALS (Liu et al., 2004). Interestingly, the anti-apoptotic protein Bcl-2 binds to mutant SOD1 and aggregates in spinal cord mitochondria from patients and a mouse model of ALS, suggesting that mutant SOD1 may be toxic by depleting motor neurons of this anti-apoptotic protein (Pasinelli et al., 2004). Mutant SOD1 targeted to the mitochondrial intermembrane space in NSC34 cells induces cell death upon exposure of the cells to hydrogen peroxide (Magrane et al., 2009). In addition, the increase in carbonylated proteins and lipid hydroperoxides in mitochondria, as well as the abnormally high rates of production of hydrogen peroxide in $SOD1^{G93A}$ transgenic mice (Mattiazzi et al., 2002; Panov et al., 2011) support the mutant SOD1 aberrant catalytic gain-of-function. Indeed, it was shown that metal-deficient SOD1s are prone to mitochondrial translocation and are found in the mitochondrial intermembrane space (Okado-Matsumoto and Fridovich, 2002). The mitochondria contain the majority of the cellular copper because is required by the oxygen-consuming proteins. The insertion of copper into the translocated metal-deficient SOD would result in the formation of Zn-deficient SOD inside the mitochondria (Figure 1A). This could explain why the mitochondria are affected early in the onset of the disease (Beckman et al., 2002). The ROS-linked toxic gain-of-function of mutant SOD1 would produce hydroxyl radical from H_2O_2 as well as peroxynitrite in the mitochondria. The mutant enzyme could then catalyze the nitration of mitochondrial proteins such as cyclophilin D and the adenine nucleotide translocator (Martin, 2010). Due to these toxic effects of mutant SOD1 on mitochondria, it has been proposed that the abnormal activity of the mitochondria in ALS may account for the initiation and progression of the disease. However, whether the mitochondrial localization of mutant SOD1 is cause or a consequence of pathology needs to be established.

5. Expression of mutant SOD1 in motor neurons and neighboring cells

A new mechanism integrating the autonomous and non-autonomous induction of motor neuron death in ALS is emerging. In this scenario, the role of motor neurons and surrounding cells in the onset and progression of ALS is temporally determined. Several studies were conducted where mutant SOD1 was selectively expressed *in vivo* either in motor neurons or microglia of chimeric mice, or in culture in embryonic primary or stem cell-based models, allowing the study of the role of individual population of cells in the onset and progression of ALS. The cell-autonomous degeneration of motor neurons expressing mutant SOD1 seems to be more relevant for the onset and early progression of the disease, while microglia, peripheral macrophages, and astrocytes would play a role in the late disease progression.

5.1. Expression of mutant SOD1 in motor neurons

ALS is a motor neuron disease characterized by the gradual and selective loss of both, upper and lower motor neurons. Expression of mutant SOD1 in spinal motor neurons and interneurons of chimeric mice is enough to induce neuronal degeneration (Boillee et al., 2006; Wang et al., 2008). The mice do not develop clinical ALS but the motor neurons expressing mutant SOD1 exhibit pathological and immunohistochemical abnormalities, while motor neurons negative for mutant SOD1 expression do not. These observations indicate that in the chimeric mice the degeneration of motor neurons can be cell-autonomous. The fact that only some of the motor neurons express mutant SOD1 in this model may explain why the animals do not develop the disease (Wang et al., 2008). Indeed, normal motor neurons can prevent or delay the degeneration of mutant SOD1-expressing motor neurons (Clement et al., 2003). In addition, decreased expression of mutant SOD1 in motor neurons has a modest effect on the duration of the disease but significantly delay the onset and early phase of the disease progression (Wang et al., 2008). Similar results were observed in culture, where primary spinal motor

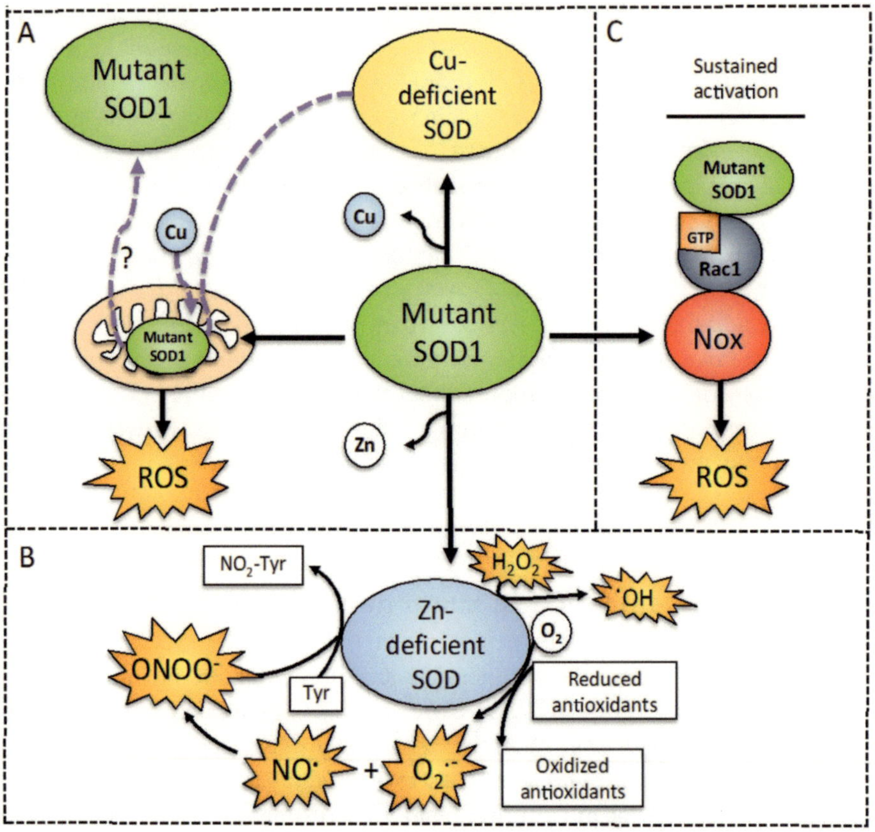

Figure 1. Role of oxidative stress in mutant SOD1 toxic gain-of-function. A. The toxic gain-of-function depends on the redox properties of the enzyme and relies on the copper atom. The mutant SOD1 translocates to mitochondria, while the metal-deficient enzyme may translocate and bind copper in the organelle. B. Zn-deficient SOD1 as catalyst of ROS production and tyrosine nitration. C. Mutant SOD1 regulation of ROS production by Noxs. NO_2-Tyr: nitrotyrosine, HO·: hydroxyl radical, O_2: molecular oxygen, ONOO·: peroxynitrite, NO·: nitric oxide, O2·: superoxide.

neurons as well as embryonic stem cell-derived motor neurons expressing mutant SOD1 showed changes characteristic of neurodegeneration (Di Giorgio et al., 2007; Raoul et al., 2002). Primary embryonic motor neurons from $SOD1^{G93A}$ and $SOD1^{G85R}$ transgenic animals exposed to endogenously produced or exogenously added nitric oxide show an increased susceptibility to cell death in culture (Raoul et al., 2002). Thus, motor neurons expressing mutant SOD1 are susceptible to cell death stimulated by oxidative stress.

5.2. Expression of mutant SOD1 in glial cells

Neighboring cells also seem to play a role in mutant SOD1 toxicity. Normal motor neurons in the context of a mutant SOD1-expressing chimera show signs of neurodegeneration, while non-neuronal cells negative for mutant SOD1 expression delay neuronal degeneration and significantly extend survival of mutant-expressing motor neurons (Clement et al., 2003). In the last few years, a role for microglia and astrocytes in the induction of motor neuron death has become evident.

5.2.1. Role of microglia in the induction of motor neuron death

Activated microglia is found in the spinal cord of SOD1^{G93A} transgenic mice, suggesting that it may play a role in the neurodegeneration of neighboring motor neurons (Beers et al., 2006). Reducing the expression of mutant SOD1 in microglia and peripheral macrophages in chimeric mice leads to a delay in the late progression of ALS but has little effect on the onset and early disease progression (Boillee et al., 2006). Likewise, in the PU.1$^{(-/-)}$/SOD1^{G93A} mice unable to synthesize myeloid cells, the replacement of microglia, monocyte, and macrophage lineages with genotypically identical wild type cells slows disease progression and extends overall survival (Beers et al., 2006), suggesting that non cell-autonomous effects contribute to ALS progression independently of disease onset. Comparable findings were observed in co-culture studies where glial cells expressing mutant-SOD1 had a direct adverse effect on motor neuron survival (Di Giorgio et al., 2007). Microglia expressing G93A-SOD1 is toxic to primary motor neurons *in vitro*. In addition, SOD^{G93A} microglia show an increase in superoxide and nitric oxide production and release respect to wild type microglia. Treatment with lipopolysaccharide further increases SOD^{G93A} microglia activation and induction of motor neuron death (Beers et al., 2006). Hence, mutant SOD1-expressing microglia is activated, is more susceptible to activation, and it is capable of inducing motor neuron death *in vitro* (Beers et al., 2006). Interestingly, PU.1$^{(-/-)}$ mice transplanted with bone marrow from a SOD1^{G93A} donor do not develop clinical or pathological evidence of ALS, suggesting that expression of mutant SOD1 in microglia is not enough to induce motor neuron disease *in vivo* (Beers et al., 2006). The fact that expression of mutant SOD1 in microglia alone does not induce motor neuron degeneration suggests that motor neurons and other glial cells play a role in the pathological process. Indeed, motor neurons expressing mutant SOD1 are more susceptible to cell death induced by exposure to nitric oxide or Fas activation (Raoul et al., 2002).

5.2.2. Role of astrocytes in the induction of motor neuron death

Astrocytes are the most abundant non-neuronal cells in the nervous system. The co-culture of normal primary embryonic or stem cell-derived motor neurons with astrocytes expressing mutant SOD1 result in motor neuron death. The death pathway is triggered by a toxic factor released by the astrocytes (Aebischer et al., 2011; Nagai et al., 2007). A population of phenotypically aberrant astrocytes was recently described in the SOD1^{G93A} mouse model of ALS (Diaz-Amarilla et al., 2011). These astrocytes, referred to as "AbA cells", have an increased proliferative capacity and secrete soluble factors that are 10 times more potent than neonatal SOD1^{G93A} astrocytes for the induction of motor neuron death. AbA cells are present in degenerating spinal cord of SOD^{G93A} rats surrounding affected motor neurons, and their number increases dramatically after disease onset, highlighting the importance of this finding. Interestingly, the levels of interferon-γ (IFNγ) are significantly increased in mutant SOD1-expressing astrocytes, and IFNγ induces motor neuron death (Aebischer et al., 2011), suggesting that this cytokine may be one of the toxic factors mediating induction of cell death (Figure

2). The role of astrocytes in the induction of motor neuron death was recently confirmed in astrocytes generated from post-mortem tissue of familial and sporadic ALS patients, additionally providing an *in vitro* model system for the study of these mechanisms (Haidet-Phillips et al., 2011).

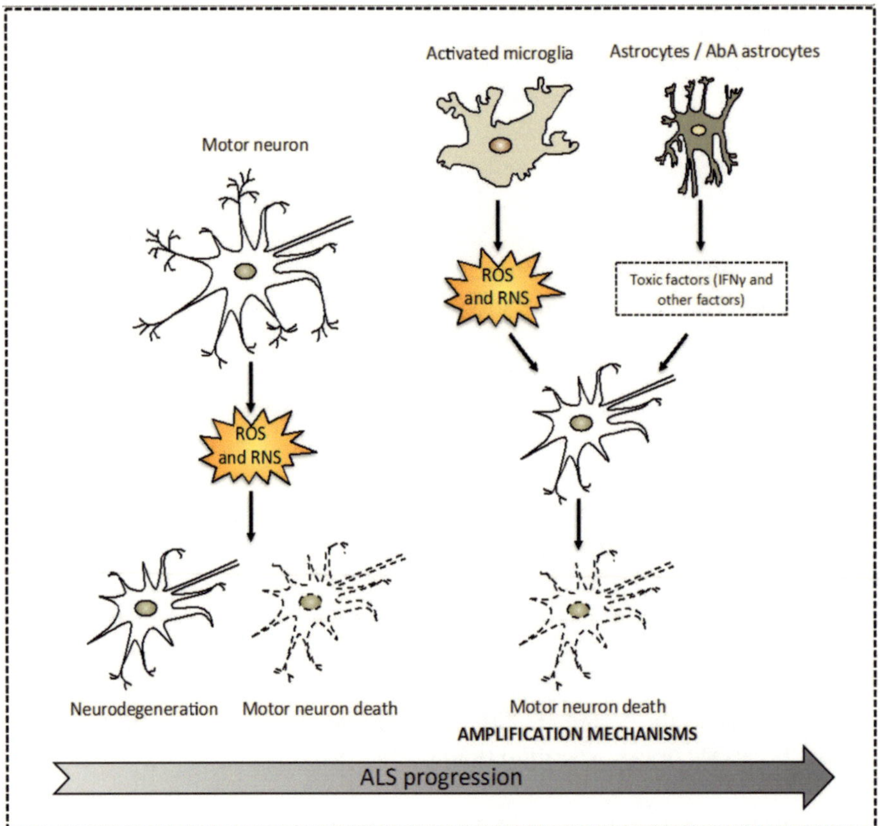

Figure 2. Model for the role of motor neurons and glia in the ROS-mediated ALS progression. Different cell types are affected and play a role at different stages of the disease. During the onset and early disease progression, motor neurons undergo degeneration and cell death by cell-autonomous mechanisms. Later in the disease progression, activated microglia and astrocytes release ROS, RNS, and toxic factors that magnify the injury (cell death amplification mechanisms).

6. Conclusion

In summary, the mechanism of mutant SOD1 toxicity is unknown and highly controversial but there is strong evidence suggesting that the mutant SOD1 toxic gain-of-function is related to an alteration of its redox properties and the induction of oxidative stress. In this scenario, the aberrant chemistry of mutant SOD1 turns the enzyme from antioxidant to pro-oxidant. Zn-

http://dx.doi.org/10.5772/56488

deficient SOD1 reacts with hydrogen peroxide, produces superoxide and peroxynitrite, and is able to catalyze tyrosine nitration, altering the cellular redox balance. In addition, although not related to the redox properties of the enzyme, the interaction of mutant SOD1 with mitochondria and Nox, the two major sources of cellular ROS, further support the involvement of oxidative stress in the toxic gain-of-function. The cell type affected by mutant SOD1 is also controversial. A picture in which several cell types are affected and play a role at different stages of the disease seems to be emerging. In this context, during onset and early stages of the disease SOD1-expressing motor neurons undergo neurodegeneration and cell death by cell-autonomous processes. The activation of microglia and astrocytes may work as an amplification mechanism in the induction of motor neuron death in the late progression of the disease (Figure 2).

Author details

María Clara Franco[1,2], Cassandra N. Dennys[1,2], Fabian H. Rossi[1,2] and Alvaro G. Estévez[1,2]

1 Burnett School of Biomedical Sciences, College of Medicine, University of Central Florida, Orlando, FL, USA

2 Orlando VA Healthcare System, Orlando, USA

References

[1] Aebischer, J, Cassina, P, Otsmane, B, Moumen, A, Seilhean, D, Meininger, V, Barbeito, L, Pettmann, B, & Raoul, C. (2011). IFNgamma triggers a LIGHT-dependent selective death of motoneurons contributing to the non-cell-autonomous effects of mutant SOD1. *Cell death and differentiation* , 18, 754-768.

[2] Barber, S. C, & Shaw, P. J. (2010). Oxidative stress in ALS: key role in motor neuron injury and therapeutic target. *Free radical biology & medicine* , 48, 629-641.

[3] Beal, M. F, Ferrante, L. J, Browne, S. E, Matthews, R. T, Kowall, N. W, & Brown, R. H. (1997). Increased 3-nitrotyrosine in both sporadic and familial amyotrophic lateral sclerosis. *Ann Neurol* , 42, 644-654.

[4] Beckman, J. S, Carson, M, Smith, C. D, & Koppenol, W. H. (1993). ALS, SOD and peroxynitrite. *Nature* 364:584.

[5] Beckman, J. S, Estévez, A. G, Barbeito, L, & Crow, J. P. (2002). CCS knockout mice establish an alternative source of copper for SOD in ALS. *Free Rad. Biol. Med.* , 33, 1433-1435.

[6] Beckman, J. S, Estevez, A. G, Crow, J. P, & Barbeito, L. (2001). Superoxide dismutase and the death of motoneurons in ALS. *Trends in neurosciences* 24:S, 15-20.

[7] Beers, D. R, Henkel, J. S, Xiao, Q, Zhao, W, Wang, J, Yen, A. A, Siklos, L, Mckercher, S. R, & Appel, S. H. (2006). Wild-type microglia extend survival in PU.1 knockout mice with familial amyotrophic lateral sclerosis. *Proceedings of the National Academy of Sciences of the United States of America* , 103, 16021-16026.

[8] Bernard-marissal, N, Moumen, A, Sunyach, C, Pellegrino, C, Dudley, K, Henderson, C. E, Raoul, C, & Pettmann, B. (2012). Reduced Calreticulin Levels Link Endoplasmic Reticulum Stress and Fas-Triggered Cell Death in Motoneurons Vulnerable to ALS. *The Journal of neuroscience : the official journal of the Society for Neuroscience* , 32, 4901-4912.

[9] Boillee, S, Yamanaka, K, Lobsiger, C. S, Copeland, N. G, Jenkins, N. A, Kassiotis, G, Kollias, G, & Cleveland, D. W. (2006). Onset and progression in inherited ALS determined by motor neurons and microglia. *Science* , 312, 1389-1392.

[10] Borchelt, D. R, Lee, M. K, Slunt, H. S, Guarnieri, M, Xu, Z. S, Wong, P. C, Brown, R. H, Jr, D. L, Price, S. S, & Sisodia, D. W. Cleveland. (1994). Superoxide dismutase 1 with mutations linked to familial amyotrophic lateral sclerosis possesses significant activity. *Proceedings of the National Academy of Sciences of the United States of America* , 91, 8292-8296.

[11] Brown, D. I, & Griendling, K. K. (2009). Nox proteins in signal transduction. *Free radical biology & medicine* , 47, 1239-1253.

[12] Bruijn, L. I, & Cleveland, D. W. (1996). Mechanisms of selective motor neuron death in ALS: insights from transgenic mouse models of motor neuron disease. *Neuropathology and applied neurobiology* , 22, 373-387.

[13] Clement, A. M, Nguyen, M. D, Roberts, E. A, Garcia, M. L, Boillee, S, Rule, M, Mcmahon, A. P, Doucette, W, Siwek, D, Ferrante, R. J, Brown, R. H, Jr, J. P, Julien, L. S, & Goldstein, D. W. Cleveland. (2003). Wild-type nonneuronal cells extend survival of SOD1 mutant motor neurons in ALS mice. *Science* , 302, 113-117.

[14] Crow, J. P, Sampson, J. B, Zhuang, Y, Thompson, J. A, & Beckman, J. S. (1997a). Decreased zinc affinity of amyotrophic lateral sclerosis-associated superoxide dismutase mutants leads to enhanced catalysis of tyrosine nitration by peroxynitrite. *J. Neurochem.* , 69, 1936-1944.

[15] Crow, J. P, Strong, M. J, Zhuang, Y, Ye, Y, & Beckman, J. S. (1997b). Superoxide dimutase catalyzes nitration of tyrosines by peroxinitrite in the rod and head domains of neurofilament L. *J Neurochem* , 69, 1945-1953.

[16] Deng, H, Shi, X. , Y, Furukawa, Y, Zhai, H, Fu, R, Liu, E, Gorrie, G. H, Khan, M. S, Hung, W. -Y, Bigio, E. H, & Lukas, T. M.C. Dal Canto, T.V. O'Halloran, and T. Siddique. (2006). Conversion to the amyotrophic lateral sclerosis phenotype is associated

with intermolecular linked insoluble aggregates of SOD1 in mitochondria. *PNAS* , 103, 7142-7147.

[17] Deng, H. X, Hentati, A, Tainer, J. A, Iqbal, Z, Cayabyab, A, Hung, W. Y, Getzoff, E. D, Hu, P, Herzfeldt, B, Roos, R. P, et al. (1993a). Amyotrophic lateral sclerosis and structural defects in Cu,Zn superoxide dismutase. *Science* , 261, 1047-1051.

[18] Deng, H. X, Hentati, A, Tainer, J. A, Iqbal, Z, Cayabyab, A, Hung, W. Y, Getzoff, E. D, Hu, P, Herzfeldt, B, Roos, R. P, Warner, C, Deng, G, Soriano, E, Smyth, C, Parge, H. E, Ahmed, A, Roses, A. D, Hallewell, R. A, Prericak-vance, M. A, & Siddique, T. (1993b). Amyotrophic lateral sclerosis and structural defects in Cu,Zn superoxide dismutase. *Science* , 261, 1047-1051.

[19] Di GiorgioF.P., M.A. Carrasco, M.C. Siao, T. Maniatis, and K. Eggan. (2007). Non-cell autonomous effect of glia on motor neurons in an embryonic stem cell-based ALS model. *Nature neuroscience* , 10, 608-614.

[20] Diaz-amarilla, P, Olivera-bravo, S, Trias, E, Cragnolini, A, Martinez-palma, L, Cassina, P, Beckman, J, & Barbeito, L. (2011). Phenotypically aberrant astrocytes that promote motoneuron damage in a model of inherited amyotrophic lateral sclerosis. *Proceedings of the National Academy of Sciences of the United States of America* , 108, 18126-18131.

[21] Ermilova, I. P, Ermilov, V. B, Levy, M, Ho, E, Pereira, C, & Beckman, J. S. (2005). Protection by dietary zinc in ALS mutant G93A SOD transgenic mice. *Neuroscience letters* , 379, 42-46.

[22] Estévez, A. G, Crow, J. P, Sampson, J. B, Reiter, C, Zhuang, Y. -X, Richardson, G. J, Tarpey, M. M, Barbeito, L, & Beckman, J. S. (1999). Induction of nitric oxide-dependent apoptosis in motor neurons by zinc-deficient superoxide dismutase. *Science* , 286, 2498-2500.

[23] Ferrante, R. J, Shinobu, L. A, Schulz, J. B, Mathews, R. T, Thomas, C. E, Kowall, N. W, Gurney, M. E, & Beal, M. F. (1997). Increased 3-nitrotyrosine and oxidative damage in mice with a human copper/zinc superoxide dismutase mutation. *Ann Neurol* , 42, 326-334.

[24] Franco, M. C, & Estévez, A. G. (2011). Reactive Nitrogen Species in Motor Neuron Apoptosis. In: Amyotrophic Lateral Sclerosis, edited by Martin H. Mauer. InTech, Rijeka, Croatia. pp., 313-334.

[25] Fukada, K, Nagano, S, Satoh, M, Tohyama, C, Nakanishi, T, Shimizu, A, Yanagihara, T, & Sakoda, S. (2001). Stabilization of mutant Cu/Zn superoxide dismutase (SOD1) protein by coexpressed wild SOD1 protein accelerates the disease progression in familial amyotrophic lateral sclerosis mice. *Eur J Neurosci* , 14, 2032-2036.

[26] Furukawa, Y, Fu, R, Deng, H. -X, Siddique, T, & Halloran, T. V. O. (2006). From the Cover: Disulfide cross-linked protein represents a significant fraction of ALS-associ-

ated Cu, Zn-superoxide dismutase aggregates in spinal cords of model mice. *PNAS* , 103, 7148-7153.

[27] Getzoff, E. D, Tainer, J. A, Stempien, M. M, Bell, G. I, & Hallewell, R. A. (1989). Evolution of CuZn superoxide dismutase and the Greek key beta-barrel structural motif. *Proteins* , 5, 322-336.

[28] Gurney, M. E, Pu, H, Chiu, A. Y, Canto, M. C. D, Polchow, C. Y, Alexander, D. D, Caliendo, J, Hentati, A, Kwon, Y. W, Deng, H. -X, Chen, W, Zhai, P, Sufit, R. L, & Siddique, T. (1994). Motor neuron degeneration in mice that express a human Cu,Zn superoxide dismutase mutation. *Science* , 264, 1772-1775.

[29] Haidet-phillips, A. M, Hester, M. E, Miranda, C. J, Meyer, K, Braun, L, Frakes, A, Song, S, Likhite, S, Murtha, M. J, Foust, K. D, Rao, M, Eagle, A, Kammesheidt, A, Christensen, A, Mendell, J. R, Burghes, A. H, & Kaspar, B. K. (2011). Astrocytes from familial and sporadic ALS patients are toxic to motor neurons. *Nature biotechnology* , 29, 824-828.

[30] Harraz, M. M, Marden, J. J, Zhou, W, Zhang, Y, Williams, A, Sharov, V. S, Nelson, K, Luo, M, Paulson, H, Schoneich, C, & Engelhardt, J. F. (2008). SOD1 mutations disrupt redox-sensitive Rac regulation of NADPH oxidase in a familial ALS model. *J Clin Invest* , 118, 659-670.

[31] Higgins, C. M, Jung, C, Ding, H, & Xu, Z. (2002). Mutant Cu, Zn superoxide dismutase that causes motoneuron degeneration is present in mitochondria in the CNS. *The Journal of neuroscience : the official journal of the Society for Neuroscience* 22:RC215.

[32] Ischiropoulos, H, Zhu, L, Chen, J, Tsai, M, Martin, J. C, Smith, C. D, & Beckman, J. S. (1992). Peroxynitrite-mediated tyrosine nitration catalyzed by superoxide dismutase. *Archives of Biochemistry and Biophysics* , 298, 431-437.

[33] Lin, M. T, & Beal, M. F. (2006). Mitochondrial dysfunction and oxidative stress in neurodegenerative diseases. *Nature* , 443, 787-795.

[34] Liu, D, Wen, J, Liu, J, & Li, L. (1999). The roles of free radicals in amyotrophic lateral sclerosis: reactive oxygen species and elevated oxidation of protein, DNA, and membrane phospholipids. *FASEB journal : official publication of the Federation of American Societies for Experimental Biology* , 13, 2318-2328.

[35] Liu, J, Lillo, C, Jonsson, P. A, Velde, C. V, Ward, C. M, Miller, T. M, Subramaniam, J. R, Rothstein, J. D, Marklund, S, Andersen, P. M, Brannstrom, T, Gredal, O, Wong, P. C, Williams, D. S, & Cleveland, D. W. (2004). Toxicity of Familial ALS-Linked SOD1 Mutants from Selective Recruitment to Spinal Mitochondria. *Neuron* , 43, 5-17.

[36] Lyons, T. J, Liu, H, Goto, J. J, Nersissian, A, Roe, J. A, Graden, J. A, Cafe, C, Ellerby, L. M, Bredesen, D. E, Gralla, E. B, & Valentine, J. S. (1996). Mutations in copper-zinc superoxide dismutase that cause amyotrophic lateral sclerosis alter the zinc binding

site and the redox behavior of the protein. *Proceedings of the National Academy of Sciences of the United States of America*, 93, 12240-12244.

[37] Magrane, J, Hervias, I, Henning, M. S, Damiano, M, Kawamata, H, & Manfredi, G. (2009). Mutant SOD1 in neuronal mitochondria causes toxicity and mitochondrial dynamics abnormalities. *Hum Mol Genet*, 18, 4552-4564.

[38] Manfredi, G, & Xu, Z. (2005). Mitochondrial dysfunction and its role in motor neuron degeneration in ALS. *Mitochondrion*, 5, 77-87.

[39] Marden, J. J, Harraz, M. M, Williams, A. J, Nelson, K, Luo, M, Paulson, H, & Engelhardt, J. F. (2007). Redox modifier genes in amyotrophic lateral sclerosis in mice. *J Clin Invest*, 117, 2913-2919.

[40] Marklund, S. L, Andersen, P. M, Forsgren, L, Nilsson, P, Ohlsson, P. I, Wikander, G, & Oberg, A. (1997). Normal binding and reactivity of copper in mutant superoxide dimutase isolated from amyotrophic lateral sclerosis patients. *J Neurochem*, 69, 675-681.

[41] Martin, L. J. (2010). The mitochondrial permeability transition pore: a molecular target for amyotrophic lateral sclerosis therapy. *Biochimica et biophysica acta*, 1802, 186-197.

[42] Mattiazzi, M, Aurelio, M. D, Gajewski, C. D, Martushova, K, Kiaei, M, Beal, M. F, & Manfredi, G. (2002). Mutated human SOD1 causes dysfunction of oxidative phosphorylation in mitochondria of transgenic mice. *The Journal of biological chemistry*, 277, 29626-29633.

[43] Mccord, J. M, & Fridovich, I. (1969). Superoxide dismutase. An enzymic function for erythrocuprein (hemocuprein). *The Journal of biological chemistry*, 244, 6049-6055.

[44] Nagai, M, Re, D. B, Nagata, T, Chalazonitis, A, Jessell, T. M, Wichterle, H, & Przedborski, S. (2007). Astrocytes expressing ALS-linked mutated SOD1 release factors selectively toxic to motor neurons. *Nature neuroscience*, 10, 615-622.

[45] Nauser, T, & Koppenol, W. H. (2002). The rate constant of the reaction of superoxide with nitrogen monoxide: Approaching the diffusion limit. *J Phys Chem A*, 106, 4084-4086.

[46] Okado-matsumoto, A, & Fridovich, I. (2002). Amyotrophic lateral sclerosis: a proposed mechanism. *Proceedings of the National Academy of Sciences of the United States of America*, 99, 9010-9014.

[47] Panov, A, Kubalik, N, Zinchenko, N, Hemendinger, R, Dikalov, S, & Bonkovsky, H. L. (2011). Respiration and ROS production in brain and spinal cord mitochondria of transgenic rats with mutant G93a Cu/Zn-superoxide dismutase gene. *Neurobiol Dis*, 44, 53-62.

[48] Pasinelli, P, Belford, M. E, Lennon, N, Bacskai, B. J, Hyman, B. T, Trotti, D, & Brown, R. H. Jr. (2004). Amyotrophic lateral sclerosis-associated SOD1 mutant proteins bind and aggregate with Bcl-2 in spinal cord mitochondria. *Neuron* , 43, 19-30.

[49] Pasinelli, P, Borchelt, D. R, Houseweart, M. K, & Cleveland, D. W. and R.H. Brown Jr. (1998). Caspase-1 is activated in neural cells and tissue with amyotrophic lateral sclerosis-associated mutations in copper-zinc superoxide dismutase. *Proc Natl Acad Sci USA* , 95, 15763-15768.

[50] Perry, J. J, Shin, D. S, Getzoff, E. D, & Tainer, J. A. (2010). The structural biochemistry of the superoxide dismutases. *Biochimica et biophysica acta* , 1804, 245-262.

[51] Prudencio, M, Durazo, A, Whitelegge, J. P, & Borchelt, D. R. (2009). Modulation of Mutant Superoxide Dismutase 1 Aggregation by Co-Expression of Wild-Type Enzyme. *J Neurochem* , 108, 1009-1018.

[52] Prudencio, M, Lelie, H, Brown, H. H, Whitelegge, J. P, Valentine, J. S, & Borchelt, D. R. (2012). A novel variant of human superoxide dismutase 1 harboring amyotrophic lateral sclerosis-associated and experimental mutations in metal-binding residues and free cysteines lacks toxicity in vivo. *Journal of neurochemistry* , 121, 475-485.

[53] Raoul, C, Estévez, A. G, Nishimune, H, Cleveland, D. W, Delapeyrière, O, Henderson, C. E, Haase, G, & Pettmann, B. (2002). Motoneuron death triggered by a specific pathway downstream of Fas: potentiation by ALS-linked SOD1 mutations. *Neuron* , 35, 1067-1083.

[54] Reaume, A. G, Elliott, J. L, Hoffman, E. K, Kowall, N. W, Ferrante, R. J, Siwek, D. F, Wilcox, H. M, Flood, D. G, Beal, M. F, Brown, R. H, Jr, R. W, & Scott, W. D. Snider. (1996). Motor neurons in Cu/Zn superoxide dismutase-deficient mice develop normally but exhibit enhanced cell death after axonal injury. *Nature genetics* , 13, 43-47.

[55] Rhoads, T. W, Lopez, N. I, Zollinger, D. R, Morre, J. T, Arbogast, B. L, Maier, C. S, Denoyer, L, & Beckman, J. S. (2011). Measuring copper and zinc superoxide dismutase from spinal cord tissue using electrospray mass spectrometry. *Analytical biochemistry* , 415, 52-58.

[56] Roberts, B. R, Tainer, J. A, Getzoff, E. D, Malencik, D. A, Anderson, S. R, Bomben, V. C, Meyers, K. R, Karplus, P. A, & Beckman, J. S. (2007). Structural characterization of zinc-deficient human superoxide dismutase and implications for ALS. *Journal of molecular biology* , 373, 877-890.

[57] Rosen, D. R, Siddique, T, Patterson, D, Figlewicz, D. A, Sapp, P, Hentati, A, Donaldson, D, Goto, J, Regan, J. P. O, Deng, H. -X, Rahmani, Z, Krizus, A, Mckenna-yasek, D, Cayabyab, A, Gaston, S. M, Berger, R, Tanszi, R. E, Halperin, J. J, Herzfeldt, B, Bergh, R. V. d, Hung, W. -Y, Bird, T, Deng, G, Mulder, D. W, Smyth, C, Lang, N. G, Soriana, E, Pericak-vance, M. A, Haines, J, Rouleau, G. A, Gusella, J. S, Horvitz, H. R, & Brown, R. H. J. (1993). Mutations in Cu/Zn superoxide dimutase gene are associated with familial amyotrophic lateral sclerosis. *Nature* , 362, 59-62.

[58] Rothstein, J. D, Patel, S, Regan, M. R, Haenggeli, C, Huang, Y. H, Bergles, D. E, Jin, L, Dykes, M, Hoberg, S, Vidensky, D. S, Chung, S. V, Toan, L. I, Bruijn, Z. Z, & Su, P. Gupta, and P.B. Fisher. (2005). Beta-lactam antibiotics offer neuroprotection by increasing glutamate transporter expression. *Nature* , 433, 73-77.

[59] Sahawneh, M. A, Ricart, K. C, Roberts, B. R, Bomben, V. C, Basso, M, Ye, Y, Sahawneh, J, Franco, M. C, Beckman, J. S, & Estevez, A. G. (2010). Cu,Zn superoxide dismutase (SOD) increases toxicity of mutant and Zn-deficient superoxide dismutase by enhancing protein stability. *The Journal of biological chemistry* , 285, 33885-33897.

[60] Subramaniam, J. R, Lyons, W. E, Liu, J, Bartnikas, T. B, Rothstein, J, Price, D. L, Cleveland, D. W, Gitlin, J. D, & Wong, P. C. (2002). Mutant SOD1 causes motor neuron disease independent of copper chaperone-mediated copper loading. *Nature Neurosci* , 5, 301-307.

[61] Tanaka, K, Watase, K, Manabe, T, Yamada, K, Watanabe, M, Takahashi, K, Iwama, H, Nishikawa, T, Ichihara, N, Kikuchi, T, Okuyama, S, Kawashima, N, Hori, S, Takimoto, M, & Wada, K. (1997). Epilepsy and exacerbation of brain injury in mice lacking the glutamate transporter GLT-1. *Science* , 276, 1699-1702.

[62] Trotti, D, Rolfs, A, Danbolt, N. C, Brown, R. H. J, & Hediger, M. A. (1999). SOD 1 mutants linked to amyotrophic lateral sclerosis selectivity inactivate a glial glutamate transporter. *Nature Neurosci* , 2, 427-433.

[63] Trotti, D, Rossi, D, Gjesdal, O, Levy, L. M, Racagni, G, Danbolt, N. C, & Volterra, A. (1996). Peroxynitrite inhibits glutamate transporter subtypes. *J Biol. Chem.* , 271, 5976-5979.

[64] Trumbull, K. A, & Beckman, J. S. (2009). A role for copper in the toxicity of zinc-deficient superoxide dismutase to motor neurons in amyotrophic lateral sclerosis. *Antioxidants & redox signaling* , 11, 1627-1639.

[65] Vijayvergiya, C, Beal, M. F, Buck, J, & Manfredi, G. (2005). Mutant superoxide dismutase 1 forms aggregates in the brain mitochondrial matrix of amyotrophic lateral sclerosis mice. *The Journal of neuroscience : the official journal of the Society for Neuroscience* , 25, 2463-2470.

[66] Wang, H, Ying, Z, & Wang, G. (2012). Ataxin-3 Regulates Aggresome Formation of Copper-Zinc Superoxide Dismutase (SOD1) by Editing K63-linked Polyubiquitin Chains. *The Journal of biological chemistry* , 287, 28576-28585.

[67] Wang, J. J, Slunt, H. H, Gonzales, V. V, Fromholt, D. D, Coonfield, M. M, Copeland, N. G. N. G, Jenkins, N. A. N. A, & Borchelt, D. R. D. R. (2003). Copper-binding-site-null SOD1 causes ALS in transgenic mice: aggregates of non-native SOD1 delineate a common feature. *Human molecular genetics* 12:2753.

[68] Wang, L, Deng, H. X, Grisotti, G, Zhai, H, Siddique, T, & Roos, R. P. (2009). Wild-type SOD1 overexpression accelerates disease onset of a G85R SOD1 mouse. *Hum Mol Genet* , 18, 1642-1651.

[69] Wang, L, Sharma, K, Deng, H. X, Siddique, T, Grisotti, G, Liu, E, & Roos, R. P. (2008). Restricted expression of mutant SOD1 in spinal motor neurons and interneurons induces motor neuron pathology. *Neurobiol Dis* , 29, 400-408.

[70] Watanabe, M, Dykes-hoberg, M, Culotta, V. C, Price, D. L, Wong, P. C, & Rothstein, J. D. (2001). Histological evidence of protein aggregation in mutant SOD1 transgenic mice and in amyotrophic lateral sclerosis neural tissues. *Neurobiol Dis* , 8, 933-941.

[71] Watanabe, S, Nagano, S, Duce, J, Kiaei, M, Li, Q. -X, Tucker, S. M, Tiwari, A, Brown, J. R. H, Beal, M. F, Hayward, L. J, Culotta, V. C, Yoshihara, S, Sakoda, S, & Bush, A. I. (2007). Increased affinity for copper mediated by cysteine 111 in forms of mutant superoxide dismutase 1 linked to amyotrophic lateral sclerosis. *Free Radical Biology and Medicine* , 42, 1534-1542.

[72] Wiedau-pazos, M, Gato, J. J, Rabizadeh, S, Gralla, E. B, Roe, B, Lee, C. K, Valentine, J. S, & Bredesen, D. E. (1996). Alterd reactivity of superoxide dismutase in familial amyotrophic lateral sclerosis. *Science* , 271, 515-518.

[73] Witan, H, Gorlovoy, P, Kaya, A. M, Koziollek-drechsler, I, Neumann, H, Behl, C, & Clement, A. M. (2009). Wild-type Cu/Zn superoxide dismutase (SOD1) does not facilitate, but impedes the formation of protein aggregates of amyotrophic lateral sclerosis causing mutant SOD1. *Neurobiol Dis* , 36, 331-342.

[74] Yim, M. B, Chock, P. B, & Stadtman, E. R. (1990). Copper, zinc superoxide dismutase catalyzes hydroxyl radical production from hydrogen peroxide. *Proceedings of the National Academy of Sciences of the United States of America* , 87, 5006-5010.

[75] Yim, M. B, Kang, J. H, Yim, H. S, Kwak, H. S, Chock, P. B, & Stadtman, E. R. function of an amyotrophic lateral sclerosis-associated Cu,Zn-superoxide dismutase mutant: An enhancement of free radical formation due to a decrease in Km for hydrogen peroxide. *Proceedings of the National Academy of Sciences of the United States of America* , 93, 5709-5714.

Chapter 6

The Use of Human Samples to Study Familial and Sporadic Amyotrophic Lateral Sclerosis: New Frontiers and Challenges

Laura Ferraiuolo, Kathrin Meyer and Brian Kaspar

Additional information is available at the end of the chapter

http://dx.doi.org/10.5772/56487

1. Introduction

Amyotrophic lateral sclerosis (ALS) is a fatal neurodegenerative disease characterized by death of upper and lower motor neurons, which results in muscle wasting and death from respiratory failure typically within 2-5 years from diagnosis.

ALS is a multifactorial disease [1] where different cell types, i.e. astrocytes, microglia and oligodendrocytes, contribute to the pathologic mechanism [2, 3]. For a long time ALS was thought to be a pure motor neuron disease, however, thorough pathological investigations and recent findings linking mutations in transactive response DNA-binding protein gene (TARDBP) to familial and sporadic cases of ALS have relocated this disease within a spectrum of neurological disorders, ranging from pure motor neuron disease to frontotemporal dementia [4, 5].

Since 1993, when the first mutation in the Cu/Zn superoxide dismutase (SOD1) enzyme was linked to familial forms of ALS, researchers have tried to unravel the mechanisms underlying this disease by interrogating *in vivo* and *in vitro* models overexpressing human SOD1. Although these models have highly contributed to understanding the pathogenic mechanisms involved in motor neuron degeneration, they only account for less than 2% of all cases. Hence, the ALS field is still lacking effective therapies and a deep understanding of the etiology of the sporadic disease.

For 15 years the SOD1 models have been the only available, until, in 2008, mutations in TARDBP were found to be responsible for familial and sporadic forms of ALS [6, 7]. This led to the discovery that mutations in a second RNA/DNA-binding protein called fused in sarcoma (FUS) or translocated in liposarcoma (TLS) were also cause of the disease [8, 9]. More recently, the field of ALS has seen a breakthrough with the association of GGGGCC-hexanucleotide repeat expansion in chromosome 9 open reading frame 72 (C9ORF72) to 35-40% of familial cases and 5-7% of sporadic cases [10-12].

In the same years, from 2007 to present, *in vitro* technologies to model neurological disorders have also undergone an impressive development.

With the discovery that adult human fibroblasts could be reprogrammed to induced pluripotent stem (iPS) cells with the use of selected transcription factors [13], the field of ALS saw the opportunity to finally model not only the familial, but especially the sporadic disease *in vitro*. In fact, in 2008, the first human iPS-derived motor neurons from patients were cultured in a petri dish [14]. Since then, several iPS lines have been produced from patients and healthy individuals and they have been made commercially available (http://www.coriell.org/stem-cells).

Moreover, in 2011, neural progenitors cells (NPCs) were isolated from post-mortem spinal cord samples of ALS patients and successfully cultured and differentiated into motor neurons, astrocytes and oligodendrocytes *in vitro* [15]. This technology provided for the first time the possibility to model all forms of ALS *in vitro* without inducing major epigenetic alterations in the cells used.

In this chapter we will give an overview of how human tissues have been used so far, what discoveries they have led to since 2007, and how the recent advances in technology combined with the recent genetic discoveries, have tremendously widened the horizon of ALS research.

2. Latest genetic discoveries

Even though Jean-Martin Charcot initially described ALS in 1869, it took more than a century until the first disease-causing gene – the Cu/Zn superoxide dismutase (SOD1) - was identified [16]. Mutations in this gene account for approximately 10-20% of the familial ALS (FALS) cases (Anderson 2006) and about 1% of the sporadic (SALS). Up to now, mutations in 21 different genes have been linked to ALS, although some of them present with atypical disease characteristics [17]. FALS is usually inherited in an autosomal-dominant manner, but in rarer cases, it appears also recessive or X-linked. Along with the rising number of genes and mutations involved, the differentiation between sporadic and familial ALS becomes increasingly difficult and depends on the definition applied. With the most stringent classification, a patient is considered to suffer from the familial form if he/she has at least one first- or second-degree relative affected by ALS [18]. However, other studies define FALS when at least one relative is affected by motor neuron disease, i.e. ALS, primary lateral sclerosis (PLS) or progressive muscular atrophy (PMA) [19]. In addition, several indications exist that mutations leading to ALS are also involved in the development of other neurodegenerative diseases such as different types of dementia or Parkinsons disease. This further broadens the range of possible familial linkage [19]. Missing family history data and the existence of mutations with incomplete penetrance, thus masking inherited genetic forms of the disease as sporadic, further contribute to complicate the discrimination between FALS and SALS.

In the last 20 years, most efforts were concentrated on studying the effect of SOD1 mutations, resulting in the generation of over 30 different animal models including *Drosophila, C. elegans, D. rerio, mice, rats* and *dogs* [20]. In most cases, expression of human mutant SOD1 in the animal models led to astrogliosis, inflammation and degeneration of motor neurons in a similar manner as observed in patients.

The generated SOD1 animal models highly contributed to the understanding of SOD1 functions in the central nervous system (CNS) leading to the development of potential therapeutic strategies targeting these pathways. Unfortunately, most of the therapeutics that show an effect in rodent models, fail in human clinical trials. Overall, SOD1 only accounts for about 2% of all ALS cases, therefore the question arose how applicable the findings from these models really are for other familial cases and especially for the huge majority of sporadic ALS cases.

In 2006, the transactive response DNA-binding protein (TDP-43) was identified as a major component of intraneuronal inclusions, a form of protein aggregates representing a hallmark of SALS and non-SOD1-FALS cases [21]. Soon after, researchers found ALS causing mutations in this gene [6, 7]. One year later, mutations in a second RNA/DNA-binding protein called fused in sarcoma (FUS) or translocated in liposarcoma (TLS) were published [8, 9]. While TDP-43 mutations account for 4% of FALS, FUS mutations are less frequent and account for approximately 1-2% [22]. The discovery of the involvement of these two genes can be considered a milestone in ALS research, not necessarily because of the mutation frequency, but rather because of the wide presence of these proteins in the aggregates characterizing tissues from sporadic ALS cases. Mutations in TDP-43 and FUS can also be found in some forms of frontotemporal dementia (FTD), while aggregates of the non-mutated protein seem to be an even more common feature for neurodegenerative diseases including Huntington's, Alzheimer's and Parkinson's [23]. As both proteins are involved in RNA metabolism, a common disease mechanism underlying sporadic and familial forms of ALS might exist. This link rises hope that a common therapeutic strategy could be developed benefitting a broad patient population.

The TARDBP gene encoding TDP-43 lies on chromosome 1p36.2. The TDP-43 protein consists of 414 amino acids and is highly conserved among species [7]. The expression pattern is almost ubiquitous with high levels during development. Loss of TDP-43 is detrimental in rodents as knockouts in mice are lethal in both cases, either when performed during embryonic stages, or also as conditional knockouts in the adult mouse [24-26]. As mentioned above, the protein is involved in RNA metabolism, but therein, various functions including regulation of alternative splicing, transcription, miRNA levels, RNA stabilization, as well as formation of stress and RNA granules have been described. TDP-43 seems to preferentially bind RNAs with unusually long introns and/or such that are involved in neuronal function like synaptic activity and neuronal development. Some of these RNAs encode proteins which have previously been shown to be involved in neurodegenerative diseases [27]. Although TDP-43 depletion affects the expression and splicing of many different RNAs in the CNS, the vast majority of the more than 40 ALS causing mutations identified so far, lie within the C-terminal domain encoding a glycine rich stretch that is important for protein-protein interaction. While in healthy individuals TDP-43 is mainly localized in the nucleus, it gets mislocalized and trapped in cytoplasmic aggregates in ALS patients, leading to reduced levels in the nucleus [22]. The trapped TDP-43 seems to be heavily modified displaying ubiquitination, phosphorylation and cleavage and in some cases, misfolding. The exact meaning of TDP-43 mislocalization in ALS and other neurodegenerative diseases remains to be elucidated, as so far, it is unclear whether the inclusions actively participate in the disease development and progression or rather represent a mere indicator of other dysregulated cellular mechanisms. The observed changes in RNA regulation could arise from both, the mislocalization itself, leading to a reduced abundance in the nucleus, or function altering mutations or modifications of the protein. In addition, it was reported that certain mutations increase the stability of the protein and therefore its overall abundance in the cell [28], which might lead to the visible accumulations and alterations in RNA metabolism.

Until now, a plethora of different animal models including Drosophila, mouse and rats has been generated. Unfortunately at present, TDP-43 models have originated controversial results. In fact, overexpressing wild type TDP-43 in the CNS appears to be toxic by itself, while the effects of the mutant protein vary broadly ranging from no symptoms to severe neurodegeneration in different regions of the mouse brain [20]. Mostly, it is unclear whether the toxicity is due to the mutation or the simple presence of the transgene.

The gene encoding FUS lies on chromosome 16 in a region that was already linked to familial ALS before the first mutations were identified. After the discovery of TDP-43 mutations, the focus on genes encoding RNA/DNA-binding proteins increased leading to the fast discovery of mutations in FALS patients by two independent groups [8, 9]. Similar to TDP-43, more than 40 different FUS mutations have been identified in FALS patients or patients suffering from FTD. The FUS protein consists of 526 amino acids and like TDP-43, it is widely expressed amongst different tissues. Knockout of FUS in different mouse strains led to differing results, indicating that the genetic background of the used mouse strain plays an important role as disease modifier. In the inbred strains (C57BL/6 and 129), the knockout causes death at birth, whereas outbred strains survive until adulthood. In all cases, FUS depletion seems not to induce classical neurodegeneration as a primary effect. Interestingly, unlike TDP-43, the ALS related mutations in the FUS gene do not cluster in the glycine-rich region of the protein, but rather at the very end of the highly conserved C-terminus of the protein that contains the nuclear localization signal [22]. FUS is also mainly localized in the nucleus of cells in healthy individuals, but its mislocalization and aggregation in cytoplasmic granules in ALS patients leads to a less severe reduction in the nucleus than TDP-43 [22]. Up to now, only few binding partners of FUS (RNA or proteins) are known, making it further challenging to speculate about the function of the protein, which remains mostly unknown. In general, FUS is thought to be involved in regulation of gene expression, transcription, RNA splicing, RNA transport, translation, miRNA processing as well as DNA damage repair [29]. Interestingly, TDP-43 and FUS might directly interact with each other as they were detected in the same complex in cultured cells [28, 30]. Even though further data from patients and animal models are needed to confirm this finding, it is an interesting observation, as TDP-43 does not seem to be mislocalized in ALS cases that have accumulation of FUS containing aggregates in the cytoplasm [28].

Following TDP-43 and FUS, the thorough analysis of the cytoplasmic aggregates found in ALS patients led to the identification of additional common components such as optineurin and ubiquilin-2. Several of these proteins were afterwards identified to be mutated in a smaller portion of ALS patients as well [31].

In 2011, the identification of a new ALS gene harboring a different type of mutation was achieved. The association of the chromosomal locus 9p21.2 with ALS and FTD had already been described in 2006 [32]. The improvement of sequencing techniques and continuous research finally led to the identification of the disease causing gene: C9ORF72. While the function of this widely expressed protein is unknown, the type of mutation differs from other ALS related genes. It consists of a massive GGGGCC-hexanucleotide repeat expansion in intron 1 between two non-coding exons. Whereas healthy individuals carry up to about 23 repeats, affected patients have at least 30, but in some cases, many hundred copies of it [11, 12].

The first reports about the mutation in this gene came from two independent studies analyzing relatively small cohorts respectively of sporadic and familial ALS cases in Finland and Europe and ALS/FTD cases in the USA. Both studies started off with re-sequencing of the 9p21.2 locus from well defined families, in which the linkage of the disease to this chromosome 9 location had been previously demonstrated [11, 12]. After the detection of the repeat, the analyses were expanded to larger cohorts.

The most striking discovery of these studies is the high frequency of mutations in this gene in the analysed cohorts. Between 9 and 20% of American patients suffering from familial FTD and up to 38% of familial ALS cases from different European countries resulted positive for the new mutation. For the sporadic cases, the percentage lies around 7% for the American FTD patient population and 21% of sporadic ALS patients in the genetically homogenous Finnish population. With these initially published percentages, C9ORF72 mutations appeared to be the so far most frequent known cause of ALS and FTD. However, the cohorts were recruited through only few institutions and were rather small. Recently, a cross-sectional study including more patients from various different countries and with differing genetic background has been published. In this study, a total of 588 familial ALS cases and 403 familial FTD cases were screened for the mutation. For FALS, 37.6% of patients were identified to carry the pathological repeat, for FTD the percentage was 25.1% [33]. Although further studies are needed to confirm these findings, they are truly exciting, considering the fact that together with SOD1, which accounts for approximately 10-20% of FALS, almost 50% of the familial disease cases can now be explained by mutations in one of these two genes.

The observation that C9ORF72 mutations not only cause ALS, but also FTD and clinically mixed syndromes such as ALS-FTD, is in line with the clinical spectrum caused by TDP-43 and FUS mutations as well as wild type aggregations in both diseases. This further strengthens the indications that these two clinically distinct syndromes share a common pathogenic link [19, 34].

Interestingly, the pathological features of C9ORF72 related ALS seem very unusual and distinct up to the point that the mutation itself can actually be predicted from the observed pathology [35]. While the spinal cord shows the typical neuronal loss and TDP-43 positive cytoplasmic inclusions, other regions of the brain seem to accumulate aggregates that are widely devoid of TDP-43 and contain p62.

The mechanism through which this expansion repeat conveys toxicity to neurons still has to be elucidated. Two major hypotheses can be distinguished: 1) The expansion repeat alters or abolishes expression of all or certain C9ORF72 protein isoforms leading to reduced protein levels and a loss of functionality, 2) the expanded repeat itself conveys toxicity by sequestration of other RNA binding proteins and aggregate formation inside the nucleus, thus inhibiting proper functionality of the bound proteins. To date, it is not known which hypothesis applies in the case of C9ORF72 expansions, but the experience from various other toxic expansion repeat diseases like Huntington's disease are favoring the second. While Renton et. al demonstrate the presence of aggregates in the nucleus of fibroblasts from affected patients, the results from the second study by DeJesus et al are less clear concerning accumulation of RNA granules. The latter study also lies more emphasis on a change in the expression levels of different C9ORF72 mRNA isoforms, which would support the first hypothesis rather than the second. Currently, the tools for a detailed analysis of protein expression and function are still lacking, but considering the importance of the mutation, huge efforts are put into the development of better antibodies, probes and assays.

Overall, the finding that mutations in TDP43, FUS and C9ORF72 might cause ALS by altering the normal interaction of these proteins with RNA or might cause a toxic gain of function leading to unexpected protein-RNA interaction opens new avenues for ALS research. These recent genetic discoveries have shifted the attention to cellular processes, i.e. RNA metabolism, transport and processing, that were not under investigation in the SOD1 models. These pathways might represent a common mechanism for different forms of ALS, as well as creating a link between ALS and a wider spectrum of neurodegenerative conditions.

3. The role of wild type SOD1 in ALS

In 1993 for the first time mutations in SOD1 were identified as cause of familial ALS and were found to be responsible for about 20% of familial cases [16]. Since that discovery nearly twenty years ago, more than 160 mutations in SOD1 have been identified (http://alsod.iop.kcl.ac.uk/) and cellular and animal models of the disease carrying different forms of mutant SOD1 have been generated [36, 37]. Experiments using animal models revealed that the toxicity of mutant SOD1 is not related to a loss of function of the enzyme [38], but

http://dx.doi.org/10.5772/56487

rather a gain of toxic function. In the past twenty years different forms of mutant SOD1 have been characterized for their biochemical properties, however no common characteristics between mutations have been found. In fact, different mutations seem to cause different changes in enzymatic function or no change at all [39-41], leading to the conclusion that SOD1 dismutase activity is not responsible for protein toxicity. Although the nature of the toxic function gained by mutant SOD1 is still obscure, there is clear evidence that the mutant enzyme undergoes conformational changes leading to its misfolding and subsequent aggregation [41, 42]. SOD1 aggregates are, in fact, one of the histological hallmarks of SOD1-related FALS, as well as sporadic cases carrying SOD1 mutations.

Although SOD1 mutations are responsible for less than 2% of ALS cases and this disease is mainly of sporadic origin, sporadic and familial cases are clinically undistinguishable. Moreover, with the exception of patients carrying C9ORF72 mutation, which seem to define a specific clinical subgroup [35], other genetic mutations do not determine different clinical characteristics. This observation has led to the conclusion that familial and sporadic ALS must share common pathogenic mechanisms [1]. Consequently, in recent years, efforts have been made in understanding whether the genes causing familial ALS can be responsible or can be involved in the pathophysiology of sporadic cases. Recently, strong evidence has been gathered suggesting that SOD1 might play a crucial role also in SALS.

Wild-type human SOD1 is a 32KDa homodimer known to be one of the most stable proteins with a melting temperature around 90°C. However, its stability is highly dependent upon post-translational processes including binding of copper and zinc ions and the formation of an intramolecular disulfide bond. Impairment or retardation of these post-translational processes can disrupt SOD1 stability, causing the formation of misfolded structures and aggregates. Indeed, in 2007, it was shown that oxidised wild-type SOD1 could acquire *in vitro* aberrant properties leading to association with poly-ubiquitin, Hsp70 and chromogranin B, similarly to the mutant enzyme [43]. The same year, another group used covalent chemical modification to show that spinal cord samples from both familial and sporadic ALS cases displayed a form of SOD1 that was absent in non-neurological controls as well as in spinal cord samples from patients affected by other neurodegenerative disorders [44]. Recently, Guareschi et al [45] managed to immunoprecipitate SOD1 from sporadic and familial ALS patients' lymphoblasts and then analysed the presence of oxidized carbonyl groups. A form of over-oxidized wild-type SOD1 was indeed found in a subset of SALS patients. This post-translationally modified form of the wild-type enzyme recapitulates some of the toxic properties attributed to mutant SOD1, i.e. the ability to cause mitochondrial damage through interaction with Bcl-2 [45]. Altogether, these findings supported the hypothesis that SOD1 could be a link between familial and sporadic ALS.

On another front, the use of the SOD1 mouse model also provided important clues as to whether normal SOD1 can play a role in the disease. Surprisingly, overexpression of wild-type human SOD1 accelerated disease onset in several transgenic mouse models of ALS [46, 47], supporting the involvement of wild type SOD1 in the disease mechanism. However, these results have to be interpreted with caution, as they might derive by the toxicity of transgene accumulation rather than a specific SOD1-related mechanism.

In order to determine whether *in vivo* wild-type SOD1 can undergo misfolding and can be detected without altering the original sample, recent studies have focused on the production and investigation of new antibodies able to distinguish mutant/misfolded/monomeric SOD1 as opposed to its wild-type form. Although some of these antibodies have been tested only on limited samples and their ability to discriminate between aberrant conformations of SOD1 is debatable, their use has led to potentially interesting findings. One of the first antibodies produced to detect abnormalities in SOD1 post-translational processing was the SOD1-exposed dimer interface (SEDI). This antibody was prepared with the peptide at the dimer interface of SOD1. When SOD1 is folded as a homodimer in its active state, this site is inaccessible, while it is exposed upon monomerization [48]. This antibody successfully stained inclusions in motor neurons from SALS samples, however it did not detect positive inclusions in SALS spinal cords where no SOD1 mutations were detected [49]. Similarly, an antibody developed against the region Leu^{42}-His^{48}, which specifically recognizes SOD1 in which the beta barrel is unfolded, failed to detect misfolded SOD1 in SALS spinal cord samples, but succeeded in recognizing aggregates in the FALS samples [50]. Despite these results, it could not be concluded that wild-type SOD1 does not contribute to the pathogenic mechanisms occurring in SALS. Indeed, Forsberg et al. have produced a series of polyclonal antibodies against several SOD1 peptides that react with the denaturated enzyme, but not with the wild-type form. Using these antibodies, small inclusions were detected in the motor neurons of SALS patients [51] as well as in the nuclei of astrocytes, microglia and oligodendrocytes [52]. These studies supported the hypothesis that wild-type SOD1, although not involved in the formation of Lewy body-like inclusions in SALS, is likely to undergo conformational changes, thus contributing to the pathologic mechanism.

Another antibody that has been used to detect misfolded SOD1 is C4F6. This peptide was raised against metal depleted (apo) SOD1 with G93A mutation [53]. Although this antibody was raised against a specific mutant form of SOD1, it successfully recognised skein-like inclusions in FALS spinal cord samples, as well as inclusions in SALS [54].

Recently, a monoclonal antibody, called 3H1, was used to detect misfolded SOD1 in a subset of SALS cases displaying TDP-43/FUS-positive inclusions. This antibody recognizes a peptide corresponding to a structurally disrupted SOD1 electrostatic loop, detectable only when the protein is misfolded. Spinal cord immunocytochemistry showed that, in some SALS samples, TDP-43/FUS-positive inclusions were also positive for 3H1 antibody, suggesting that the pathologic mechanisms involved in ALS might trigger SOD1 misfolding, thus triggering toxic pathways common to both sporadic and familial ALS [55].

Besides the efforts to generate antibodies able to detect misfolded SOD1, no consensus has been reached on which antibodies, if any, can reliably and consistently detect the different forms of misfolded SOD1. Other studies have, therefore, used a different approach, trying to understand whether normal SOD1 shares common characteristics with the mutant form of the enzyme. Recently, a novel rare mutation in SOD1 (L117V) was identified in two Syrian ALS families [39]. Unusually, the disease showed uncommon low penetrance and slow progression. Biochemical analysis of L117V SOD1 showed that its properties were indistinguishable from the wild-type form and yet causing the disease. This study highlights that normal SOD1 is in the range of protein stability that can cause disease and suggests that mutant forms of SOD1 with high stability might be related to low penetrance and be therefore categorized as sporadic forms of ALS. The authors suggest that, similarly, other complex genetic, environmental and lifestyle factors can influence the stability of normal SOD1 causing its misfolding in SALS cases. However, this does not exclude that the toxicity related to L117V mutation could derive by the interaction with other proteins and not by its stability.

The importance of finding common pathways or players between sporadic and familial ALS is crucial for therapeutic approaches. One recent study explored this possibility [15]. The authors assessed the toxicity of astrocytes derived from neural progenitors isolated from the spinal cord of sporadic and familial ALS patients. This study showed for the first time that astrocytes from sporadic cases of disease are as toxic to motor neurons as astrocytes carrying mutations in SOD1. As expected, the shRNA mediated reduction of mutated SOD1 led to a complete rescue of motor neurons in this co-culture system. Of particular interest however, was the finding that even the knock down of wild type SOD1 in astrocytes from sporadic patients markedly attenuated toxicity towards motor neurons.

The data summarized in this section provide strong evidence for a pathologic role of wild-type SOD1 in sporadic disease. This hypothesis opens new frontiers for future therapeutic approaches in the treatment of ALS.

4. Human samples to study ALS

In ALS the cells mainly affected by the disease, the motor neurons and the glia, are located in the motor cortex and the spinal cord, which are accessible only post-mortem. The scarce availability of CNS samples, along with post-mortem delay and different preservation techniques that can affect the quality of the tissue and limit its use, are great challenges when studying this disease. Moreover, post-mortem material is only representative of the end stage of disease and, although used in microarray studies to unravel the mechanisms of neurodegeneration, it is unlikely to help identify early biomarkers. For these reasons, peripheral tissues, i.e. blood, fibroblasts and cerebrospinal fluid (CSF) have been preferentially used in high-throughput screening assays for biomarkers identification as well as gene expression profiling.

4.1. Gene expression profiling

Multiple research groups have used post-mortem samples to identify the pathways involved in the neurodegenerative process of ALS. The studies utilizing complex tissues, representative of a mixed cell population, i.e. motor cortex [56] or spinal cord [57], have mainly recorded gene expression changes indicating the presence of an aggressive inflammatory reaction and active astrogliosis. These processes are prevalent in the spinal cord of ALS patients and have masked the transcriptional changes occurring in motor neurons. However, the motor cortex seems to be affected to a lesser extent by astrogliosis and this enabled Lederer and colleagues to identify important changes in transcripts involved in the cytoskeletal, mitochondrial and proteasomal functions, as well as ion homeostasis and glycolysis [56], in agreement with other lines of research in ALS [1].

In order to determine those genes differentially expressed in the cell type most affected in ALS, i.e. spinal motor neurons, laser capture microdissection (LCM) has been used to isolate single cells from human post mortem spinal cord samples.

Gene expression profiling of motor neurons has been performed on sporadic ALS cases [58], as well as ALS cases carrying mutations in the SOD1 and chromatin modifying protein 2B (*CHMP2B*) genes [59, 60]. The three studies highlighted the activation of different pathogenic pathways. The motor neurons isolated from sporadic cases showed decreased expression of genes associated with the cytoskeleton and transcription, whilst cell death-associated transcripts were increased. Moreover, genes involved in cell cycle activation and progression were found to be upregulated, supporting the theory that inappropriate activation of the cell cycle in these post-mitotic cells can lead to cell death [58].

In contrast, microarray analysis of motor neurons isolated from *SOD1*-related ALS cases highlighted the activation of a cell survival pathway in the motor neurons that were spared by the disease. The study, in fact, revealed differential expression of genes involved in the protein kinase B/phosphatidylinositol-3 kinase (AKT/PI3K) pathway, along with decrease in phophastase and tensin homologue (*PTEN*) gene, a negative regulator of AKT [60]. The authors also showed that inhibition of PTEN led to increased activation of the AKT/PI3K pathway, with beneficial effects on primary motor neuron survival. Thus, activation of the AKT/PI3K pathway is a potential candidate for future therapeutic strategies.

Finally, the transcriptional profiles from motor neurons isolated from the *CHMP2B*-related ALS cases showed dysregulation of genes involved in p38 MAPK signalling pathway, reduced autophagy and repression of translation [59]. The significant impairment of the autophagy pathway reflects the function of *CHMP2B*, the gene mutated in these patient samples.

In spite of the differences between the pathways described above, dysregulation of calcium handling and cell cycle, as well as transcription, cytoskeleton assembly and metabolism, were common between the different genetic subtypes and SALS. Taking into account that these results derive from end-stage tissues, they support the evidence that etiologically diverse forms of ALS converge into common mechanisms involved in motor neuron death.

4.1.1. Results from use of human peripheral tissue

Gene expression profiling has also been conducted on blood cells from ALS patients in order to identify biomarkers and/or achieve a better classification of disease subtypes through the identification of common transcriptional patterns [61-63]. In the study conducted by Saris and colleagues, microarray analysis of SALS and control whole blood samples was followed by hierarchical clustering of all differentially expressed transcripts [61]. This approach successfully identified different clusters that were able to differentiate between ALS and control samples. Interestingly, this study showed that peripheral blood can be used to investigate the pathways activated during disease, as the blood from ALS patients reveals decrease in transcripts involved in RNA processing as well as upregulation of inflammatory genes. This suggests that the mechanisms affecting motor neurons, also strike other cell type. However, because of their post-mitotic characteristics and their unique function, motor neurons are the most susceptible.

A more recent study performed gene expression profiling on peripheral blood mononuclear cells (PBMCs) from patients with SALS [62]. The results show upregulation of LPS/TLR4-signaling associated genes in response to elevated LPS plasma levels. A similar transcription pattern was obtained by culturing PBMCs from normal controls with LPS for a short time *in vitro*.

Similarly, Mougeot et al. found that peripheral blood lymphocytes (PBLs) display dysregulation of the ubiquitin/proteasome system (UPS) [63]. In particular, microarray analysis revealed upregulation of the ubiquitin-protein ligase E3-alpha-2 (UBR2) expression. UBR2 is known to act in synergy with UBR1 in a quality control mechanism for degradation of unfolded proteins. UBR2 upregulation correlated inversely with time since onset of disease and directly with the ALS functional rating scale (ALSFRS-R), suggesting that UBR2 is increased early in the disease course and decreases as disease progresses. The authors confirmed with *in vitro* experiments that cultured PBMCs from ALS patients accumulated more ubiquitinated proteins than PBMCs from healthy controls in a serum-dependent manner, as expected from the transcription data.

Very recently, human samples have been used to interrogate micro RNA (miRNA) expression [64, 65]. Two studies successfully identified dysregulation of miRNAs in peripheral leukocytes [64] and monocytes [65] from SALS samples compared to controls. These miRNA are involved in pathways relevant to the CNS and, in particular, Butovsky et al. identified changes relevant for the inflammatory response, similarly to the expression pattern displayed by monocytes isolated from multiple sclerosis (MS) patients. These results suggest that miRNAs profiles found in the peripheral blood cells can be relevant to understand the pathogenesis of ALS and/or used as biomarkers of the disease.

4.2. Biomarkers in ALS

ALS is fatal rapidly progressive neurodegenerative disorder, characterized by the activation of an intricate network of pathways and still lacking an effective treatment beside Riluzole [1]. The diagnosis of ALS is still mainly based on clinical assessment of progression of symptoms, which results in a delay of about a year from symptom onset to diagnosis. Although the clinical course of disease can considerably vary from case to case, in the majority of cases death occurs within 2-5 years [66].

In this scenario, significant effort has been spent trying to identify molecules that could help classify different forms of ALS and lead to early diagnosis, as well as monitor disease progression.

The tissues mainly utilized for biomarker screening in the past five years have been peripheral blood mononuclear cells (PBMCs) and cerebrospinal fluid (CSF). PBMCs have already been shown to display some of the traits of the disease, such as increase in inflammatory genes [65] and downregulation of Bcl-2 [67] and might, therefore, be used to investigate the disease during its progression as well as provide unique biomarkers.

Recently, Nardo et al. performed proteomic analysis of PBMCs isolated from 60 sporadic ALS patients and 30 healthy controls [68]. The authors identified and validated in a second cohort 14 protein biomarkers, that could discriminate between ALS patients and controls regardless of age and gender. Remarkably, of these 14 biomarkers, 5 were able to discriminate between ALS patients and individuals with other neuropathies and 3, among which TDP43, were markers of disease severity. Notably, these results are consistent with a CSF biomarker study reporting that TDP43 levels were increased in ALS patients [69]. The value of this result goes beyond the finding of a disease biomarker, as it supports the even more interesting hypothesis that TDP43 could be a common player in early disease in familial as well as sporadic ALS cases. This would confirm what is already suggested by the presence of TDP-43 positive aggregates in SALS biopsy samples.

Although there is still no consensus on valid biomarkers for ALS [70], proteome analysis has recently led to the identification of fetuin-A and transthyretin (TTR) as candidates to distinguish ALS patients with rapid versus slow disease progression. The upregulation of TTR and fetuin-A, involved in immune regulatory functions, could be associated with the inflammatory state of the CNS. At present, these markers were tested in two independent cohorts of 18 and 20 patients with a follow up of 2 years [71] and TTR had already been identified as a potential biomarker for ALS compared to controls in a previous study [72]. Although further validation is needed, these results are encouraging and would provide an invaluable tool to discriminate between patients with different disease progression rates. This would help clinician determine the timing for clinical intervention such as gastrostomy and non-invasive ventilation [73].

5. Stem cell technology for ALS research

Stem cells are defined as a population of cells that maintains the ability to self-renew and differentiate into several cell types of the adult body. In mammals, several tissues such as muscle, brain and bone marrow, harbor subtypes of stem cells that can give rise to a relatively small variety of different cell types. These adult stem cells are committed to certain cell lineages and do not produce cells from other tissue types under normal conditions. Unlike adult stem cells, embryonic stem cells that can be isolated from the inner cell mass of early stage embryos are pluripotent and can, therefore, still differentiate into virtually any cell type of the human body. While the collection of embryonic stem cells from mice is a widely accepted approach used for disease modeling, the use of human embryonic stem cells is controversial and rises severe ethical concerns. With the discovery that adult human fibroblasts can be reprogrammed to an embryonic stem cell like state, new hope arose for stem cell based approaches in human research. Induced pluripotent stem cells (iPS) are usually generated by the introduction of 2-5 defined pluripotency transcription factors into fibroblasts or other readily available differentiated cell types. These transcription factors drastically alter gene expression in the target cells until some of them eventually become pluripotent and can then be isolated and amplified. Initially, the transcription factors were introduced by retroviral or lentiviral constructs leading to the integration of the transgene into the target genome. As the random integration of additional genes can disrupt/alter the expression of endogenous genes, more recent approaches rely on less invasive techniques such as transposons or RNA transfection [74]

The use of stem cell technologies in ALS research started in 2007 when mouse embryonic stem cells from the most prominent SOD1 model carrying the G93A mutation were established [75]. When differentiated into motor neurons, mild phenotypic differences between motor neurons expressing human wild type SOD1 or the G93A mutation could be observed. After several weeks in culture, SOD1 containing inclusions as well as the overall level of ubiquitinated proteins were more frequent in the motor neurons expressing the mutant human protein. In 2009, a human embryonic stem cell line was used to generate motor neurons that were then transfected with different SOD1 mutation containing constructs [76]. The researchers observed a reduction in neurite length and in line with the study of the mouse G93A embryonic stem cell derived motor neurons, reduced survival. However, in the human study, it is unclear whether the observed phenotype arises from the mutations or the increase of SOD1 abundance itself, as a control overexpressing wild type SOD1, was not generated.

Since the discovery of the iPS technology, huge efforts were put in the generation of patient specific iPS lines. Up to now, several hundred lines with various mutations have been generated and some are now becoming commercially available thereby getting accessible to a broad scientific community.

In 2008, Dimos et al reported the successful generation of motor neurons and glial cells from an ALS patient derived iPS line carrying a SOD1 mutation causing a mild disease phenotype [14]. Surprisingly, unlike the previous studies with mouse and human embryonic stem cells, no disease related phenotype was reported from these cells until now. This potential lack of phenotype could in part be explained by the patient's late onset and mild disease form. Another report from 2011, where motor neurons were generated from a patient harboring a VAPB mutation, did also not mention any phenotype despite reduced levels of VAPB. As the levels of this protein were already reduced in the fibroblasts used for the reprogramming, the lower levels in the resulting motor neurons could either be due to mutation induced expression or translational changes or could also be explained by an incomplete reprogramming of this genomic locus in the generated iPS lines [77]. Recently, the first report of an iPS line harboring a TDP-43 mutation was published [78]. The motor neurons generated from this line showed elevated TDP-43 levels, but no change in localization or signs of aggregate formation. In addition, motor neurons from both, control and TDP-43 mutant were phenotypically and functionally similar despite an elevated sensitivity to PI3K signaling inhibition and elevated cell death. These data suggest that the toxicity of this TDP-43 mutation might arise from its increased stability leading to a higher overall protein amount in the cell.

Despite the growing number of iPS lines from ALS patients available, no further reports of disease relevant phenotypes or major discoveries of disease mechanisms from the use of these cells were reported so far. In addition, observations from other neurological disorders show a similar trend: cells differentiated from embryonic stem cells or induced pluripotent stem cells often reflect only certain aspects of the disease and sometimes it takes several weeks before such differences can be recorded and/or the observed symptoms are very mild [79, 80]. The problems to reproduce patient phenotypes have ameliorated the initial excitement about this new method to model neurological diseases. More recently, it became clear that even cells differentiated from individual embryonic stem cell clones or iPS clones from the same patient can show substantial phenotypic differences, a phenomenon called clonal variation [81]. Similar observations were made in a study using iPS lines of ALS patients carrying TDP-43 mutations. After differentiation of individual iPS clones from the same patient into motor neurons, the levels of TDP-43 expression as well as aggregate formation and oxidative stress induced cell death showed substantial variation [82]. Considering the confusing reports, it has to be assumed that the reprogramming as well as the following differentiation mechanisms are not yet fully under control and more mechanistic research and standardization of the protocols will hopefully soon lead to more pronounced and reproducible results. Initial steps to improve reproducibility and differentiation are already under way. The main focus lies on the standardization of the initial characterization of the iPS clones prior to use as well as the improvement of differentiation protocols by addition of various small molecules and growth factors [83, 84].

While these approaches emerge, sporadic and familial forms of ALS can be modeled with cells isolated from human post mortem spinal cord or brain samples. A recent report demonstrated that post-mortem isolated neuronal progenitor cells from patients with sporadic or familial ALS, can be differentiated into astrocyte-like cells *in vitro*. Astrocytes from patients, but not from healthy controls conveyed toxicity to wild type mouse motor neurons in a co-culture [15]. This system provides a promising tool for testing of potential therapeutic approaches.

5.1. The promises and limitations of stem cells for therapeutic approaches

The disease modeling described in the upper section is in particular important for the huge proportion of ALS cases, where no causing mutation is known. Until the discovery of the iPS technology, this lack of knowledge made it impossible to model such cases *in vitro* in a cell based assay or with animal models, unless post-mortem cells could be collected. Now we can use skin fibroblasts or other readily available cell types from affected patients during different time points of disease progression prior to end stage. From these fibroblasts, various cell types that are known to play a crucial role in ALS can be generated and their behavior and interplay in a cell culture dish can be studied in-depth.

Despite emerging into an invaluable tool to study disease mechanisms, stem cells also hold a huge potential for the development of therapeutic approaches for ALS and many other neurodegenerative diseases. On the one hand, the generated cells can now be used in drug screenings to identify new target mechanisms or to assess potential new therapeutics. On the other hand, the stem cells can be used for cell replacement approaches. For patients with known mutations, the cells can be genetically modified or corrected prior to reprogramming and differentiation. Such individualized strategies would allow the use of the patient's own cells for transplantation, thereby reducing the risk of graft rejection.

In ALS, a major future goal would be to produce and replace dying motor neurons. A proof of principle that motor neuron transplantation might become possible came from the observation that mouse embryonic stem cell derived motor neurons transplanted into the lumbar part of paralysed adult rats can actually survive and form functional neuromuscular junctions leading to phenotypical improvements [85]. However, in human ALS patients, the replacement of motor neurons might be more complicated due to the size differences, amount of cells needed and distance that the axon would have to grow out. In addition, it becomes more and more evident that ALS is a non-cell autonomous disease in which astrocytes, microglia and oligodendrocytes play a crucial role in modulating disease onset and progression [3, 15, 86]. In this context, a strategy approaching several cell types at a time might be more successful than bringing in healthy motor neurons alone into a heavily diseased environment. A promising candidate that can generate various cell types in the CNS and at the same time positively stimulate the neuronal environment by producing neuroprotective factors, are neuronal progenitor cells (also called neuronal stem cells). Several reports indicate that transplanted neuronal progenitor cells are able to differentiate into different cell types *in vivo* [87, 88]. Further, injection of NPCs has been shown to ameliorate disease progression in ALS rodent models even if most of the cells do not migrate or differentiate into other cell types in various neurodegenerative diseases [89]. However, it is not known how these cells would behave and survive when transplanted into a diseased environment.

One of the largest limitations for cell replacement strategies to date is the lack of efficiency as well as specificity during the amplification and differentiation step. The differentiation of ES or iPS cells into various different neurons or neuronal progenitor cells is guided by the application of different growth factors and small molecules. However, this process usually generates a mixed population containing many different cell types. The cell type of interest often represents only 30% or even less of the total population. Therefore, it might be difficult to generate enough cells for therapeutic applications.

When using ES or iPS lines to generate the cell type of interest, a further drawback is that a small portion of cells remains undifferentiated and immature, thereby representing a major risk factor for transplantation [90]. When neuronal progenitor cells derived from mouse iPS cells were injected into adult mouse brains, they formed tumors in up to 60% of the injected animals [88]. The use or more restricted cell types such as NPCs on the opposite, appears to be safer.

Finally, the generation and maintenance of a stable iPS lines from human adult cells is expensive and very time consuming [74]. If clinical applications are considered, a thorough characterization of several individual clones needs to be undertaken prior to use, making a widespread application of this approach today unlikely. Very recent reports indicate that fibroblasts can be directly differentiated into several types of neurons and even neuronal progenitor cells in a much faster and more efficient way than through iPSing [91]. It remains to be evaluated to which extent these cells recapitulate neurodegenerative disease phenotypes, although a first report from fibroblast derived neurons from a familial Alzheimer's patient seem promising [92].

In summary, the technique of reprogramming holds great promises in terms of disease modeling and unraveling of underlying mechanisms of sporadic neurodegenerative diseases such as ALS. Despite the current confusion due to the various methods used to generate the lines, the observed clonal variations as well as the limited reflection of disease phenotypes, the field has advanced with tremendous speed if one considers that the first report about reprogramming of mouse fibroblasts was published only 6 years ago. With combined efforts and improved methods, a better understanding and control of the reprogramming mechanisms can be achieved, thereby facilitating the interpretation and usage of the generated cells.

6. Future trends in modeling ALS and discovering new therapies

The recent remarkable advancement in the cell biology field that adult fibroblasts can be reprogrammed to virtually originate all cell types have created a unique opportunity to model neurological disorders *in vitro*. iPS technology has already been applied to several neurodegenerative conditions, from Alzheimer's disease [93] to Down syndrome [94], as well schizophrenia [80], Rett syndrome [95] and ALS [14].

Although a large number of iPS cell lines from patients affected by various diseases have been made commercially available, it is still not clear how robustly these recapitulate the characteristics specific of each disease. Although the promises of iPS technology are to lead to high-throughput screenings to find new efficacious therapeutic targets, they are subject to some main limitations that have already been addressed in other sections of this book chapter. It is, therefore, of paramount importance that the properties of the differentiated cells are well characterized and it is verified that they are representative of the disease they are modeling.

However, some promising results have been obtained from a very recent study suggesting that iPS-derived motor neurons originated from patients carrying TDP-43 mutations display abnormalities typical of TDP-43 proteinopathy. These cells display elevated levels of soluble and detergent-resistant TDP-43 protein, decreased survival, and increased vulnerability to inhibition of phosphatidylinositol 3-kinase (PI3K) pathway [78] as well as shorter neurites and TDP-43 cytoplasmic aggregates [82]. These parameters can be used as readout for high-throughput drug screenings as well as short hairpin RNA (shRNA) library screenings. Indeed, Egawa and colleagues performed microarray analysis on iPS-derived motor neurons transduced with lentivirus expressing green fluorescent protein (GFP) under the control of the HB9 promoter. Based on the results obtained from gene expression analysis, the authors tested 4 drugs known to modulate transcription through histone modification and RNA splicing. Using the high content imaging analyzer InCell 6000, Egawa and colleagues found that anacardic acid had protective effects against arsenite-induced motor neuron death and was able to decrease TDP-43 cytoplasmic aggregates as well as increase neurite length [82].

A different approach was taken in 2011 by Haidet-Phillips and colleagues [15], producing cells from patients without the use of viral vectors or induction of major epigenetic modifications. In this study, astrocytes were derived from NPCs isolated from ALS patients and it was observed that, regardless of their familial or sporadic origin, these cells were toxic to wild type murine motor neurons expressing GFP under HB9 promoter [15]. The authors found that SOD1 knockout via shRNA could rescue motor neurons at different extents depending on whether these were co-cultured on astrocytes from familial or sporadic cases. This study overcomes some of the major issues related to iPS cells and sets the premises for drug and shRNA screening to target pathways and single genes involved in astrocyte toxicity.

Concluding, it is clear that in the past five years the ALS field has seen a major change of scenario, where more tools are available to study more forms of FALS as well as the striking majority of SALS. As the recent genetic discoveries have highlighted the importance of previously unexplored pathways, i.e. RNA metabolism, also common targets linking sporadic and familial ALS have been identified, i.e. TDP-43 and SOD-1. Moreover, the advances in highthroughput screening technology with the advent of new gene profiling techniques, i.e. deep-sequencing, and high content imaging systems are bound to determine the beginning of a new era for ALS research.

Author details

Laura Ferraiuolo*, Kathrin Meyer and Brian Kaspar

Research Institute at Nationwide Children's Hospital, Columbus, OH, USA

References

[1] Ferraiuolo, L., et al., Molecular pathways of motor neuron injury in amyotrophic lateral sclerosis. Nature reviews. Neurology, 2011. 7(11): p. 616-30.

[2] Ilieva, H., M. Polymenidou, and D.W. Cleveland, Non-cell autonomous toxicity in neurodegenerative disorders: ALS and beyond. The Journal of cell biology, 2009. 187(6): p. 761-72.

[3] Lee, Y., et al., Oligodendroglia metabolically support axons and contribute to neurodegeneration. Nature, 2012. 487(7408): p. 443-8.

[4] Geser, F., V.M. Lee, and J.Q. Trojanowski, Amyotrophic lateral sclerosis and frontotemporal lobar degeneration: a spectrum of TDP-43 proteinopathies. Neuropathology : official journal of the Japanese Society of Neuropathology, 2010. 30(2): p. 103-12.

[5] Hammad, M., et al., Clinical, electrophysiologic, and pathologic evidence for sensory abnormalities in ALS. Neurology, 2007. 69(24): p. 2236-42.

[6] Kabashi, E., et al., TARDBP mutations in individuals with sporadic and familial amyotrophic lateral sclerosis. Nature genetics, 2008. 40(5): p. 572-4.

[7] Sreedharan, J., et al., TDP-43 mutations in familial and sporadic amyotrophic lateral sclerosis. Science, 2008. 319(5870): p. 1668-72.

[8] Kwiatkowski, T.J., Jr., et al., Mutations in the FUS/TLS gene on chromosome 16 cause familial amyotrophic lateral sclerosis. Science, 2009. 323(5918): p. 1205-8.

[9] Vance, C., et al., Mutations in FUS, an RNA processing protein, cause familial amyotrophic lateral sclerosis type 6. Science, 2009. 323(5918): p. 1208-11.

[10] Majounie, E., et al., Frequency of the C9orf72 hexanucleotide repeat expansion in patients with amyotrophic lateral sclerosis and frontotemporal dementia: a cross-sectional study. Lancet neurology, 2012. 11(4): p. 323-30.

[11] DeJesus-Hernandez, M., et al., Expanded GGGGCC hexanucleotide repeat in noncoding region of C9ORF72 causes chromosome 9p-linked FTD and ALS. Neuron, 2011. 72(2): p. 245-56.

[12] Renton, A.E., et al., A hexanucleotide repeat expansion in C9ORF72 is the cause of chromosome 9p21-linked ALS-FTD. Neuron, 2011. 72(2): p. 257-68.

[13] Takahashi, K., et al., Induction of pluripotent stem cells from adult human fibroblasts by defined factors. Cell, 2007. 131(5): p. 861-72.

[14] Dimos, J.T., et al., Induced pluripotent stem cells generated from patients with ALS can be differentiated into motor neurons. Science, 2008. 321(5893): p. 1218-21.

[15] Haidet-Phillips, A.M., et al., Astrocytes from familial and sporadic ALS patients are toxic to motor neurons. Nature biotechnology, 2011. 29(9): p. 824-8.

[16] Rosen, D.R., Mutations in Cu/Zn superoxide dismutase gene are associated with familial amyotrophic lateral sclerosis. Nature, 1993. 364(6435): p. 362.

[17] Al-Chalabi, A., et al., The genetics and neuropathology of amyotrophic lateral sclerosis. Acta neuropathologica, 2012. 124(3): p. 339-52.

[18] Byrne, S. and O. Hardiman, Familial aggregation in amyotrophic lateral sclerosis. Annals of neurology, 2010. 67(4): p. 554.

[19] van Rheenen, W., et al., Hexanucleotide repeat expansions in C9ORF72 in the spectrum of motor neuron diseases. Neurology, 2012. 79(9): p. 878-82.

[20] Joyce, P.I., et al., SOD1 and TDP-43 animal models of amyotrophic lateral sclerosis: recent advances in understanding disease toward the development of clinical treatments. Mammalian genome : official journal of the International Mammalian Genome Society, 2011. 22(7-8): p. 420-48.

[21] Neumann, M., et al., Ubiquitinated TDP-43 in frontotemporal lobar degeneration and amyotrophic lateral sclerosis. Science, 2006. 314(5796): p. 130-3.

[22] Mackenzie, I.R., R. Rademakers, and M. Neumann, TDP-43 and FUS in amyotrophic lateral sclerosis and frontotemporal dementia. Lancet neurology, 2010. 9(10): p. 995-1007.

[23] Lagier-Tourenne, C. and D.W. Cleveland, Rethinking ALS: the FUS about TDP-43. Cell, 2009. 136(6): p. 1001-4.

[24] Sephton, C.F., et al., TDP-43 is a developmentally regulated protein essential for early embryonic development. The Journal of biological chemistry, 2010. 285(9): p. 6826-34.

[25] Wu, L.S., et al., TDP-43, a neuro-pathosignature factor, is essential for early mouse embryogenesis. Genesis, 2010. 48(1): p. 56-62.

[26] Chiang, P.M., et al., Deletion of TDP-43 down-regulates Tbc1d1, a gene linked to obesity, and alters body fat metabolism. Proceedings of the National Academy of Sciences of the United States of America, 2010. 107(37): p. 16320-4.

[27] Polymenidou, M., et al., Long pre-mRNA depletion and RNA missplicing contribute to neuronal vulnerability from loss of TDP-43. Nat Neurosci, 2011. 14(4): p. 459-68.

[28] Ling, S.C., et al., ALS-associated mutations in TDP-43 increase its stability and promote TDP-43 complexes with FUS/TLS. Proceedings of the National Academy of Sciences of the United States of America, 2010. 107(30): p. 13318-23.

[29] Buratti, E. and F.E. Baralle, Multiple roles of TDP-43 in gene expression, splicing regulation, and human disease. Frontiers in bioscience : a journal and virtual library, 2008. 13: p. 867-78.

[30] Kim, S.H., et al., Amyotrophic lateral sclerosis-associated proteins TDP-43 and FUS/TLS function in a common biochemical complex to co-regulate HDAC6 mRNA. The Journal of biological chemistry, 2010. 285(44): p. 34097-105.

[31] Maruyama, H., et al., Mutations of optineurin in amyotrophic lateral sclerosis. Nature, 2010. 465(7295): p. 223-6.

[32] Vance, C., et al., Familial amyotrophic lateral sclerosis with frontotemporal dementia is linked to a locus on chromosome 9p13.2-21.3. Brain : a journal of neurology, 2006. 129(Pt 4): p. 868-76.

[33] Majounie, E., et al., Large C9orf72 repeat expansions are not a common cause of Parkinson's disease. Neurobiology of aging, 2012. 33(10): p. 2527 e1-2.

[34] Ince, P.G., et al., Molecular pathology and genetic advances in amyotrophic lateral sclerosis: an emerging molecular pathway and the significance of glial pathology. Acta neuropathologica, 2011. 122(6): p. 657-71.

[35] Murray, M.E., et al., Clinical and neuropathologic heterogeneity of c9FTD/ALS associated with hexanucleotide repeat expansion in C9ORF72. Acta neuropathologica, 2011. 122(6): p. 673-90.

[36] Gurney, M.E., et al., Motor neuron degeneration in mice that express a human Cu,Zn superoxide dismutase mutation. Science, 1994. 264(5166): p. 1772-5.

[37] Menzies, F.M., et al., Mitochondrial dysfunction in a cell culture model of familial amyotrophic lateral sclerosis. Brain : a journal of neurology, 2002. 125(Pt 7): p. 1522-33.

[38] Reaume, A.G., et al., Motor neurons in Cu/Zn superoxide dismutase-deficient mice develop normally but exhibit enhanced cell death after axonal injury. Nature genetics, 1996. 13(1): p. 43-7.

[39] Synofzik, M., et al., Mutant superoxide dismutase-1 indistinguishable from wild-type causes ALS. Human molecular genetics, 2012. 21(16): p. 3568-74.

[40] Wang, L., et al., The effect of mutant SOD1 dismutase activity on non-cell autonomous degeneration in familial amyotrophic lateral sclerosis. Neurobiology of disease, 2009. 35(2): p. 234-40.

[41] Chattopadhyay, M. and J.S. Valentine, Aggregation of copper-zinc superoxide dismutase in familial and sporadic ALS. Antioxidants & redox signaling, 2009. 11(7): p. 1603-14.

[42] Prudencio, M., et al., Variation in aggregation propensities among ALS-associated variants of SOD1: correlation to human disease. Human molecular genetics, 2009. 18(17): p. 3217-26.

[43] Ezzi, S.A., M. Urushitani, and J.P. Julien, Wild-type superoxide dismutase acquires binding and toxic properties of ALS-linked mutant forms through oxidation. Journal of neurochemistry, 2007. 102(1): p. 170-8.

[44] Gruzman, A., et al., Common molecular signature in SOD1 for both sporadic and familial amyotrophic lateral sclerosis. Proceedings of the National Academy of Sciences of the United States of America, 2007. 104(30): p. 12524-9.

[45] Guareschi, S., et al., An over-oxidized form of superoxide dismutase found in sporadic amyotrophic lateral sclerosis with bulbar onset shares a toxic mechanism with mutant SOD1. Proceedings of the National Academy of Sciences of the United States of America, 2012. 109(13): p. 5074-9.

[46] Wang, L., et al., Wild-type SOD1 overexpression accelerates disease onset of a G85R SOD1 mouse. Human molecular genetics, 2009. 18(9): p. 1642-51.

[47] Deng, H.X., et al., Conversion to the amyotrophic lateral sclerosis phenotype is associated with intermolecular linked insoluble aggregates of SOD1 in mitochondria. Proceedings of the National Academy of Sciences of the United States of America, 2006. 103(18): p. 7142-7.

[48] Rakhit, R., et al., An immunological epitope selective for pathological monomer-misfolded SOD1 in ALS. Nature medicine, 2007. 13(6): p. 754-9.

[49] Liu, H.N., et al., Lack of evidence of monomer/misfolded superoxide dismutase-1 in sporadic amyotrophic lateral sclerosis. Annals of neurology, 2009. 66(1): p. 75-80.

[50] Kerman, A., et al., Amyotrophic lateral sclerosis is a non-amyloid disease in which extensive misfolding of SOD1 is unique to the familial form. Acta neuropathologica, 2010. 119(3): p. 335-44.

[51] Forsberg, K., et al., Novel antibodies reveal inclusions containing non-native SOD1 in sporadic ALS patients. PloS one, 2010. 5(7): p. e11552.

[52] Forsberg, K., et al., Glial nuclear aggregates of superoxide dismutase-1 are regularly present in patients with amyotrophic lateral sclerosis. Acta neuropathologica, 2011. 121(5): p. 623-34.

[53] Urushitani, M., S.A. Ezzi, and J.P. Julien, Therapeutic effects of immunization with mutant superoxide dismutase in mice models of amyotrophic lateral sclerosis. Proceedings of the National Academy of Sciences of the United States of America, 2007. 104(7): p. 2495-500.

[54] Bosco, D.A., et al., Wild-type and mutant SOD1 share an aberrant conformation and a common pathogenic pathway in ALS. Nature neuroscience, 2010. 13(11): p. 1396-403.

[55] Pokrishevsky, E., et al., Aberrant localization of FUS and TDP43 is associated with misfolding of SOD1 in amyotrophic lateral sclerosis. PloS one, 2012. 7(4): p. e35050.

[56] Lederer, C.W., et al., Pathways and genes differentially expressed in the motor cortex of patients with sporadic amyotrophic lateral sclerosis. BMC Genomics, 2007. 8: p. 26.

[57] Offen, D., et al., Spinal cord mRNA profile in patients with ALS: comparison with transgenic mice expressing the human SOD-1 mutant. J Mol Neurosci, 2009. 38(2): p. 85-93.

[58] Jiang, Y.M., et al., Gene expression profile of spinal motor neurons in sporadic amyotrophic lateral sclerosis. Ann Neurol, 2005. 57(2): p. 236-51.

[59] Cox, L.E., et al., Mutations in CHMP2B in lower motor neuron predominant amyotrophic lateral sclerosis (ALS). PLoS ONE, 2010. 5(3): p. e9872.

[60] Kirby, J., et al., Phosphatase and tensin homologue/protein kinase B pathway linked to motor neuron survival in human superoxide dismutase 1-related amyotrophic lateral sclerosis. Brain, 2011. 134(Pt 2): p. 506-17.

[61] Saris, C.G., et al., Weighted gene co-expression network analysis of the peripheral blood from Amyotrophic Lateral Sclerosis patients. BMC Genomics, 2009. 10: p. 405.

[62] Zhang, R., et al., Gene expression profiling in peripheral blood mononuclear cells from patients with sporadic amyotrophic lateral sclerosis (sALS). J Neuroimmunol, 2011. 230(1-2): p. 114-23.

[63] Mougeot, J.L., et al., Microarray analysis of peripheral blood lymphocytes from ALS patients and the SAFE detection of the KEGG ALS pathway. BMC medical genomics, 2011. 4: p. 74.

[64] De Felice, B., et al., A miRNA signature in leukocytes from sporadic amyotrophic lateral sclerosis. Gene, 2012.

[65] Butovsky, O., et al., Modulating inflammatory monocytes with a unique microRNA gene signature ameliorates murine ALS. The Journal of clinical investigation, 2012.

[66] Turner, M.R., et al., Biomarkers in amyotrophic lateral sclerosis. Lancet Neurol, 2009. 8(1): p. 94-109.

[67] Mantovani, S., et al., Immune system alterations in sporadic amyotrophic lateral sclerosis patients suggest an ongoing neuroinflammatory process. Journal of neuroimmunology, 2009. 210(1-2): p. 73-9.

[68] Nardo, G., et al., Amyotrophic lateral sclerosis multiprotein biomarkers in peripheral blood mononuclear cells. PloS one, 2011. 6(10): p. e25545.

[69] Kasai, T., et al., Increased TDP-43 protein in cerebrospinal fluid of patients with amyotrophic lateral sclerosis. Acta neuropathologica, 2009. 117(1): p. 55-62.

[70] Tarasiuk, J., et al., CSF markers in amyotrophic lateral sclerosis. Journal of neural transmission, 2012. 119(7): p. 747-57.

[71] Brettschneider, J., et al., Proteome analysis reveals candidate markers of disease progression in amyotrophic lateral sclerosis (ALS). Neuroscience letters, 2010. 468(1): p. 23-7.

[72] Ranganathan, S., et al., Proteomic profiling of cerebrospinal fluid identifies biomarkers for amyotrophic lateral sclerosis. Journal of neurochemistry, 2005. 95(5): p. 1461-71.

[73] Andersen, P.M., et al., EFNS guidelines on the clinical management of amyotrophic lateral sclerosis (MALS)--revised report of an EFNS task force. European journal of neurology : the official journal of the European Federation of Neurological Societies, 2012. 19(3): p. 360-75.

[74] Robinton, D.A. and G.Q. Daley, The promise of induced pluripotent stem cells in research and therapy. Nature, 2012. 481(7381): p. 295-305.

[75] Di Giorgio, F.P., et al., Non-cell autonomous effect of glia on motor neurons in an embryonic stem cell-based ALS model. Nature neuroscience, 2007. 10(5): p. 608-14.

[76] Karumbayaram, S., et al., Human embryonic stem cell-derived motor neurons expressing SOD1 mutants exhibit typical signs of motor neuron degeneration linked to ALS. Disease models & mechanisms, 2009. 2(3-4): p. 189-95.

[77] Mitne-Neto, M., et al., Downregulation of VAPB expression in motor neurons derived from induced pluripotent stem cells of ALS8 patients. Human molecular genetics, 2011. 20(18): p. 3642-52.

[78] Bilican, B., et al., Mutant induced pluripotent stem cell lines recapitulate aspects of TDP-43 proteinopathies and reveal cell-specific vulnerability. Proceedings of the National Academy of Sciences of the United States of America, 2012. 109(15): p. 5803-8.

[79] Soldner, F., et al., Parkinson's disease patient-derived induced pluripotent stem cells free of viral reprogramming factors. Cell, 2009. 136(5): p. 964-77.

[80] Brennand, K.J., et al., Modelling schizophrenia using human induced pluripotent stem cells. Nature, 2011. 473(7346): p. 221-5.

[81] Osafune, K., et al., Marked differences in differentiation propensity among human embryonic stem cell lines. Nature biotechnology, 2008. 26(3): p. 313-5.

[82] Egawa, N., et al., Drug Screening for ALS Using Patient-Specific Induced Pluripotent Stem Cells. Science translational medicine, 2012. 4(145): p. 145ra104.

[83] Boulting, G.L., et al., A functionally characterized test set of human induced pluripotent stem cells. Nature biotechnology, 2011. 29(3): p. 279-86.

[84] Kim, D.S., et al., Robust enhancement of neural differentiation from human ES and iPS cells regardless of their innate difference in differentiation propensity. Stem cell reviews, 2010. 6(2): p. 270-81.

[85] Deshpande, D.M., et al., Recovery from paralysis in adult rats using embryonic stem cells. Annals of neurology, 2006. 60(1): p. 32-44.

[86] Yamanaka, K., et al., Astrocytes as determinants of disease progression in inherited amyotrophic lateral sclerosis. Nature neuroscience, 2008. 11(3): p. 251-3.

[87] Darsalia, V., T. Kallur, and Z. Kokaia, Survival, migration and neuronal differentiation of human fetal striatal and cortical neural stem cells grafted in stroke-damaged rat striatum. The European journal of neuroscience, 2007. 26(3): p. 605-14.

[88] Ring, K.L., et al., Direct reprogramming of mouse and human fibroblasts into multipotent neural stem cells with a single factor. Cell stem cell, 2012. 11(1): p. 100-9.

[89] Suzuki, M., et al., GDNF secreting human neural progenitor cells protect dying motor neurons, but not their projection to muscle, in a rat model of familial ALS. PloS one, 2007. 2(8): p. e689.

[90] Cohen, J.D., et al., Use of human stem cell derived cardiomyocytes to examine sunitinib mediated cardiotoxicity and electrophysiological alterations. Toxicology and applied pharmacology, 2011. 257(1): p. 74-83.

[91] Kim, D.S., et al., Highly Pure and Expandable PSA-NCAM-Positive Neural Precursors from Human ESC and iPSC-Derived Neural Rosettes. PloS one, 2012. 7(7): p. e39715.

[92] Qiang, L., et al., Directed conversion of Alzheimer's disease patient skin fibroblasts into functional neurons. Cell, 2011. 146(3): p. 359-71.

[93] Israel, M.A., et al., Probing sporadic and familial Alzheimer's disease using induced pluripotent stem cells. Nature, 2012. 482(7384): p. 216-20.

[94] Mou, X., et al., Generation of disease-specific induced pluripotent stem cells from patients with different karyotypes of Down syndrome. Stem cell research & therapy, 2012. 3(2): p. 14.

[95] Marchetto, M.C., et al., A model for neural development and treatment of Rett syndrome using human induced pluripotent stem cells. Cell, 2010. 143(4): p. 527-39.

Chapter 7

The Role of the Statistical Method of Motor Unit Number Estimation (MUNE) to Assess the Potential Therapeutic Benefits of Riluzole on Patients with Pre-symptomatic Familial Amyotrophic Lateral Sclerosis

Arun Aggarwal

Additional information is available at the end of the chapter

http://dx.doi.org/10.5772/56559

1. Introduction

Amyotrophic lateral sclerosis (ALS) is a fatal neurodegenerative disease which attacks the motor system. There is a family history in approximately 10% percent of cases and 20% of such families have point mutations in the Cu, Zn superoxide dimutase 1 (SOD1) gene. Pre-symptomatic loss of motor neurons has been identified prior to the onset of symptoms in SOD1 mice. This loss was biphasic with initial loss in the pre-symptomatic phase followed by a period of stabilisation and then gradual loss at time of weakness to death. (Kong & Xu, 1998).

In order to determine the time course of motor neurone loss prior to symptomatic onset of disease, a longitudinal study of at-risk asymptomatic individuals (i.e. SOD1 mutation carriers with no neurological symptoms or signs as determined by a neurologist) was performed. There was no detectable difference in the number of motor units in SOD1 mutation carriers compared to their SOD1 negative family controls. (Aggarwal & Nicholson, 2001). This may indicate that mutation carriers have undetectable loss of motor neurones until rapid and widespread cell death of motor neurones occurs, coinciding with the onset of symptomatic features. This implies that the disease is not the end result of the slow attrition of motor neurones. (Aggarwal, 2009).

This longitudinal study was extended on 20 asymptomatic carriers of the Cu, Zn superoxide dimutase 1 (SOD1) point mutation. There was a sudden reduction in MUNE, several months prior to the onset of weakness. (Aggarwal & Nicholson 2002) and (Aggarwal, 2009). This suggests that gradual pre-clinical loss of motor neurones does not occur in asymptomatic SOD1 mutation carriers and supports the observation that sudden, catastrophic loss of motor neurones occurs immediately prior to the onset of symptoms and the development of the disease, rather than a gradual attrition of motor neurones over time. These results suggest that there may be a biological trigger initiating rapid cell loss, just prior to the onset of symptoms.

Current treatment for sporadic ALS or Cu, Zn superoxide dimutase 1 (SOD 1 mutation) familial ALS, produces only a modest increase in survival. The excitatory amino acid neurotransmitter, glutamate, may be involved in the pathogenesis of ALS. Riluzole, an anti-glutamate agent, remains the only disease modifying therapy available for ALS and has been used since 1995. (Cheah et al, 2010). Treatment of human ALS patients or transgenic Cu, Zn superoxide dimutase 1 (SOD 1) mice, most commonly produce a modest but significant increase in survival. (Bensimon et al, 1994). It has also been shown to have a small beneficial effect on bulbar function, but not muscle strength.

Using the statistical motor unit number estimation (MUNE) technique, (Daube, 1995), a longitudinal study was performed to determine whether early institution of Riluzole can reduce that rate of motor unit loss in familial amyotrophic lateral sclerosis (fALS). Motor unit numbers were estimated from the right abductor pollicis brevis (APB) and right extensor digitorum brevis (EDB) muscles. Our subjects had a presumptive diagnosis of fALS, as electromyography (EMG) was "normal" with an absence of fasciculation and fibrillation potentials, normal motor unit potentials and normal recruitment. MUNE is more sensitive that EMG and once changes occur on conventional EMG studies, the window of opportunity to influence the progression of this condition has been missed. They were all commenced on Riluzole therapy in the pre-symptomatic phase, as soon as loss of motor units was detected using motor unit number estimation (MUNE). After commencing Riluzole, "symptomatic" improvement occurred, especially a decrease in muscle fasciculations and an improvement in MUNE. Riluzole is not a disease altering agent but possibly if given early in the pre-symptomatic phase of the disease, before significant motor neurone loss has occurred, it may have some therapeutic benefit.

This effect may have implications for the management of asymptomatic carriers of the SOD 1 gene, as these subjects are at risk of developing ALS.

Regular follow-up of SOD1 carriers with MUNE may lead to early diagnosis, creating an opportunity for future approaches and therapies aimed at preserving motor neurones rather than replacing lost motor neurones. Detecting the onset of motor neurone loss in asymptomatic individuals will identify those who may benefit from early institution of an active management program to improve their quality of life, until more effective treatment modalities are available for this devastating condition.

2. Background

Amyotrophic lateral sclerosis (ALS) is a group of fatal, neurodegenerative disorders, which is characterised pathologically by progressive degeneration and loss of motor neurones in the

http://dx.doi.org/10.5772/56559

anterior horn cells of the spinal cord, motor nuclei of the brainstem and the descending pathways within the corticospinal tracts. The term amyotrophic lateral sclerosis (ALS) is used synonymously with motor neurone disease (MND) in the USA, but in the UK and Australia is used only to refer to patients who have a combination of upper and lower motor neurone dysfunction. (Talbot, 2002).

It is primarily a condition of middle to late life, with onset of symptoms between the ages of 50 and 70 and a mean age of onset of 57.4 years. (Ringel et al., 1993). Occasionally, it arises as early as the 2nd decade or as late as the 9th decade. In a natural history study, the overall median survival is 4.0 years from the onset of symptoms, but only 2.1 years from the time of diagnosis. (Ringel et al., 1993). In a study performed at the Mayo clinic, approximately 50% of patients died within 3 years of referral, but 20% were still alive at 5 years and 10% were still alive at 10 years. (Mulder & Howard, 1976).

Aging, motor neurone diseases and many peripheral neuropathies are all associated with loss of motor neurones or axons. When the disorders are recent or rapidly progressive, the extent of the loss may be indicated by weakness and wasting. In slowly progressive denervating conditions, like MND, loss of more than 50-80% of motor units may occur with little or no clinically apparent weakness.

It has been showed that patients with substantial chronic denervation could maintain normal muscle twitch tension until loss of about 70-80% of motor units occurred. (McComas, 1971). The surviving motor neurones enlarge their territories, through collateral sprouting (reinnervation) to keep pace with cell loss, to maintain the muscle maximum compound muscle action potential (CMAP), until late in the disease. At this point, collateral reinnervation is no longer able to provide full functional compensation. (Campbell et al., 1973).

In MND, needle electromyography often reveals evidence of chronic reinnervation (increased motor unit action potential amplitudes and duration with reduced recruitment), but provides little direct evidence to the extent of motor neurone and axonal loss. The supramaximal CMAP amplitude also provides little direct evidence of the extent of motor neurone loss. Normal CMAP amplitudes might mistakenly suggest that motor neurone loss has not occurred yet. (Shefner, 2001).

Motor unit number estimation (MUNE) is a more reliable method for following changes in neurogenic disorders than the CMAP amplitude. It estimates the number of functioning lower motor neurones innervating a muscle or a group of muscles i.e. the number of motor units, which can be excited by electrical stimulation. It is therefore an indirect measure of motor neurone loss, rather than a measure of primary pathology. It can identify that the number of motor units may be well below normal, in the presence of normal CMAP amplitudes. (Brown, 1972).

Pre-symptomatic loss of motor neurones has been identified in an animal model of the disease (transgenic mice expressing mutant human SOD1-G93A). The initial loss in the pre-symptomatic phase related to severe motor axonal degeneration due to vacuolar changes in motor neurones and a slow decrease in CMAP amplitudes. After a period of stabilisation, there was a gradual loss of motor neurones and a rapid decrease in CMAP amplitude, at the onset of weakness due to myelin alteration. At this point, there was a striking loss of motor units. There was also decrease in evoked motor potentials (an indirect measure of the number of motor units), prior to the onset of symptoms. The onset of disease in transgenic G93A mice involves a sharp decline of muscle strength and a transient explosive increase in vacuoles derived from degenerating mitochondria, but little motor neurone death. These did not die until the terminal stage. (Kong & Xu, 1998). The decline exhibited kinetics consistent with both a constant and exponentially decreasing risk of neuronal death. An escalating risk forced by cumulative damage was not responsible for cell death. (Azzouz et al., 1997).

It is possible that the high metabolic activity in motor neurones, combined with the toxic oxidative properties of the mutant SOD1, causes massive mitochondrial vacuolation in motor neurones, resulting in degeneration, earlier than other neurones, triggering the onset of weakness. The involvement of mitochondrial degeneration in the early stages is consistent with a direct effect of toxicity, mediated by properties gained by the mutant enzyme in catalysing redox reactions. (Beckman et al., 1993).

Until recently, it has not been possible to address this in humans, as pre-symptomatic diagnosis was not possible. Now, with the ability to identify Cu, Zn superoxide dismutase 1, (SOD1) mutation carriers, a group of human pre-symptomatic subjects can be studied to determine whether there was gradual lifelong pre-symptomatic loss of motor neurones or whether sudden catastrophic loss of motor neurones occurs just prior to the onset of clinical symptoms.

3. Familial ALS

The only forms of MND in which a clear cause has been established are the genetic variants. 20% of all familial cases are the dominantly inherited adult onset form of MND, which is clinically indistinguishable from the sporadic form of MND. These are due to a point mutation in the cytosolic Cu, Zn superoxide dismutase 1, (SOD1) gene on long arm of chromosome 21 (21q22.1). (Siddique & Deng, 1996). Mutations in other genes, alsin and the heavy subunit of neurofilament (NEFH) can also result in motor neurone degeneration in humans. Two other genes that have been investigated are the other isoforms of SOD. MnSOD (SOD2) maps to chromosome 6q25 and is primarily located in mitochondria and extracellular SOD (SOD3) maps to chromosome 4p15.2. Neither of these genes have yet to be linked to FALS. (Hand & Rouleau, 2002). There is however genetic heterogeneous and other causal genes remain to be found to explain the vast majority of FALS cases. (Siddique et al., 1989).

The initial study to establish a causal link between the SOD1 gene and familial MND (FALS) identified a total of 11 missense mutations in two exons studied in 13 autosomal dominant MND families. (Rosen et al., 1993). This led to an explosion of SOD1 gene screening in MND pedigrees. To date 112 different mutations in the SOD1 have been found which can lead to changes throughout the protein. There have been 99 substitutions, 5 polymorphisms, 3 insertions, 4 deletions and 1 compound mutation types identified. Mutations have been identified in all five exons of the gene. These include 20 on exon 1, 13 on exon 2, 8 on exon 3, 39 on exon 4 and 29 on exon 5 (Figure 1). There have also been 2 non-exon mutations identified on intron 4 and intron 1 and 14 'apparently' sporadic cases described with 6 different SOD1 mutations. (Shaw et al., 1998).

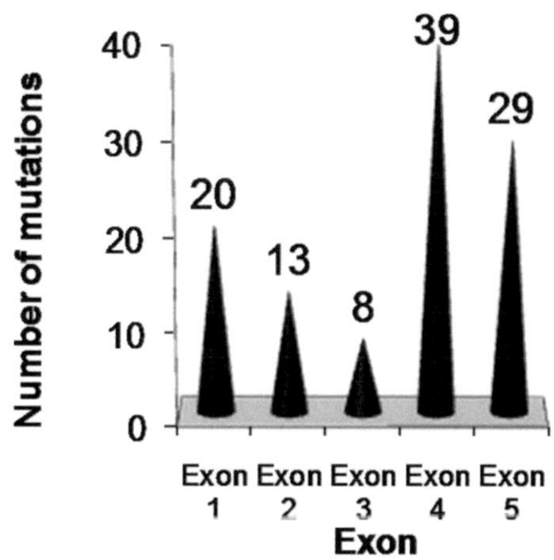

Figure 1. Number of SOD1 mutations identified for each exon

Most are autosomal dominant in inheritance, but there is one confirmed autosomal recessive mutation, the D90A mutation in exon 4. This is unique in that it exists in dominant families in a heterozygous state, but in a number of pedigrees, specifically those of Scandinavian ancestry, homozygous mutations are required for disease. (Andersen et al., 1997).

Mutations in the heavy polypeptide 200kDa subunit of neurofilaments (NEFH) have been identified in sporadic MND cases, (Figlewicz et al., 1994) and in one FALS case. (Al-Chalabi et al., 1999). Accumulation of neurofilaments in cell bodies and axons of motor neurons is a pathological hallmark of early stages of many neurodegenerative diseases. These mutations lie in the region of the protein involved in cross-linking and thus may disrupt normal aggregation of filaments. Thus far, 1 insertion and 5 deletion mutations have been identified on exon 4. Analysis of the NEFH locus on chromosome 22 however has failed to detect linkage in MND families. (Vechio et al., 1996). Genome search on a large pedigree with autosomal dominant juvenile onset MND found strong evidence for linkage to chromosome 9q34 (ALS4). The average age of onset is 17 years, with slow progression of disease. (Chance et al., 1998). There is also an autosomal recessive, juvenile onset MND, with linkage to a locus on chromosome 15 (ALS5). (Hentati et al., 1998).

The other 90% of all MND patients have the sporadic form. There is no recognisable phenotypic difference between FALS and sporadic MND. The male: female ratio is 1:1 in FALS and 1.7:1 in sporadic MND. (De Belleroche et al., 1995). This decreases with increasing age of onset and approaches 1:1 after the age of 70. (Haverkamp et al., 1995). The site of onset is variable. Survival does not seem to be affected by age or gender, but rather the site of symptom onset. Generally, bulbar onset disease has a worse prognosis, and upper limb onset is more favourable. (Mulder et al., 1986).

It has be postulated that sporadic MND may be the final development of a chain of events that may be set in motion at one or more places in the central nervous system by endogenous and exogenous causes, or both. The aetiology of MND however remains unknown and is probably multifactorial. (Eisen 1995). There is no evidence to support the cause of sporadic MND being due to accumulation of heavy metals in the environment, (Needleman, 1997), deficiencies or excess of essential trace metals, (Mena et al., 1967) or exposure to environmental poisons and industrial solvents. (Leigh, 1997). There is also no evidence to support the cause of sporadic MND being due excessive physical activity or antecedent trauma.

4. Possible patterns of motor neurone loss

In normal healthy individuals, it has been shown that there is little loss of functioning motor neurones before the age of 60. The normal aging process then accounts for loss of approximately 3.9% of the original motor neurone pool per annum after the age of 60. (Brown, 1972). In this situation, the number of motor neurones remain fairly constant up to the age of 60, after which there is a gradual steady decline with age.

MND may be due to a slow attrition of motor neurones over time (Pattern 1 in Figure 2). If this were the case, pre-symptomatic motor neurone loss may be identifiable in SOD1 mutation carriers, as eventually there may be a gradual decline over time (Figure 2).

Another possible course of MND is that normal numbers of motor neurones are maintained until sudden, rapid multi-focal cell death of motor neurones occurs, corresponding with the development of symptoms (Pattern 2 in Figure 2). If this situation, it would be expected that SOD1 mutation carriers have a normal number of motor neurones during the pre-symptomatic phase. In this case, cell death occurs as neurones gradually accumulate damage, secondary to the mutation, which ultimately overwhelms cellular homeostasis. This is the cumulative damage hypothesis. (Clarke et al., 2000).

One of the mechanisms most frequently proposed to underlie cumulative damage is oxidative stress, in which an imbalance between the production of reactive oxygen species and cellular antioxidant mechanisms results in chemical modifications of macromolecules, thereby disrupting cellular structure and function. (Robberecht, 2000). A key prediction of the cumulative damage hypothesis is that the probability that any individual neurone will become committed to apoptosis increases as damage accrues within it. A mutant neurone in an older patient will have accumulated a greater amount of damage and is therefore be more likely to die than in a younger patient. Consequently, early in the course of disease, the chance of a cell containing a sufficient amount of damage to initiate apoptosis is small, and the rate of cell loss is correspondingly low. However, as the amount of intracellular damage increases, the chance that a cell will die also increases

It has been shown that the kinetics of neuronal death in a number of inherited neurodegenerative diseases was best explained by models in which the risk of cell death remains constant throughout life of the neurone and that cell death occurred randomly in time and was

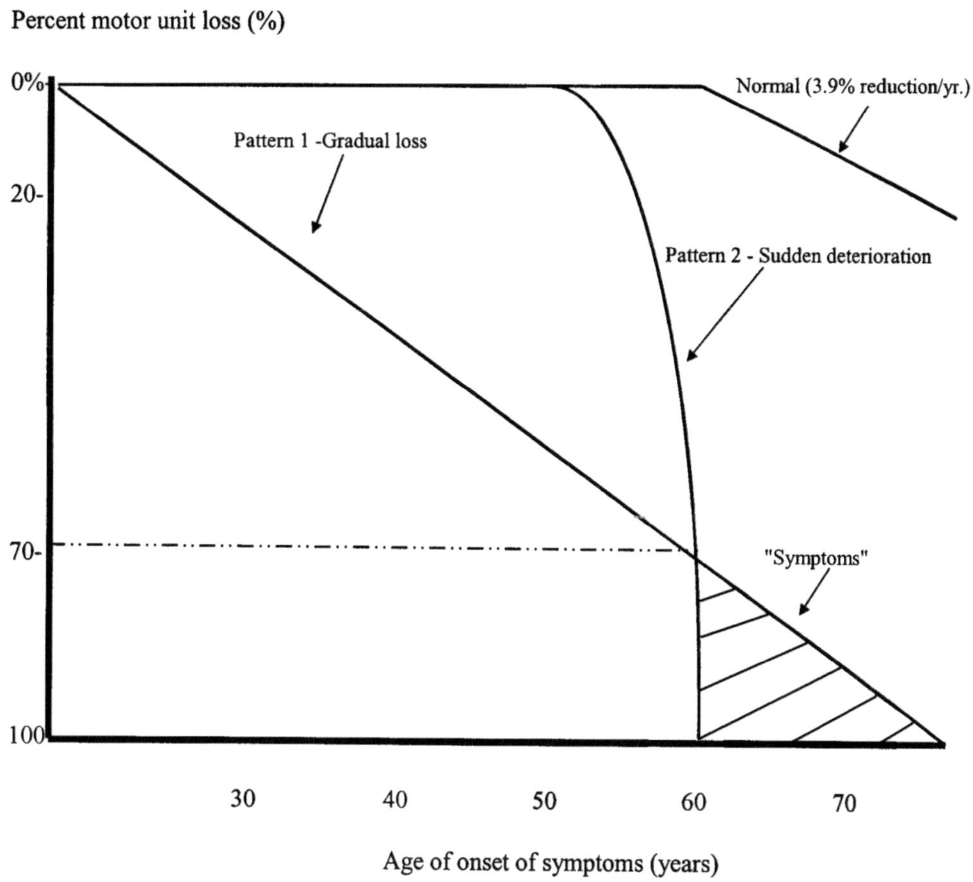

Figure 2. Diagrammatic representation of possible patterns for motor neurone loss in an individual.

independent of any other neurone. This implies a "one-hit" biochemical phenomenon in which the mutant imposes an abnormal mutant steady state on the neurone and a single catastrophic event randomly initiates cell death and apoptosis. The principal features of the mutant steady state are that the living mutant neurones function very well for years or even decades and that the predominant feature of the mutant neurones is that they are all at a risk of death. This argues against the multiple environmental factors hypothesis as a cause of MND, as a random process is probably responsible for the initiation of disease. (Clarke et al., 2001).

5. Cu/Zn Superoxide Dismutase (SOD1) mutations

Linkage studies for familial MND (FALS) on chromosome 21q22.1 led to the identification of point mutations in the gene for Cu/Zn superoxide dismutase (SOD1) as a cause of MND. (Siddique 1991). Superoxide (O2-) is an unstable and highly active molecule, which causes oxidation of cell constituents either directly or through toxic and stable derivatives. The major superoxide dismutase activity in cytoplasm is from SOD1, which consists of 5 small exons that encode 153 highly conserved amino acids with a molecular weight of 16Kda. SOD1 is a homodimer. Within each monomer, there is an active site containing one atom each of copper and zinc. (Radunovic & Leigh, 1996).

The most common SOD1 gene mutation seen in FALS is an alanine to valine shift at codon 4 (Ala4Val). This accounts for 50% of all mutations in the USA. (Rosen, 1993). Of all the clinical variables, only bulbar onset and three specific mutations seem to influence age of onset of MND. Bulbar patients are older when their illness begins, whereas the Gly37Arg and Leu38Val mutations predict an earlier age of onset.). Leu38Val is associated with the earliest onset (mean 35.5 years) and Ile113Thr with the latest onset (mean 58.9 years).

In terms of survival, Ala4Val correlated with the shortest survival of 1.5 years. Whereas, Gly37Arg, Gly41Asp, and Gly93Ala mutation predicted longer survival. The mutations that predict earlier onset are not the same as those that correlate with shortest duration of disease. (Cudkowicz et al., 1997). This suggests that the factors that influence onset of disease differ from those that influence the rate of progression of the disease.

Determining the mechanism by which mutations in the Cu/Zn superoxide dismutase (SOD1) gene triggers the destruction of motor neurones causing MND remains a challenging and complex problem. Five primary hypotheses have been postulated for the pathogenesis of FALS (Figure 3). (Hand & Rouleau, 2002). At present the favoured hypotheses is that the mutation causes disease as a result of a toxic gain of function by the mutant SOD1 provoking selective neurotoxicity, probably disrupting the intracellular homeostasis of copper and/or protein aggregation. (Clevland, 1999).

The mutant SOD1 enzyme has altered reactivity with certain substrates, (Noor et al., 2003), in addition to the major superoxide dismutase activity. The SOD1 enzyme catalyses the reduction of hydrogen peroxide (H_2O_2), therefore acting as a peroxidase. This leads to the formation of hydoxyl radicals that can also alter the neurofilament network. Motor neurones have high-energy requirements and thus contain many mitochondria that generate superoxide radials (O_2-) through normal metabolism. SOD1 is an anti-oxidant defence which catalyses conversion of superoxide free radical anion (O2-) to hydrogen peroxide (H_2O_2), which is reduced to H_2O and O_2 by catalse. Mutations at SOD1 binding sites, alter the redox behaviour of the enzyme and destabilise the SOD1 ligand, leading to increased oxidative damage as hydrogen peroxide and its derivatives are toxic to the cell. (Yim et al., 1990).

This supports the hypothesis that the pathogenesis of SOD1 related FALS may be due to increased peroxidase activity of mutant SOD1 resulting in oxidative damage mainly to lipids of the cell membrane.

Mapping of the mutation sites predicted that these mutations destabilise the protein structure, leading to a less active enzyme i.e. "loss of function". This is however not supported by the fact that transgenic mice over expressing SOD1 gene developed disease similar to MND in humans, while those over-expressing normal SOD1 remained unaffected. This suggests that the mutant mice develop the disease independent of the level of SOD1 activity and suggests

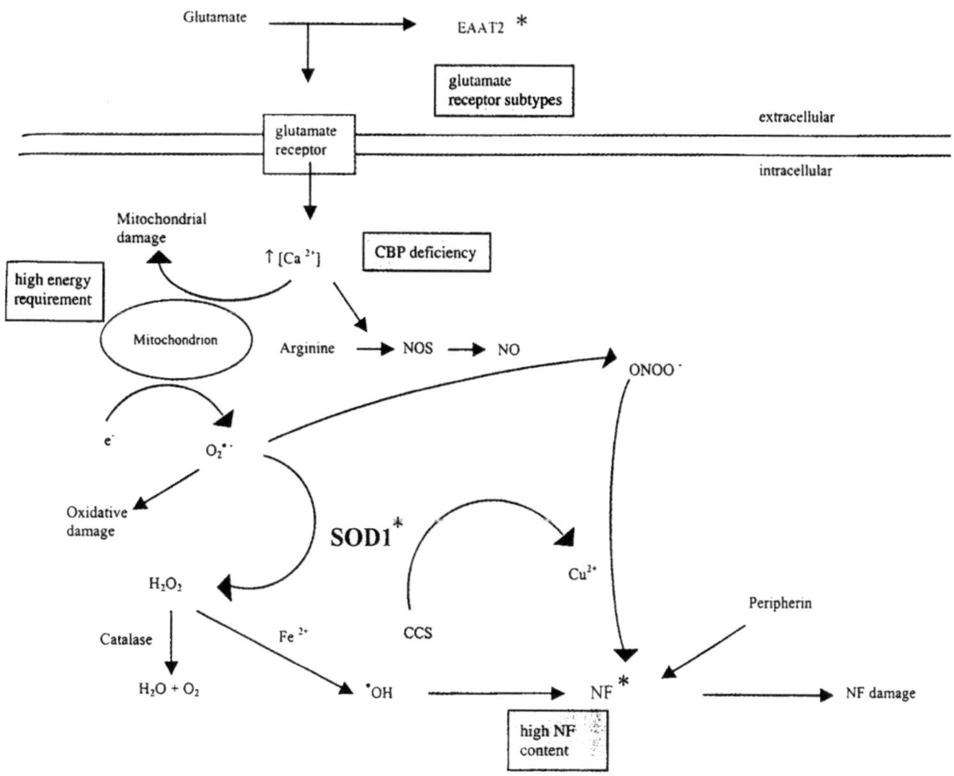

Figure 3. Pathways that have been implicated in motor neurone cell death in amyotrophic lateral sclerosis (Reproduced from Hand CK. Familial Amyotrophic Lateral Sclerosis. Muscle Nerve 2002; 25:137).

that the mutant protein itself is selectively toxic to motor neurones and that there is a "gain of toxic function" rather than a "loss of function". (Gurney et al., 1994). Also, although most mutations in SOD1 gene cause decrease in steady state of cytosolic SOD1 activity, Gly37Arg and Asp90Ala, have no significant decrease in SOD1 activity. (Shaw et al., 1998).

As most SOD1 mutations destabilise SOD1 protein (except Asp90Ala), it is possible that the mutant protein, with altered conformation may become unstable and precipitate to form aggregates or inclusions in motor neurons. These aggregates may then disturb normal cell function and lead to cell death. They are easily formed when SOD1 protein stability is decreased because this protein exists in large amounts accounting for 0.5-1% of total cytosolic protein in neurons. Alternations in the length of the coding sequence, folding, solubility or degradation results in the formation of aggregates. (Yim et al., 1990). Structural changes of mutant SOD1 may distort the rim of the electrostatic guidance channel and allow the catalytic site to become exposed and shallow. Molecules that are normally excluded may gain access to the catalytic reactive site. This results in less buffering of copper and zinc, which then become neurotoxic. (Radunovic & Leigh, 1996).

The nitric oxide (NO) produced by nitric oxide synthase (NOS) reacts spontaneously with O_2- to generate peroxynitrite ($ONOO^-$), which nitrosylates proteins leading to damage. Excess NO may also cause an increase in O_2- production by inhibition of mitochondrial electron flow, resulting in further generation of peroxynitrite. This facilitates nitrosylation of tyrosine residues of critical cytosolic proteins thus injuring cells. This reaction is copper dependent. The source of free copper may be mutant SOD1, which cannot accept the ion from the copper chaperone (CCS) protein. Mutant SOD1 possibly exhibit metal mediated cytotoxicities by disrupting the intracellular homeostasis of Cu and Zn, which are potential neurotoxins. (Gurney & Tomasselli, 1994).

The target proteins for nitrosylation include the neurofilament (NF) subunits, which may result in abnormal NF accumulation and subsequent disruption of the NF network and axonal transport, as there is a high neurofilament content in motor neurones. It has also been demonstrated that transgenes encoding mutant NF subunits can directly cause selective degeneration and death of motor neuones. (Cleveland, 1999). Conformational changes have been described in the mutations, Ala4Val, Gly37Arg and His6Arg that may affect the rim of the electrostatic guidance channel coded by exon 3. (Sjalander et al., 1995).

Glutamate is released from the presynaptic terminal activates the glutamate receptor on the postsynaptic cell membrane. It is then cleared from the synaptic cleft by specific glutamate transporters such as EAAT2. (Trotti et al., 1999). Astrocyte (glial cell) dysfunction may result in selective loss of EAAT2, interfering with the normal clearance of glutamate and allowing it to accumulate in the cell membrane and continue to activate the receptor. (Bruijin et al., 1997). Once activated, the glutamate receptor causes a calcium influx and a cascade of toxicity. The neurone does not have the capacity to buffer this efficiently due to a deficiency in calcium binding proteins (CBP's). This results in disturbances in mitochondrial metabolism and as a consequence, motor neurone cell death. (Beal, 1996).

To date, the only effective approved treatment for amyotrophic lateral sclerosis is Riluzole, (Cheah et al., 2010), which has a neuroprotective role, possibly due to pre-synaptic inhibition of glutamate release. (Doble, 1996). Treatment of human ALS patients or transgenic Cu, Zn superoxide dimutase 1 (SOD 1) mice, most commonly produce a modest but significant increase in survival. (Bensimon et al., 1994). It has also been shown to have a small beneficial effect on bulbar function, but not muscle strength. (Miller et al., 2007).

Apoptosis is characterised by a series of cellular changes leading to non-inflammatory cell death. Mitochondrial involvement in the apoptotic pathway also leads to the release of cytochrome c, an activator of the initiator caspase-9, which in turn activates caspase-3, which are executioners in the breakdown of essential cellular proteins. There is evidence that the mutant SOD1 transgene causes motor neurone death in mice through caspase-mediated programmed cell death. (Li et al., 2000). This may then be a target for inhibiting the apoptotic cascade, as it has been shown in a SOD1 transgenic mouse model that a small peptide caspase inhibitor (*zVAD-fmk*), prolonged survival after onset of disease by nearly 70%. (Kosti et al., 1997). It has also been reported that there are elevated levels of *bax* protein in MND spinal motor neurones, which promotes apoptosis. (Mu et al., 1996).

6. Methods

The Department of Molecular Medicine at Concord hospital had a large database of family members with a known family history of MND, who had blood samples collected for DNA, as part of a previous linkage study. From this database, family members were contacted by telephone by the department's genetic counsellor and informed about the study.

The regional committees for Ethics in Medical Research from Central Sydney Area Health Service, Royal North Shore Hospital and Prince Charles Hospital, approved this study.

All individuals participated without knowledge of their mutation status and on the understanding that this would not be revealed to them. Subjects were also aware that the results obtained from the study would not be available to them and that the information would only be used for research purposes. New consents were obtained from all individuals who participated in the study. The neurologist performing the MUNE studies also had no knowledge of their mutation status. The mutation status was only used in the final analysis of results. Subsequently, they were divided into "SOD1 negative family controls" and "asymptomatic SOD1 mutation carriers".

In addition, studies were also carried out on normal individuals, such as department technicians, spouses of SOD1 family members and individuals from the general population who attended MND support meeting and had an interest in helping to advance research into MND. This group was used as "population controls", to test the validity and reproducibility of the MUNE technique used.

Sporadic MND subjects were also initially studied once the MUNE technique had been validated to demonstrate that the MUNE technique used was able to detect a loss of motor neurones, when present. These were used as "positive controls".

6.1. Motor unit number estimation

Motor unit number estimation (MUNE) estimates the number of functioning lower motor neurones innervating a muscle or a group of muscles and is a measure of the primary pathologic process of motor neurone loss. The concept of motor unit number estimation (MUNE) originated in 1967. At the time there was no satisfactory method of assessing the extent of denervation in muscles during life. Analysis of the density of the electromyographic interference pattern during maximal effort was not quantitative, and required the full co-operation of the patient.

The principle of MUNE is that if one can measure the mean single motor unit amplitude (SMUP), it is possible to obtain an estimate of the total number of motor units in the muscle. The results achieved were comparable with estimates of alpha motor fibres obtained by counting axons in specimens of motor nerves. (McComas, 1971).

MUNE has been performed in a number of different ways, each with their advantages and limitations. (Stein & Yang, 1990). The choice of technique depends on the speed and simplicity of the technique, as well as its accuracy and reproducibility. Some methods sample a very small proportion of the number of motor units innervating a muscle (typically 10-20). The coefficient of variation associated with different methods range from 10-45%. (McComas, 1991). If the variability is too large, then the technique cannot be used to follow motor unit loss reliably over time.

The way the average single motor unit potential (SMUP) size is obtained distinguishes the several techniques available. Most employ electrical stimulation of the motor nerve to determine the sizes of the SMUP, but a few use needle EMG.

Each method measures both the average size of the potentials generated by single motor units - single motor unit potentials (SMUP) and the size of the compound muscle action potential (CMAP) obtained with maximal stimulation of a motor nerve.

The motor unit number estimate is calculated by:

$$\text{MUNE}=\frac{\text{Maximum CMAP amplitude (or area)}}{\text{Average single motor unit potential (SMUP) amplitude or area.}}$$

Whereas the methods of measuring the average SMUP differ, they have common assumptions about the measurement of the supramaximal CMAP and the measurement of the average SMUP.

i. Maximal stimulation of any peripheral motor nerve activates all the muscles innervated by that nerve distal to the point of stimulation. Therefore, measurements of the CMAP are the summation of activity from multiple muscles and the MUNE is more accurately an estimate of the number of motor units in a group of muscles rather than in a single muscle.

For example, the median CMAP recorded at abductor pollicis brevis (APB) is more correctly a "thenar MUNE", as it is a summation of the activity of APB, opponens pollicis, flexor pollicis brevis, and to a lesser extent, the lateral lumbricals.

Extensor digitorum brevis (EDB) on the other hand, is a muscle innervated by the deep peroneal nerve. The only source of interfering muscle action potential is from extensor hallucis longus, which can be reduced by correct position of the stimulating electrodes. The muscle belly is flat in profile, eliminating deeper motor units as a cause of small potentials. The recording electrode is placed transversely across the innervation zone, resulting in a simple biphasic negative-positive M wave.

ii. The motor unit potentials used in the calculation of the average SMUP are representative of those generated by the total population of units. All methods, select a subset of the total population of motor units, measure their sizes and calculate an average SMUP for that subgroup.

iii. Finally, there is a phenomenon caused "alternation". This refers to fluctuations in the CMAP amplitude of the same motor unit with similar stimulation intensities. The thresholds of the first few motor axons excited are not sufficiently separate from one another, so that when graded increases in the stimulus intensity occur, the motor axons excited often overlap and add more than one SMUP to the CMAP being recorded. This can result in an underestimation of the mean SMUP size, as it may appear that there are 7 or 8 motor units when there are only 2 or 3 present, which in turn results in an over-estimation of the MUNE.

6.2. Statistical MUNE method

We used the statistical electrophysiological technique of motor unit number estimation (MUNE), (Daube, 1998), was used to estimate the number of motor units in thenar and extensor digitorum brevis muscles. The statistical method estimates the average size of SMUP's and the number of motor units in a group of muscles innervated by the nerve being stimulated, based on the normal variation of the submaximal CMAP evoked with constant stimuli. No attempt is made to identify individual motor unit potentials. The method relies on the known relation between the variance of multiple measures of step functions and the size of the individual steps when the steps have a Poisson distribution. S.D. Poisson was a French mathematician (1781-1840).

Poisson statistics are useful when the distribution arising for events occur randomly in time or when small particles are distributed randomly in space. They have been used to calculate the number of quanta released from a nerve terminal at the neuromuscular junction when the individual quanta are too small to be distinguished, as in myasthenia gravis. (Lomen-Hoerth & Slawnych, 2003).

In pure Poisson statistics, the size of a series of measurements is multiples of the size of a single component. In a Poisson distribution there is a discrete asymmetrical distribution in which responses are found at some levels and others where there are no responses (Figure 4). (McNeil, 1996).

A pure Poisson distribution has decreasing numbers at higher values. In Poisson distribution, the variance of these 30 measurements is equal to the size of the individual components making up each measurement. The variance can thus provide an estimate of the average size of the SMUP's.

The statistical method looks only at variance of the CMAP and does not require identification of individual components. It can be used when the sizes of SMUP's are too small to be isolated. The statistical method assumes that each motor unit has a similar size and that it is the same size each time it is activated.

Sequences of 30 submaximal stimuli are given. The inherent variability of the threshold of individual axons causes variations in the size of the CMAP. The average change in the submaximal CMAP amplitude caused by alternation (addition and subtraction of motor axons) is derived by Poisson statistics.

The occurrence of alternation with changing units that are activated does not modify the accuracy of the statistical method, because the method is a statistical measurement, a different result is found with each series of 30 stimuli. Therefore, multiple trials are needed to obtain the most accurate measurement. (Olney et al., 2000).

Experimental testing with trials of >300 stimuli has shown that repeated measurement of groups of 30 until the standard deviation of the repeated trials is <10% provides a close estimate of the number obtained with many more stimuli.[86] Estimates of the SMUP size and of the number of motor units are also most reliable if made at multiple different stimulus intensities to test axons with different thresholds.

MUNE is calculated with the number weighted statistical method, where the mean SMUP amplitude at each level is multiplied by the number of motor units estimated at each level.

The steps in statistical MUNE are as follows:

1. Recording surface electrodes are applied as for standard nerve conduction studies.
2. An initial scan of the CMAP is performed using a series of 30 submaximal stimuli at 1 Hz, increasing in equal increments to identify unusually large steps at which further information is required.
3. On the basis of the scan, three or four 10% stimulus ranges are identified, according to an internal algorithm. Usually, one range includes the smallest step and the other ranges where the steps are >15% (Figure 4).
4. At each intensity, groups of 30 responses are captured at a rate of 3Hz. Estimates are most reliable if 10 groups of 30 responses are recorded. To minimise patient discomfort, however, repetition is repeated until the standard error of the MUNE SMUP size is less than 10%.
5. Statistical MUNE estimates the average size of SMUP's and the number of motor units in a group of muscles innervated by the nerve being stimulated, based on the normal variation of the sub-maximal CMAP evoked with constant stimuli (Figure 5).

The statistical technique of estimating the size of the SMUP was performed using proprietary software on a Nicolet Viking IV electromyography machine. This technique uses direct stimulation of the motor nerve. The low frequency filter was set at 2 Hz and the high frequency filter at 5 kHz. The gain for extensor digitorum brevis was set at 2 mV/div and for abductor pollicis brevis studies at 5 mV/div. The sweep speed was 2 ms/div. This method had excellent test-retest reproducibility (+/-2.8%). The method was quick to use and well tolerated.

This technique has been greatly modified since its original description, but numerous studies have shown that MUNE can change systematically in ALS patients when used by experienced technicians, even though evaluator bias needs to be taken into account. (Shefner et al., 2004). The statistical MUNE method has also been shown to be unreliable in the presence of clinical weakness due to motor unit instability. (Shefner, 2009).

Our study however was performed on asymptomatic patients, without clinical weakness.

6.3. MUNE Technique

Motor unit numbers were estimated in abductor pollicis brevis (resulting in a thenar MUNE) and the extensor digitorum brevis (EDB) muscle. These muscles were used, as both are easily

http://dx.doi.org/10.5772/56559

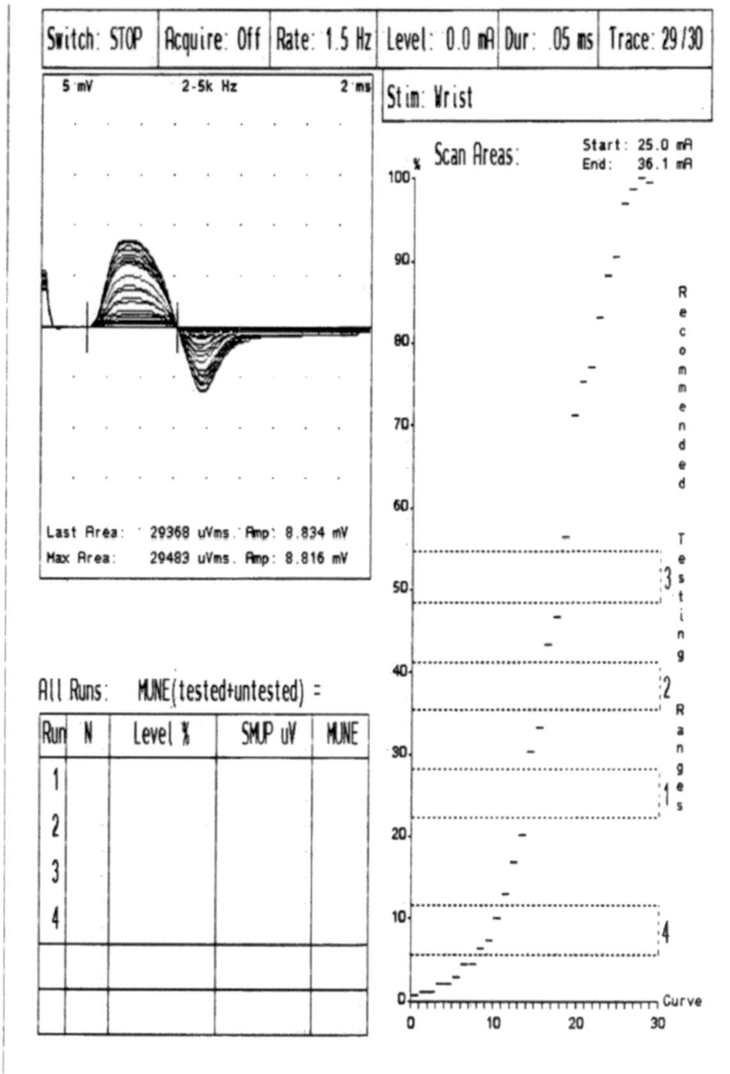

Figure 4. An initial scan of the CMAP (right) recorded from APB muscles in response to 30 sub-maximal stimuli (x-axis) with equal increments between threshold and maximum stimulation. On the basis of the scan, 10% stimulus ranges are identified, according to an internal algorithm. The CMAP increments are shown at the top left and the eventual table of results in the bottom left corner.

accessible distal muscles. The electrical activity can be recorded without interference, and in the case of EDB, the muscle belly is flat.

Self-adhesive surface recording electrodes (G1) were placed transversely across the innervation zone of each muscle, resulting in a simple biphasic negative-positive M wave, with G2 placed over a bony prominence. The deep peroneal nerve was stimulated just above the ankle and the median nerve at the wrist with a surface stimulator. This was performed by strapping

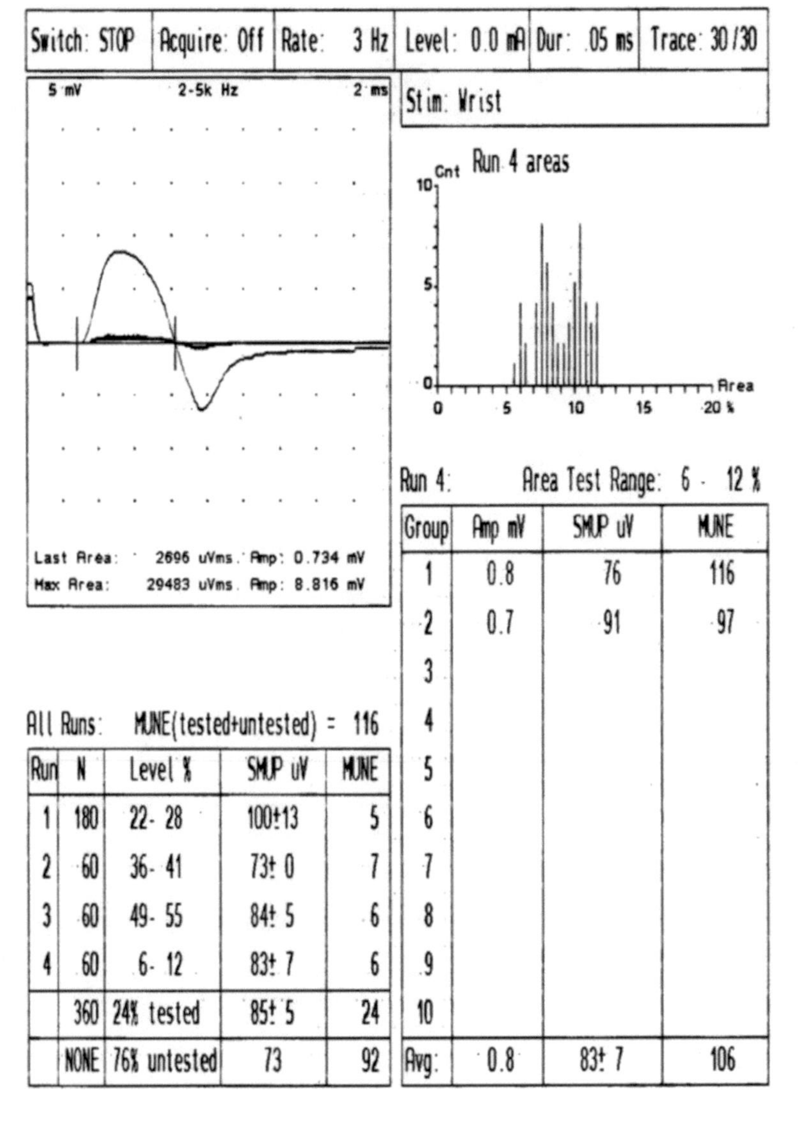

Figure 5. At each intensity level (runs 1-4), groups of 30 responses are captured at a rate of 3Hz. The CMAP amplitudes are shown at the top left, with the histogram of results at the top right. The thenar MUNE results from repeated trials are shown in the bottom left table.

the stimulating electrode onto the surface of the skin, at the point where the threshold of the nerve to electrical stimulation was at its' lowest. A hand-held stimulator was not used, as reproducibility is enhanced when the stimulating electrodes are fixed to the surface of the skin.

Initially, bilateral thenar and EDB MUNE's were obtained from all subjects. After the reproducibility phase of the study, generally only right-sided studies were performed. Once a reduction in MUNE was identified, bilateral studies were once again performed on selected subjects. The protocol was also modified depending on the subjects' tolerance to the procedure.

Median nerve stimulation at the wrist for thenar MUNE was generally well tolerated by most subjects, as the stimulation intensity required to obtain an adequate response was generally less than 20mA with duration of 0.05-0.1ms.

Peroneal nerve stimulation required for EDB MUNE resulted in slightly more discomfort, as the nerve is located further away from the surface of the skin. The stimulus intensity required, in some cases was up to 50-80mA with duration of between 0.1-0.3ms. Some subjects indicated that they were unwilling to continue to participate in the study due to the discomfort caused by performing EDB MUNE. In these subjects, only thenar MUNE's were performed.

To assess the test-retest reproducibility of the technique, SOD1 family members and population controls were followed over a 1-year period, with thenar and EDB MUNE tests repeated every 3 to 6 months. The difference between MUNE results from the first and second study, and if possible, first and third studies were divided by the MUNE of the first study, and expressed as a percentage change. The results were analysed using Pearson and Spearman correlation coefficients.

All results were entered into a database and analysed using a standard statistical software package (SPSS 9.05 for Windows). For the initial part of the study, the MUNE results from asymptomatic SOD1 mutation carriers were grouped together. Although different mutations in SOD1 have different effects on the progression of the disease once symptoms occur, these different mutations do not influence on the age of onset of symptoms.[67]

Motor unit estimates in carriers were compared to age and sex matched family controls without the SOD1 mutation, and sporadic (non-SOD1) MND patients. To determine whether groups had different numbers of motor units, an unpaired t-test was used. Although there were some outlying results, the distributions were not sufficiently skewed to contradict the use of the t-test. Statistical significance was accepted at a p-value of <0.05.

The group of asymptomatic SOD1 mutation carriers were followed over the next 2 to 5 years, depending on the volunteers' motivation, both clinically and by MUNE. Results were compared to their initial baseline MUNE and the date of the study when this reduction was first detected, was used as the date when motor neurone loss commenced.

6.4. Maximal voluntary isometric contraction testing

It has been suggested that the traditional neurological examination is inadequate for documenting motor performance impairment with reliability. (Hanten et al., 1999). Generally, manual motor testing used in a standard neurological motor examination does not allow objective documentation of change in performance, as it may be influenced by the patient's history and progress. Major changes are apparent, but subtle changes are difficult to determine with accuracy.

There are a number of methods that have been developed to quantify maximal voluntary isometric contraction (MVIC). It has been proposed that this is a clinically useful, reliable, reproducible, time efficient and quantitative measure for monitoring disease progression in MND. (Hoagland et al., 1997). This would be surprising, given that in a slowly progressive denervating process, patients with substantial chronic denervation could maintain normal muscle twitch tension until loss of about 70-80% of motor units occurs. (McComas, 1971).

The methods used to quantify maximal voluntary isometric contraction have included an electronic strain-gauge tensiometer and a hand-held Jamar hydraulic dynamometer. In this study, maximum bilateral isometric grip strength was obtained using the Jamar hydraulic dynamometer to determine whether this correlated with the number of functional motor neurones in the thenar group of muscles, as measured by MUNE. Standardised (middle handle) positioning and instructions were given to all subjects. Handgrip force was measured with subjects in the sitting position and with the arm flexed at 90 degrees. Two trials were performed on each hand, and the best result used for analysis. This method was used as previous studies of grip strength reliability showed that there was no significant difference in reliability between one attempt, the mean score of two or three attempts, or the highest score of three attempts. (Hamilton et al., 1994).

Clinical neurological examination was performed, with power of thumb abduction, finger flexion and finger abduction measured according to the Medical Research Council (MRC) grading system and compared to thenar (APB) MUNE.

Felice showed that in twenty one MND patients, changes in thenar MUNE was the most sensitive outcome measure for following disease progression, when compared to other quantitative tests, such as CMAP, isometric grip strength, forced vital capacity and Medical Research Council manual muscle testing. (Felice, 1997).

7. Results

7.1. Demographics

A total of eighty-eight (88) subjects (45 males and 43 females) gave informed consent. The subjects were divided into four test groups.

1. 24 population controls;
2. 32 SOD1 negative (normal) family controls;
3. 20 asymptomatic (pre-clinical) SOD1 mutation carriers (test group),
    a. 5 subjects with point mutation in exon 4, codon 100, GAA to GGA, Glu to Gly) – glu100gly;
    b. 5 subjects with point mutation in exon 4, codon 113, ATT to ACT, Ile to Thr) – ile113thr;
    c. 5 subjects with point mutation in exon 5; codon 148, GTA to GGA, Val to Gly) – val148gly;
    d. 5 subjects with point mutation in exon 5, codon 148, GTA to GGA, Val to Ile) val148ile.

	Thenar (APB) muscle	
	Cases	MUNE (Range)
Population Controls	24	148 (115-254)
SOD1 Negative Family Controls	32	138 (106-198)
SOD1 Mutation Carriers	20	144 (109–199)
Sporadic MND patients	12	45 (5–84)

Table 1. Thenar (APB) motor unit number estimates (MUNE number represents mean MUNE).

4. 12 sporadic symptomatic MND patients (positive controls).

There was no statistically significant difference in age distribution between these groups, with a range of 16 to 73 years of age.

7.2. Motor units in asymptomatic FALS (SOD1) carriers

For the initial part of the study, the baseline MUNE results were grouped together and the means of the groups were compared. The initial aim of the study was to determine if MND was due to a slow gradual attrition of motor neurones over time. If this were the case, the group of asymptomatic SOD1 mutation carriers, would be expected to have a reduced number of motor units, indicating the presence of pre-clinical motor neurone loss. Motor unit estimates in the group of asymptomatic SOD1 mutation carriers were compared to age and sex matched family controls without the SOD1 mutation, and sporadic (non-SOD1) MND patients. To determine whether groups had different numbers of motor units, an unpaired t-test was used. Statistical significance was accepted at a p-value of <0.05.

The numbers of motor units in the groups of population controls, SOD1 negative family controls and asymptomatic SOD1 mutation carriers were similar. In population controls the mean thenar MUNE was 148 with a range of 115 - 254, in SOD1 negative family controls was 138 with a range of 106 - 198 and in asymptomatic SOD1 mutation carriers, 144 with a range of 109 - 199. There was no detectable difference in the mean number of thenar motor units in the group of asymptomatic SOD1 mutation carriers compared to the group of SOD1 negative family controls (thenar $p>0.46$), or population controls (thenar $p>0.70$) (Table 1 and Figure 6).

In population controls the mean EDB MUNE was 138 with a range of 119 - 169, in SOD1 negative family controls was 134 with a range of 107 - 180 and in asymptomatic SOD1 mutation carriers, 136 with a range of 111 - 187.

Once again, there was no detectable difference in the mean number of EBD motor units in the group of asymptomatic SOD1 mutation carriers compared to the group of SOD1 negative family controls (EDB $p>0.95$), or population controls (EDB $p>0.50$) (Table 2 and Figure 7).

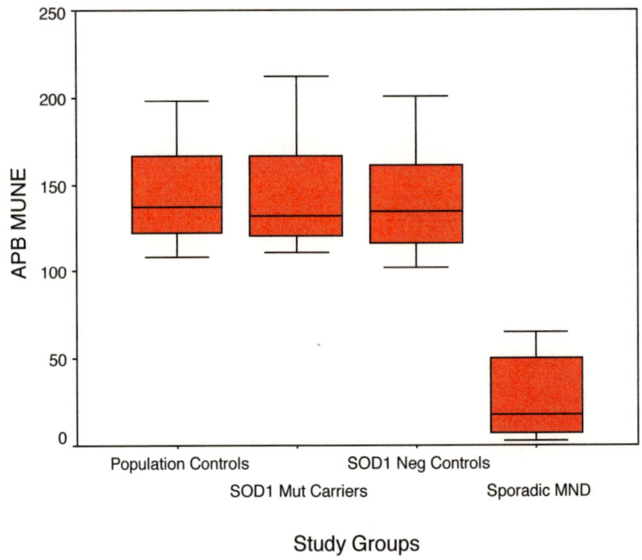

Figure 6. Baseline thenar (APB) MUNE subdivided into study groups (The lower boundary of the box is the 25th percentile, and the upper border is the 75th percentile of MUNE. The horizontal line inside the box represents the median MUNE. The whispers represent the largest and smallest observed values, i.e. the range). Data is shown in Table 1.

	Extensor Digitorum Brevis	
	Cases	**MUNE (Range)**
Population Controls	13	138 (119-169)
SOD1 Negative Family Controls	30	134 (107-180)
SOD1 Mutation Carriers	14	136 (111-187)
Sporadic MND patients	9	70 (8-82)

Table 2. EDB motor unit number estimates (MUNE number represents mean MUNE).

Symptomatic sporadic MND subjects showed a definite loss of motor units with fewer motor units compared to all other groups (p<0001) with a mean thenar MUNE of 45 with a range of 5 - 84 and a mean EDB MUNE of 70 with a range of 8 - 82 (Tables 1 and 2).

There was no cross over between thenar and EDB MUNE results in symptomatic and asymptomatic subjects.

7.3. Reproducibility of MUNE technique

To assess the test-retest reproducibility of the technique, 69 of the 88 SOD1 family members and population controls were followed over a 1-year period, with thenar and extensor

http://dx.doi.org/10.5772/56559

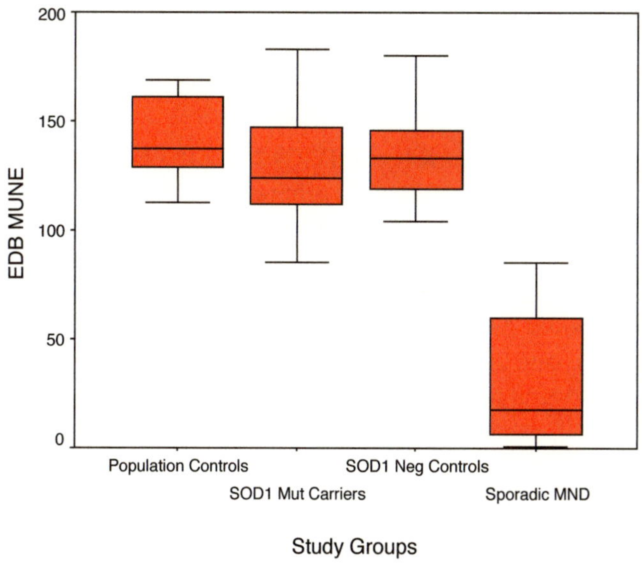

Figure 7. Baseline EDB MUNE subdivided into study groups (The lower boundary of the box is the 25th percentile, and the upper border is the 75th percentile of MUNE. The horizontal line inside the box represents the median MUNE. The whispers represent the largest and smallest observed values, i.e. the range). Data is shown in Table 2.

digitorum brevis (EDB) MUNE tests repeated every 3-6 months, depending on patient availability. The difference between MUNE results from the first and second study, and if possible, first and third studies were divided by the MUNE of the first study, and expressed as a percentage change. The results were analysed using Pearson and Spearman correlation coefficients.

The test-retest correlation of thenar MUNE in asymptomatic subjects was high with a Pearson correlation coefficient of 0.93. The mean difference between MUNE results on separate occasions on the same individual was +/- 3.6%, with a range of 0-11.7% (Table 3).

	Number of Cases	**Mean MUNE**
Thenar 1	88	145.7
Thenar 2	69	140.1
Thenar 3	33	140.0
Thenar Change	**Range (0 - 11.7%)**	**3.6%**

Table 3. Reproducibility of mean thenar (APB) motor unit number estimates in asymptomatic subjects on separate reviews over a one-year period.

For EDB MUNE, the Pearson correlation coefficient was also high, 0.88, with a mean difference between MUNE results on separate occasions on the same individual of +/- 4.6%, with a range of 0-15.7%. The test-retest correlation was high with a Pearson correlation coefficient of 0.91, when groups were broken down into the different study groups.

7.4. Maximal voluntary isometric contraction

Maximal voluntary isometric contraction (MVIC), using the Jamar hand dynamometer was used to measure isometric grip strength to determine whether this correlated with the number of functional motor neurones in the thenar group of muscles as measured by MUNE. Isometric grip strength tests, thenar MUNE and MRC power were performed on 69 asymptomatic subjects twice within a 3-6 month period to assess the test-retest reproducibility of this technique. Pearson correlation coefficients between study 1 and study 2 of right hand grip strength was 0.941, left hand grip strength 0.910 and thenar MUNE results 0.937. These results indicate that the reproducibility of these techniques was high.

Right hand grip strength correlated with left hand grip strength, with Pearson correlation coefficients of 0.959 and Spearman correlation coefficients of 0.956 Two-way analyses of variance showed a no significant difference between the right and left hands (Figure 8). There was no correlation between right grip strength and right thenar motor unit number, with Pearson correlation coefficients of 0.483 and Spearman correlation coefficient of 0.34 (Figure 9).

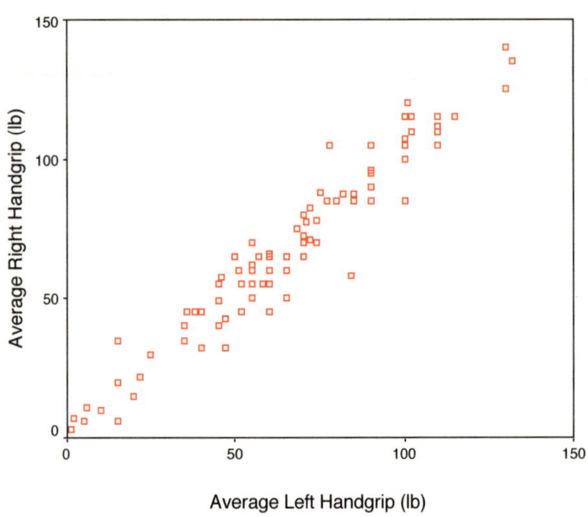

Figure 8. Graph showing the correlation between right and left handgrip

7.5. Detection of pre-symptomatic motor neurone loss in SOD1 mutation carriers

The MUNE results, after validating their reproducibility, were used as a baseline to follow the number of motor units over time in individual pre-symptomatic SOD1 mutation carriers over the next 2-5 years, to determine whether pattern of motor neurone loss is either a slow attrition of motor neurones over time or whether normal numbers of motor neurones are maintained

http://dx.doi.org/10.5772/56559

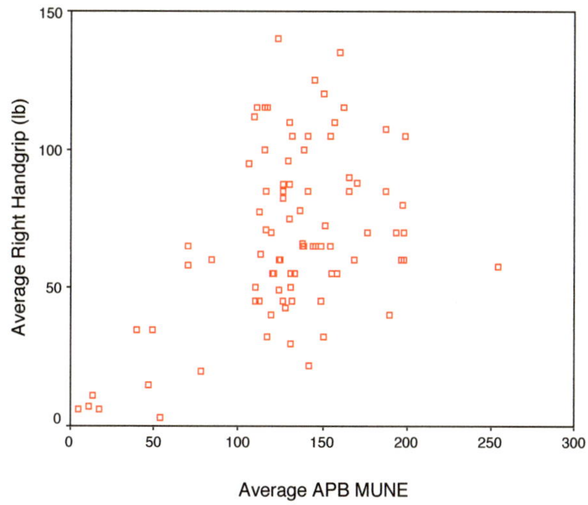

Figure 9. Scatter graph showing the lack of correlation between right handgrip and right thenar (APB) MUNE

until sudden, rapid multi-focal cell death of motor neurones occurs, corresponding with the development of symptoms.

During the course of the study, 5 of the SOD1 mutation carriers developed leg weakness. A significant fall in motor unit number was detected in these 5 SOD1 mutation carriers, were there was a detectable reduction of motor units, 4-10 months prior to the onset of weakness and the diagnosis of familial ALS being made. There was no detectable loss of motor units in the other 15 SOD1 mutation carriers or in the group of SOD1 mutation negative relatives, during the study period.

In individual cases, there was:

51% loss of motor units, 4 months prior to onset of weakness in Case 1

37% loss of motor units, 10 months prior to onset of weakness in Case 2

28% loss of motor units, 6 months prior to onset of weakness in Case 3

46% loss of motor units, 6 months prior to onset of weakness in Case 4

68% loss of motor units, 8 months prior to onset of weakness in Case 5

There was further motor unit loss as weakness progressed, at which point the diagnosis of MND was confirmed.

7.5.1. Case study 1

A 43-year-old sister of case 1. She had the same strong family history of ALS, with a point mutation in SOD1 gene at val148gly. Her pedigree is shown in Figure 10. She was asymptomatic at the time of recruitment with a normal neurological examination, and no evidence of

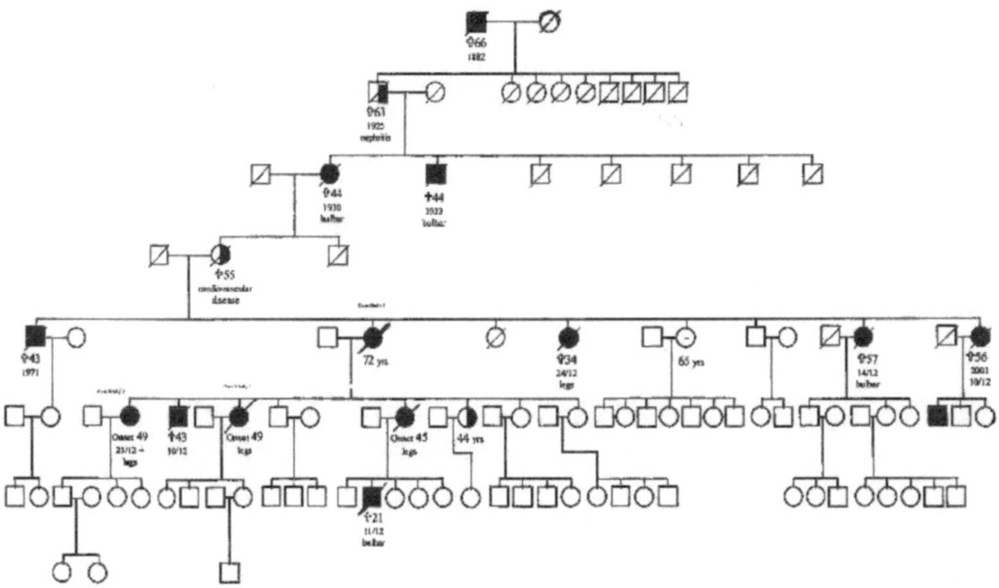

Figure 10. Pedigree of cases 1, 2 and 3

wasting, weakness or fasciculation. Her right and left thenar MUNE's remained stable for the first 2½ years of the study at around 115-120 motor units. Progress MUNE results are shown in Table 4 and Figures 11.

Over the next 6 months, there was a reduction in her right thenar MUNE to 96 (20%) and her left thenar MUNE to 89 (19%), with no detectable weakness. Her right EDB MUNE also dropped from 111 to 92 (17%), but she only had detectable weakness 10 months later of MRC grade 4+/5 in right dorsiflexors, at which time her right EDB MUNE had dropped further to 71 motor units (35%). The left EDB MUNE also dropped from a baseline of 112 (2 years previously) to 89 (20%), but with no detectable weakness.

An independent neurologist performed needle EMG examination, which showed high amplitude motor units with reduced recruitment in vastus medialis, tibialis anterior and extensor carpi radialis longus, bilaterally but no fibrillation potentials were seen. It was felt that these changes were not enough to make the diagnosis of ALS.

In view of her strong family history, a presumed diagnosis of familial ALS was made and she was commenced on Riluzole in February 2002.

Over the next 3 years, her EDB MUNE results have stabilised. Her weakness has not progressed significantly. In February 2004, she still had MRC grade 4+/5 power of her right dorsiflexors and no symptomatically apparent weakness in her left dorsiflexors or upper limbs.

Months pre and post weakness 1st detected	-42	-40	-37	-29	-20	-10	0	+11	+21	+27
Date of study	Oct-98	Dec-98	Mar-99	Nov-99	Jul-00	Jan-01	Nov-01	Oct-02	Aug-03	Feb-04
R Handgrip	60	60	65	65	60	70	65	65	65	65
R Thenar MUNE	111	111	117	119	120	114	96	97	86	85
L Handgrip	60	55	60	65	63	65	65	60	60	60
L Thenar MUNE	117				119	111	89	86	79	81
R EDB power	5/5	5/5	5/5	5/5	5/5	5/5	4+/5	4+/5	4+/5	4+/5
R EDB MUNE	104	111	119	108	104	92	71	75	75	65
L EDB power	5/5	5/5	5/5	5/5	5/5	5/5	5/5	5/5	5/5	5/5
L EDB MUNE	112						89	80	80	81

Table 4. Case 1 progressive handgrip, dorsiflexion power and thenar and EDB MUNE results

7.5.2. Case study 2

A 57-year-old man with a strong family history of ALS dating back 3 generations, had a point mutation in exon 4, codon 100, GAA to GGA, Glu to Gly) – glu100gly. He was initially recruited into the study in 1998, but as he was unable to tolerate the EDB MUNE test, he elected not to continue to participate in the study. He represented 11 years later with a 3 month history of lower limb weakness, which he noticed only when he walked long distances and up stairs. He had also been experiencing lower limb cramps and muscle fasciculations for years.

On examination, he had no evidence of wasting, but there were muscle fasciculations seen in his right quadriceps. His tone was normal in the upper and lower limbs and he had MRC grade 5/5 power in all muscle groups, proximally and distally. His sensory examination was normal to touch, vibration and position. His gait was normal.

Nerve conduction studies performed by independent neurologist were normal, with no evidence of a large fibre peripheral neuropathy and normal CMAP amplitudes. Needle EMG studies was also normal, with no evidence of active or chronic denervation in bilateral distal and proximal muscles sampled. Using the same MUNE machine and computer algorithm, as 1998, a reduction in his APB MUNE was detectable. Despite the "normal EMG" findings, a presumptive diagnosis of fALS was made. He was commenced on Riluzole therapy 50 mg twice a day. Within 3 months, he noticed an improvement in the symptoms and there was a detectable improvement in MUNE by 40-52%. He was able to walk up stairs easier, walk 100 metres without stopping and lower limb cramps and fasciculations disappeared. Unfortunately, due to poor tolerance, further studies have not been possible. MUNE results are shown in Table 5.

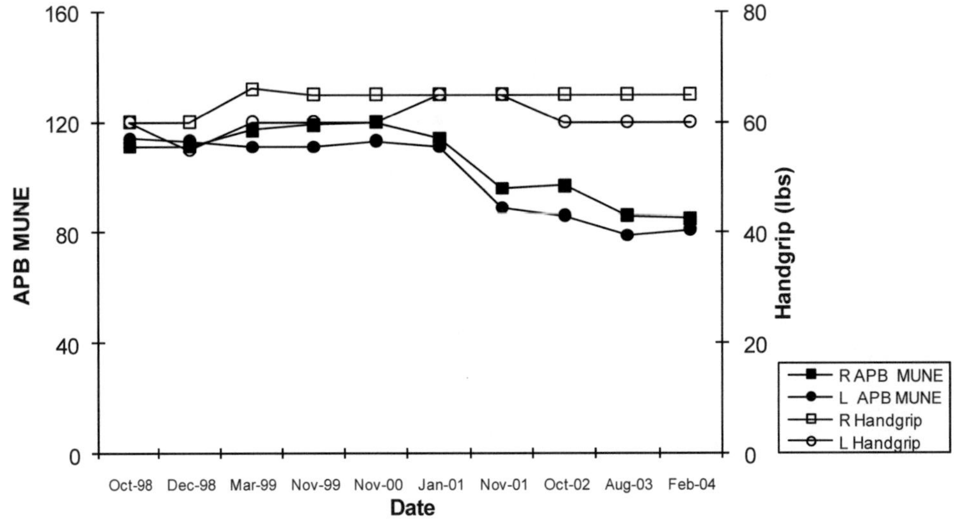

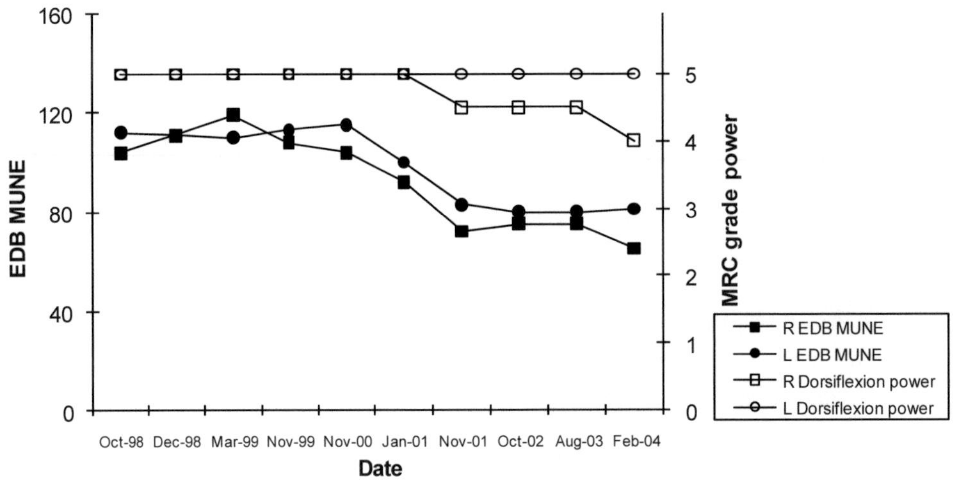

Figure 11. Progressive results of case 1 showing the change in APB and EDB motor unit estimates over time in relation to handgrip strength and power. There is a reduction of APB and EDB MUNE even though strength has remained stable.

7.5.3. Case study 3

A 43-year old lady with an extensive family history of ALS dating back 4 generations, had a point mutation in exon 5, codon 148, GTA to GGA, Val to Gly) – val148gly. She presented with generalised muscle fasciculations, but no weakness or cramps.

On examination, she had no wasting or fasciculations. Her tone, power, reflexes and sensation in the upper and lower limbs were normal. Her gait was steady and she was able to walk on her heels and toes. Tandem walking was normal and Romberg's sign was negative.

	May-98	July-09	Nov-09
Months	**Baseline**	**13 months**	**4 months**
		Riluzole commenced	
R Handgrip	105	95	80
L Handgrip	110	105	90
R APB MUNE	198	86 (56% decrease)	125 45% increase)
L APB MUNE		88	124
R ADM MUNE	110	95	
L ADM MUNE		85	
R EDB MUNE	Not tolerated	59	90 (52% increase)
L EDB MUNE		67	94 (40% increase)
Needle EMG	Normal	Normal	

Table 5. showing progressive handgrip, dorsiflexion power, thenar and EDB MUNE and needle EMG results of Case 2 (Normal EMG refers to the absence of fasciculation and fibrillation potentials, normal motor unit potentials and normal recruitment)

Nerve conduction studies performed by independent neurologist were normal, with no evidence of a large fibre peripheral neuropathy. Needle EMG studies was also normal, with no evidence of active or chronic denervation in bilateral distal and proximal muscles sampled.

On her initial MUNE testing, results were within normal values, but 5 months later, there was a detectable reduction in her MUNE's from baseline of between 13-23%. As the MUNE change was greater than our re-retest reliability limits (<5%), a presumptive diagnosis fALS was made and commenced on Riluzole therapy. This resulted in an improvement in her fasciculations and MUNE's over the next 6 months, 14-41%. Her MUNE results have remained stable over the next 12 months. Progress MUNE results are shown in Table 6.

7.5.4. Case study 4

A 47-year-old lady with a family history of dominantly inherited non-SOD 1 ALS, (father aged 68 and brother aged 45, both died of ALS). A point mutation in the SOD 1 gene has not been currently detected. She presented with a 1-year history of generalised muscle fasciculations and occasional lower limb cramps. She had generalised tiredness and muscular aches and pains, but no weakness, numbness or paraesthesia. Her gait was steady. As a result of her symptoms, she ceased work in March 2004.

	Sept-08	Feb-09	Aug-09	Aug-10
Months	**Baseline**	**5 months**	**6 months**	**12 months**
		Riluzole commenced		
R Handgrip	65	70	68	65
L Handgrip	62	70	62	65
R APB MUNE	126	109 (13% decrease)	124 (14% increase)	131
L APB MUNE	136	105 (23% decrease)	123 (17% increase)	124
R EDB MUNE	107	97 18% decrease)	134 (38% increase)	134
L EDB MUNE	104	90 (13% decrease)	127 (41% increase)	117
Needle EMG	Normal			

Table 6. showing progressive handgrip, dorsiflexion power, thenar and EDB MUNE and needle EMG results of Case 3 (Normal EMG refers to the absence of fasciculation and fibrillation potentials, normal motor unit potentials and normal recruitment)

On examination, she had no evidence of wasting, but there were generalised fasciculations, especially in the triceps and quadriceps regions. Her tone was normal in the upper and lower limbs. She had no clinical weakness with MRC grade 5/5 power in all muscle groups, proximally and distally. Her sensory examination was normal to touch, vibration and position. Her reflexes were all present and symmetrical. Her gait was normal, as she was able to walk on her heels and toes. She was able to perform tandem walking and Romberg's sign was negative.

Nerve conduction studies performed by independent neurologist were normal, with no evidence of a large fibre peripheral neuropathy. Needle EMG studies was also normal, with no evidence of active or chronic denervation in bilateral distal and proximal muscles sampled.

Initial EDB MUNE was reduced with normal APB MUNE's. Despite this, a clinical diagnosis on fALS was not made given her normal needle EMG study, and she was observed over the next 6 months. Over this time, she developed MRC grade 4/5 weakness of ankle dorsiflexion, bilaterally and her EDB MUNE dropped by 14-20%. Despite this reduction, compound muscle action potential amplitudes were maintained. Needle EMG studies were repeated and once again normal there was no spontaneous activity (fibrillation potentials) and motor unit recruitment was normal, despite the presence of weakness.

Given her family history, a presumptive diagnosis of non-SOD 1 fALS was made and commenced on Riluzole therapy. This resulted in an improvement in clinical symptoms of tiredness and fasciculations, allowing her to return to work. Her EDB MUNE improved by 34-60%, and increased further over the next year. Despite this, her treating neurologist considered this was a placebo effect and ceased Riluzole. Within 2 weeks, her generalised aches

http://dx.doi.org/10.5772/56559

and pains and fasciculations recurred. Her subsequent MUNE study was blinded, as the operator was unaware that Riluzole had been ceased and found that her EDB MUNE's had reduced once again. She then had a 3rd needle EMG study, which was once again normal. She also had a MRI scan of her brain and full spine that showed no significant abnormality. She was recommenced on Riluzole, which resulted in a slow and steady improvement in her MUNE, which she has been maintained. Progress MUNE results are shown in Table 7 and Figure 12.

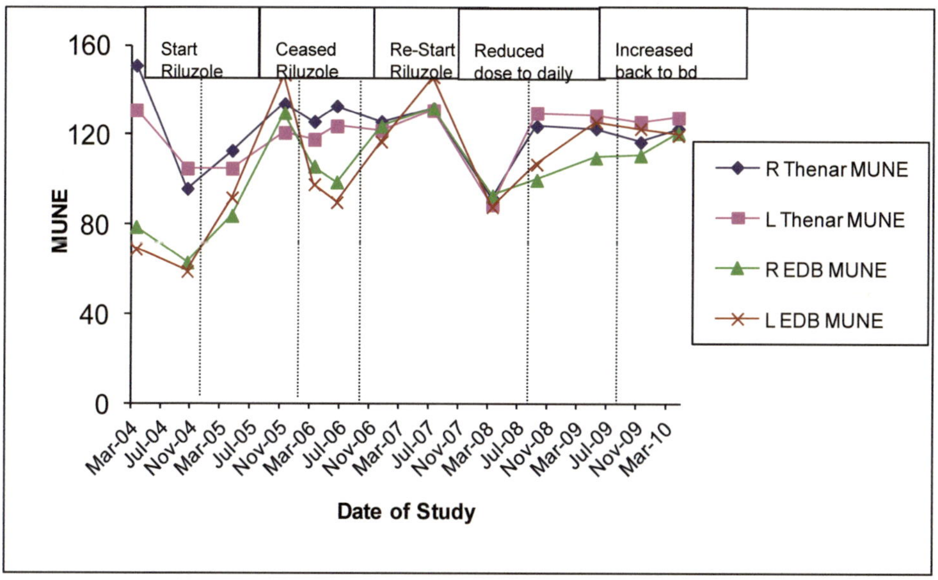

Figure 12. showing progressive thenar and EDB MUNE changes in relation to changes in the dose of Riluzole in Case 4

8. Conclusion

Motor neurone disease (MND) is a group of fatal, progressive neurodegenerative disorders, with an overall median survival is approximately 4.0 years from the onset of symptoms. By the time most patients with MND are aware of clinical weakness and seek review by their primary physician or neurologist, a significant proportion of motor units have already been lost. Early detection of motor neurone loss in clinically apparently unaffected muscles is therefore important to establish an early diagnosis of the condition.

Motor unit number estimates in the group of asymptomatic SOD1 mutation carriers were compared to age and sex matched family controls without the SOD1 mutation, and sporadic (non-SOD1) MND patients. There was no detectable difference in the number of thenar motor units in the group of asymptomatic SOD1 mutation carriers compared to the group of SOD1 negative family controls (thenar p>0.46), or population controls (thenar p>0.70).. In addition,

	Mar-04	Oct-04	Apr-05	Nov-05	Mar-06	Jun-06
Months	**Baseline**	**7 months**	**6 months**	**7 months**	**4 months**	**3 months**
Riluzole changes		**Riluzole Started**		**Riluzole Ceased**		**Riluzole Recommenced Apr-06**
R Handgrip	50	20	50	40	40	35
R Thenar MUNE	151	96 (36% decrease)	113	134	126	133
L Handgrip	40	20	40	38	40	30
L Thenar MUNE	131	105	105	121	118	124
R EDB power	5/5	4/5	4/5	4/5	4/5	4/5
R EDB MUNE	79	63 (20% decrease)	84 (33% increase)	130 (34% increase)	106	99 (23% decrease)
L EDB power	5/5	4/5	4/5	4/5	4/5	4/5
L EDB MUNE	69	59 (14% decrease)	92 (56% increase)	147 (60% increase)	98	90 (39% decrease)
Needle EMG	Normal	Normal				Normal

Date of study	**Dec-06**	**Jul-07**	**Mar-08**	**Sept-08**	**May-09**	**Nov-09**	**Apr-10**
Months	**6 months**	**7 months**	**8 months**	**6 months**	**8 months**	**6 months**	**5 months**
Riluzole changes			**Riluzole Daily**	Riluzole BD			
R Handgrip	55	45	25	34	40	40	40
R Thenar MUNE	126	132	92 (30% decrease)	124	123 (34% increase)	117	123
L Handgrip	50	45	25	35	45	30	32
L Thenar MUNE	122	131	89 (32% decrease)	130	129 (45% increase)	126	128
R EDB power	4/5	4/5	4/5	4+/5	4/5	4+/5	4+/5
R EDB MUNE	124 (25% increase)	132	93 (30% decrease)	100	110 (18% increase)	111	121
L EDB power	4/5	4/5	4/5	4+/5	4+/5	4+/5	4+/5
L EDB MUNE	117 (30% increase)	146	88 (40% decrease)	107	126 (43% increase)	123	120

Table 7. showing progressive handgrip, dorsiflexion power, thenar and EDB MUNE and needle EMG results of Case 4 (Normal EMG refers to the absence of fasciculation and fibrillation potentials, normal motor unit potentials and normal recruitment)

there was no detectable difference in the number of EBD motor units in the group of asymptomatic SOD1 mutation carriers compared to the group of SOD1 negative family controls (EDB $p>0.95$), or population controls (EDB $p>0.50$). Symptomatic sporadic MND subjects showed a definite loss of motor units with fewer motor units compared to all other groups ($p<0.001$). There was no overlap between MUNE results in symptomatic and asymptomatic subjects.

These results indicate that the group of asymptomatic carriers of the SOD1 mutation have no significant difference in the number of motor neurones, when compared to age and sex matched controls. All carriers had a full complement of motor neurones during the asymptomatic phase, indicating that mutation carriers have normal survival of motor neurones and that symptomatic MND is not the end result of a slow attrition of motor neurones. This implies that gradual pre-symptomatic loss of motor neurones does not occur in asymptomatic SOD1 mutation carriers. This supports the observation that sudden, catastrophic loss of motor neurones occurs immediately prior to the onset of symptoms and the development of the disease, rather than a gradual attrition of motor neurones over time. These results suggest that there may be a biological trigger initiating rapid cell loss, just prior to the onset of symptoms. This observation is an important contribution to the current understanding of the pathogenesis of MND. (Aggarwal & Nicholson, 2001).

The statistical MUNE technique was used for the study. This technique has been greatly modified since its original description, but numerous studies have shown that MUNE can change systematically in ALS patients when used by experienced technicians, even though evaluator bias needs to be taken into account. It has been suggested that the statistical MUNE is unreliable in the presence of clinical weakness due to motor unit instability. (Shefner, 2009). The difference is that our study was performed on asymptomatic patients, without clinical weakness.

MUNE has been performed in a number of different ways over the years, each with their advantages and limitations. The choice of technique depends largely on the speed and simplicity of the technique, as well as its accuracy and reproducibility. The way the average single motor unit potential (SMUP) size is obtained distinguishes the several techniques. Most employ electrical stimulation of the motor nerve to determine the sizes of the SMUP, but a few use needle EMG. The statistical MUNE technique was used for the study. (Daube, 1995). This technique has been compared to the multiple point stimulation method and found to be more reproducible (7% vs. 12%) and faster to administer. (Lomen-Hoeth & Olney, 2000). The technique has been greatly modified since its original description, (Shefner et al, 2004), but numerous studies have shown that MUNE can be used to monitor change in ALS patients when used by experienced technicians, even though evaluator bias needs to be taken into account. (Shefner et al., 2004).

There have been studies performed indicating that the statistical MUNE is unreliable in the presence of clinical weakness due to motor unit instability in ALS. (Shefner et al., 2011). In our previous study, we showed that there was no detectable difference in the number of motor units in 19 SOD 1 mutation carriers as a group, compared to their 34 SOD 1 negative family controls (APB $p>0.46$ and EDB $p>0.95$), or 23 population controls (APB, $p>0.70$ and EDB, $p>0.50$). (Aggarwal & Nicholson, 2001). It also showed that MUNE may be used as a reliable method of pre-symptomatic detection of motor unit loss in SOD1 mutation carriers. Following 69 SOD1 family members and population controls over a 1-year period, with thenar and EDB MUNE tests repeated every 3 to 6 months, assessed the test-retest reproducibility of the technique. The mean difference between thenar MUNE results on separate occasions in asymptomatic subjects was +/- 3.6%, with a range of 0-11.7%, and +/- 4.6%, with a range of 0-15.7% in EDB MUNE. Our test-retest correlation was high, with Pearson correlation coefficients of 0.93 for APB MUNE and 0.78 for EDB MUNE. (Aggarwal, 2009). This indicates that there is reproducibility of our statistical MUNE technique, despite recent revisions and reservations. The results can be used as a baseline for progressive MUNE studies and any change in MUNE of greater than 5% should not be considered as a variation in measurement. This is contrary to a recent report indicating that the statistical MUNE cannot be used to detect mild to moderate motor unit loss. (Blok et al., 2010).

During the course of the study, a significant fall in motor unit number was detected in 5 of the SOD1 mutation carriers, several months before the onset of weakness and the diagnosis of motor neurone disease (MND) being made. There was no detectable loss of motor units in the other 15 SOD1 mutation carriers or in the group of SOD1 mutation negative relatives. From the study, a threshold MUNE of less than 100 was considered to imply that symptoms were imminent.

In individual cases, there was a reduction of 68% 8 months prior, 51% 4 months prior, 46% 6 months prior, 35% 10 months prior and 28% 6 months prior to the onset of weakness. Further motor unit loss occurred as weakness progressed and the diagnosis of MND being made.

We followed 3 subjects with a family history of ALS, 2 of which had a documented SOD 1 point mutation, who were commenced on Riluzole therapy when loss of motor units were detected using motor unit number estimation (MUNE), before the onset of symptoms i.e. pre-symptomatic phase. A reduction in sequential MUNE was shown to improve with a therapeutic intervention, Riluzole. Currently, the only effective approved treatment for MND is Riluzole, which has a neuroprotective role, possibly due to pre-synaptic inhibition of glutamate release. Riluzole is an anti-glutamate agent that has been approved for the treatment of patients with amyotrophic lateral sclerosis in most countries. Treatment of human ALS patients or transgenic Cu, Zn superoxide dimutase 1 (SOD 1) mice, most commonly produce a modest but significant increase in survival. (Bensimon et al., 1994). There have been a least three large randomised trials involving hundreds of patients that have been unable to show that Riluzole is a disease altering agent nor does it have any restorative reports. (Miller et al., 2007).

Cases 1 and 2 are SOD 1 positive mutation carriers who developed non-specific symptoms of muscle fasciculations with no clinical weakness, but had reductions in MUNE on sequential testing. Needle EMG studies were "normal", with no evidence of active or chronic denervation in muscles sampled from bilateral distal and proximal muscles. Normal EMG was defined as the absence of fasciculation and fibrillation potentials, normal motor unit potentials and normal recruitment. A presumptive diagnosis of fALS was made, even though there are reports on incomplete penetrance. In case 3, one could argue that there is no clear evidence that she has fALS, even though she has a strong family history of ALS with an autosomal dominant pattern of inheritance. Her episodic weakness and fasciculations improved after commencing Riluzole and recurred after discontinuing Riluzole. She also had an improvement in MUNE and subsequent decline in MUNE, which are temporally associated with the administration of Riluzole.

After commencing Riluzole, there was an improvement in symptoms and MUNE. It is therefore possible that if treatment is commenced prior to significant motor neurone loss, the progression of disease can be slowed down.

In case 3, MUNE dropped when treatment was ceased on two separate occasions and improved when treatment was recommenced, with the operator being unaware of the Riluzole dose changes.

In our series, we noted an improvement in symptoms, especially a decrease in muscle fasciculations and an increase in MUNE number after commencing Riluzole. We suggest that previous trials have been performed in the symptomatic phase of the disease when 70-80% of motor units have already been lost, rather than in the pre-symptomatic phase of the disease, when the therapeutic benefit might be possible. If "treatment" is commenced prior to significant motor neurone loss occurring, the progression of disease may be able to slowed down. MUNE is believed to reduce because of remodelling of the motor units and in our study, the compound muscle action potential amplitudes were maintained despite a reduction in MUNE. This is because early in the disease, the rate of cell death is low. (Cheah et al., 2010). The increase in MUNE may be either due to reinnervation of the damaged muscles or repair of poorly functioning synapses, at the early stage of the disease, without resulting in a change in CMAP.

In one of the cases in the study, Riluzole was commenced once she developed mild weakness. At the time, there was a slight reduction in MUNE, but conventional needle EMG examination did not fulfil the criteria to make the diagnosis of MND. In view of her strong family history and positive genetic testing, a presumed diagnosis of MND was made. Since commencing Riluzole there has been no significant reduction in her EDB MUNE over the last 2 years, and her weakness of right dorsiflexors has only progressed marginally from MRC grade 4+/5 to 4/5 power. It is possible that since "treatment" was commenced prior to the loss of a significant number of motor neurones, this may have slowed down the progression of the disease in this individual case. Early in the course of ALS, the rate of cell death is low as the amount of neuronal damage caused by the mutation is small. As the amount of intracellular damage increases, a critical threshold is reached, which overwhelms cellular homeostasis, resulting in rapid apoptosis and cell death. The increase in MUNE numbers may be either due to reinnervation of the damaged muscle or repair of poorly functioning synapses, at the early stage of the disease, without resulting in a change in CMAP.

Maximum isometric grip strength was also obtained using the Jamar hydraulic dynamometer with standardised (middle handle) positioning and instructions. Maximum isometric grip strength did not reduce, even when MUNE dropped, once again supporting McComas' theory that patients can maintain normal muscle twitch tension until loss of about 70-80% of motor units, before collateral reinnervation was unable to provide functional compensation. (McComas et al., 1971). Maximum isometric grip strength using the Jamar hydraulic dynamometer also does not correlate with the number of functional motor neurones in thenar group of muscles as measured using the statistical method of MUNE, indicating that MUNE is a more sensitive test than MVIC for monitoring disease progression in MND. It has also been shown that MUNE is able to identify deterioration in functional motor units before handgrip maximal voluntary isometric contraction (MVIC).

This confirms McComas' observation that patients with substantial chronic denervation could maintain normal muscle twitch tension until loss of about 70-80% of motor units occurs. (McComas, 1971). This suggests that handgrip MVIC is not as sensitive as thenar MUNE for monitoring disease progression, as it is unable to detect early motor neurone loss due to the presence of compensatory mechanisms. The surviving motor neurones enlarge their territories, through collateral sprouting (reinnervation) until late in the disease, when collateral reinnervation is no longer able to provide full functional compensation. Thenar MUNE however does examine all of the motor units that are involved in handgrip MVIC, as forearm flexors and ulnar-innervated muscles are involved in the generation of handgrip MVIC. It also confirms Felice's study which showed that in patients with MND, changes in thenar MUNE was the most sensitive outcome measure for following disease progression, when compared to other quantitative tests, such as CMAP, isometric grip strength, forced vital capacity and Medical Research Council manual muscle testing. (Felice, 1997).

This study also shows that there can be substantial loss in MUNE and still have an essentially normal EMG with minimal signs of acute denervation or motor unit potential remodelling, as one would expected that at a minimum, the muscles with transiently reduced MUNE numbers should have reduced recruitment during EMG studies.

As there is no corroboration with needle EMG in the pre-symptomatic stage of the disease in this study, this requires a paradigm shift in the traditional concept that needle EMG is the "gold" standard for the diagnosis of ALS. McComas showed that patients with substantial chronic denervation could maintain normal muscle twitch tension until loss of about 70-80% of motor units, before collateral reinnervation was unable to provide functional compensation (McComas, 1971). The function of motor neurons remains normal because the remaining motor units incorporate more muscle fibres by collateral sprouting. This should result in larger motor unit potentials, firing at higher rates with fewer motor units active i.e. reduced recruitment. Traditional neurologists and neurophysiologists will find it hard to understand physiologically how there can be substantial loss in MUNE and still have normal EMG with no signs of acute denervation or motor unit potential remodelling.

As MUNE is a measure of the primary pathologic process of motor neurone loss and can identify that the number of motor units are reduced, even in the presence of a non-diagnostic needle EMG. Needle electromyography may reveal evidence of chronic reinnervation, but provides little direct evidence to the extent of motor neurone and axonal loss. These cases clearly indicate that loss of motor neurones is detectable in the pre-symptomatic phase, which is detectable before significant needle EMG changes of pathology. In addition, compound muscle action potential amplitudes were maintained, despite a significant reduction in MUNE. Even though some may argue that a reduction in MUNE cannot be used to support the diagnosis fALS, our previous study, suggests that once changes start to occur on conventional

EMG studies, the window of opportunity to influence the progression of this condition has been missed.

We would argue that previous trials have all be performed in the symptomatic phase of the disease when 70-80% of motor units have already been lost, rather than in the pre-symptomatic phase of the disease, when the therapeutic benefit might change, as "treatment" is commenced prior to significant motor neurone loss occurring and therefore, the progression of disease can be slowed down. MUNE numbers are believed to reduce because of remodelling of the motor unit and in our study, the compound muscle action potential amplitudes (CMAP) were retained as early in the course of the disease, the rate of cell death is low. The increase in MUNE numbers may be either due to reinnervation of the damaged muscle or repair of poorly functioning synapses, at the early stage of the disease, without resulting in a change in CMAP.

Therapies aimed at preserving motor neurones may be more feasible than trying to replace lost motor neurones. A number of treatment or preventative strategies have been suggested, such as measures to diminish SOD 1 aggregation or interactions to specifically reduce apoptosis in motor neurones. As motor neurone loss at this stage is rapid and precipitous, any potential treatment ideally should be given much earlier in SOD 1 mutation carriers. Larger randomised trials are necessary to study this question in a prospective, blinded fashion.

Even though MUNE evaluations were performed in an unblinded fashion, the statistical MUNE technique is performed with the assistance of an algorithm, which reduces operator bias. The main author has been using this technique for over 10 years and any operator bias is unintentional and unlikely to explain the marked differences in sequential MUNE.

Early in the course of ALS, the rate of cell death is low as the amount of neuronal damage caused by the mutation is small. As the amount of intracellular damage increases, a critical threshold is reached, which overwhelms cellular homeostasis, resulting in rapid apoptosis and cell death. (Clarke, 2001). The mutant neurones appear to function normally for decades, with weakness only occurring once apoptosis and cell death occurs due to a gradual accumulation of damage within the cell. (Kong & Xu, 1998).

As motor neurone loss once it occurs is rapid and precipitous, any potential treatment will need to be given early to SOD1 mutation carriers. Once the disease progresses, resulting in functional impairment and disability, restorative treatments to replace lost motor neurones becomes less feasible. To date there have been a number of drugs which have undergone clinical trials in MND, for which there is no evidence of benefit. These include creatinine, high dose vitamin E, Gabapentin and nerve growth factors such as brain derived neurotrophic factor and insulin-like growth factor-1. If effective treatment for MND were to be developed to arrest the process of degeneration, therapies aimed at preserving functional motor neurones would be more feasible. This requires the ability to be able to identify individuals at risk of developing the disease, which currently are SOD1 mutation carriers.

This longitudinal study showed that it was possible to detect loss of motor neurones in the pre-symptomatic stage of MND in humans. This study provided further evidence that considerable motor neurone loss occurred just before the onset of symptoms or weakness. (Aggarwal, 2009).

This study indicates that SOD1 mutation carriers have normal survival of motor neurones, with as carriers had a full complement of motor neurones during the asymptomatic phase. Significant pre-symptomatic loss of motor neurones did not occur in asymptomatic SOD1 mutation carriers. Sudden and widespread motor neurone death occurs at the time development of the symptomatic symptoms, rather than life-long motor neurone loss. Sudden, catastrophic and multifocal loss of motor neurons occurs immediately prior to the onset of symptoms and the development of MND. This suggests that there may be a biological trigger initiating rapid cell loss, just prior to the onset of symptoms, rather than life-long motor neurone loss. Also, if the trigger initiating motor neurone loss can be identified, it may be possible to prevent motor neurone loss in familial ALS and develop treatments for sporadic MND. The mutant SOD1 protein itself cannot be the trigger, as it is constantly expressed. There may however be a gradual accumulation of a toxic product, possibly SOD1, which has changed into a new toxic conformation or aggregate, resulting in neuronal damage. The possibility of an individual neuron undergoing apoptosis increases as damage accumulates. This cumulative damage may be due to oxidative stress, resulting in disruption of the cellular structure and function.

Neurofilament heavy polypeptide (NF-H) is an abundant stable cytoplasmic protein located in neuronal cells in large axons and may be used as a cell type marker. Abnormal accumulation of NF-H in motor neurones is associated with ALS, but it is unclear to what extent these contribute to human disease. Analysis of blood serum markers looking for increased levels of NF-H was not performed in this study, but would be interesting to be done in the future to the compare levels of NF-H in the carriers.

The results of this study indicate that the risk of cell death probably remains constant throughout life of the neurone and that cell death occurs randomly in time and is independent of that of any other neurone. This suggests a "one-hit" biochemical phenomenon in which the mutation imposes an abnormal mutant steady state on the neurone and a single catastrophic event randomly initiates cell death and apoptosis. Early in the course of MND, the rate of cell death is low as the amount of neuronal damage caused by the mutation is small. The delay in clinical onset was thought to reflect the gradual accumulation of damage within the neurones, as a result of the mutation, which ultimately overwhelms cellular homeostasis leading to cell death. The living mutant neurons function very well for years or decades but the probability that an individual neurone undergoes apoptosis increases as damage accumulates within it. A mutant neurone in an older patient will have accumulated a greater amount of damage and will therefore be more likely to die than in a younger patient. Consequently, early in the course of disease, the chance of a cell containing a sufficient amount of damage to initiate apoptosis is small, and the rate of cell loss is correspondingly low. The mutant neurones appear to function normally for decades, with weakness only occurring once apoptosis and cell death occurs due to a gradual accumulation of damage within the cell. Therapies aimed at preserving motor neurones may be more feasible than trying to replace lost motor neurones. A number of treatment or preventative strategies arise, such as measures to diminish SOD1 aggregation or interactions to specifically reduced apoptosis in motor neurones. As motor neurone loss at this stage is rapid and precipitous, any potential treatment will need to be given much earlier in SOD1 mutation carriers.

Determining the mechanism by which mutations in the Cu/Zn superoxide dismutase (SOD1) gene triggers the destruction of motor neurones causing MND remains unknown. At present, the favoured hypothesis is that the mutation causes disease as a result of a toxic gain of function by the mutant SOD1 provoking selective neurotoxicity, probably disrupting the intracellular homeostasis of copper and/or protein aggregation. However, as the amount of intracellular damage increases, the chance that a cell will die also increases. This cumulative damage may be due to oxidative stress, in which an imbalance between the production of reactive oxygen species and cellular antioxidant mechanisms results in chemical modifications of macromolecules, thereby disrupting cellular structure and function. It is possible that the high metabolic activity in motor neurones, combined with the toxic oxidative properties of the mutant SOD1, causes massive mitochondrial vacuolation in motor neurones, resulting in degeneration, earlier than other neurones, triggering the onset of weakness. Prominent cytoplasmic intracellular inclusions in motor neurones and within astrocytes surrounding them developed by the onset of clinical disease and in some cases represented the first pathological sign of disease. These aggregates increased in number as the disease progressed. This indicates that the mutant SOD1 toxicity is mediated by damage to mitochondria in motor neurones and this damage triggers the functional decline of motor neurones and the clinical onset of symptoms. The absence of motor neurone death in the early stages of the disease indicates that the majority of motor neurones could be rescued after early clinical diagnosis.

Regular follow-up of SOD1 carriers with MUNE may lead to early diagnosis, creating an opportunity for future novel approaches and therapies aimed at preserving motor neurones rather than replacing lost motor neurones. If the trigger initiating motor neurone loss can be identified, it may be possible to prevent motor neurone loss in familial ALS. At this stage, detecting the onset of motor neurone loss in asymptomatic individuals will identify those who may benefit from early institution of an active management program to improve their quality of life, until more effective treatment modalities become available for this devastating condition This observation is an important contribution to the current understanding of the pathogenesis of MND, as it shows that motor neurone disease does not seem to be the end result of slow attrition of motor neurones. MUNE may be able to be used as a method of pre-symptomatic testing of individuals who on genetic testing are SOD1 mutation carriers. Regular follow-up of SOD1 carriers with MUNE may lead to early diagnosis, creating an opportunity for future novel approaches and therapies aimed at preserving motor neurones rather than replacing lost motor neurones.

Acknowledgements

Prof. Garth Nicholson who introduced me to research into motor neurone disease and his continuing support. Prof. David Burke and Assoc. Prof. Alastair Corbett for their professional guidance and Prof. Jasper Daube for his technical assistance regarding the technique used in this research. The research was supported by the Motor Neurone Disease Association of NSW (Northern Region), ANZAC Health and Medical Research Foundation, Motor Neurone Disease Research Institute of Australia Inc. and the Nerve Research Foundation.

Author details

Arun Aggarwal

University of Sydney, Australia

References

[1] Aggarwal, A, & Nicholson, G. A. (2001). Normal complement of motor units in asymptomatic familial (SOD1 mutation) amyotrophic lateral sclerosis. J. *Neurology, Neurosurgery and Psychiatry*. 17 (4), 472-48.

[2] Aggarwal, A. (2009). Detection of pre-clinical motor unit loss in familial amyotrophic lateral sclerosis. *Supplements to Clinical Neurophysiology.* , 60, 171-179.

[3] Aggarwal, A. & G. Nicholson. ((2002). Detection Of pre-clinical motor neurone loss in SOD1 mutation carriers using motor unit number estimation. *J of Neurology, Neurosurgery & Psychiatry.* , 73(2), 199-201.

[4] Aggarwal, A. (2009). Motor unit number estimation in asymptomatic familial amyotrophic lateral sclerosis. *Supplements to Clinical Neurophysiology.* , 60, 163-169.

[5] Al-chalabi, A, Andersen, P. M, Nilsson, P, Chioza, B, Andersson, J. L, Russ, C, Shaw, C. E, Powell, J, & Leigh, P. N. (1999). Deletions of the heavy neurofilament subunit tail in amyotrophic lateral sclerosis. *Hum Mol Genet.*, 8, 157-164.

[6] Andersen, P. M, Nilsson, P, Keranen, M. L, Forsgren, L, Hagglund, J, Karlsborg, M, Ronnevi, L. O, Gredal, O, & Marklund, S. L. (1997). Phenotypic heterogenicity in motor neurone disease patients with CuZn superoxide dismutase mutations in Scandinavia. *Brain.* , 120, 1723-1737.

[7] Azzouz, M, Leclerc, N, Gurney, M, Warter, J, Poindron, M, & Borg, P. J. ((1997). Progressive motor neuron impairment in an animal model of familial amyotrophic lateral sclerosis. *Muscle Nerve.*, 20, 45-51.

[8] Beal, M. F. (1996). Mitochondria, free radicals and neurodegeneration. *Curr Opin Neurobiol.* , 6, 661-666.

[9] Beckman, J. S, Carson, M, Smith, C. D, & Koppenol, W. H. (1993). ALS, SOD and peroxinitrate. *Nature*.364: 584.

[10] Bensimon, G, Lacomblez, L, & Meiniger, V. (1994). A controlled trial of Riluzole in amyotrophic lateral sclerosis. ALS/Riluzole study group. *N Engl J Med.* , 330(9), 585-591.

[11] Blok, J. H, Van Dijk, J. P, Drenthen, J, Maathuis, E. M, & Stegeman, D. F. Size does matter: the influence of motor unit potential size on statistical motor unit number estimates in healthy subjects. *Clin Neurophysiol.* (2010). Oct; , 121(10), 1772-80.

[12] Brown, W. F. (1972). A method for estimating the number of motor units in thenar muscles and the changes in motor unit counting with aging. *J Neurol Neurosurg Psychiatry.*, 35, 845-852.

[13] Bruijn, L. I, Becher, M. W, Lee, M. K, Anderson, K. L, Jenkins, N. A, Copeland, N. G, Sisodia, S. S, Rothstein, J. D, Borchelt, D. R, Price, D. L, & Cleveland, D. W. (1997). ALS-linked SOD1 mutant G85R mediates damage to astrocytes and promotes rapidly progressive disease with SOD1-containing inclusions. *Neuron.* , 18, 327-338.

[14] Campbell, M. J, Mccomas, A. J, & Petito, F. (1973). Physiological changes in ageing muscles. *J Neurol Neurosurg Psychiatry.* , 36, 174-182.

[15] Chance, P. F, Rabin, B. A, Ryan, S. G, Ding, Y, Scavina, M, Crain, B, Griffith, J. W, & Cornblath, D. R. (1998). Linkage of the gene for an autosomal dominant form of juvenile amyotrophic lateral sclerosis to chromosome 9q34. *Am J Hum Genet.* , 62, 633-640.

[16] Cheah, B. C, Vucic, S, Krishnan, A. V, & Kiernan, M. C. (2010). Riluzole, neuroprotection and amyotrophic lateral sclerosis. *Curr Med Chem* , 17(18), 1942-49.

[17] Clarke, G, Collins, R. A, Leavitt, B. R, Andrews, D. F, Hayden, M. R, Lumsden, C. J, & Mcinnes, R. R. ((2000). A one hit model of cell death in inherited neuronal degenerations. *Nature.* , 406, 195-199.

[18] Clarke, G, Lumsden, C. J, & Mcinnes, R. R. (2001). Inherited neurodegenerative disease: the one hit model of neurodegeneration. *Human Molecular Genetics.* , 10, 2269-2275.

[19] Cleveland, D. W. (1999). From Charcot to SOD1: Mechanisms of selective motor neuron death in ALS. *Neuron.* , 24, 515-520.

[20] Cudkowicz, M. E, Mckenna-yasek, D, Sapp, P. E, Chin, W, Geller, B, Hayden, D. L, Schoenfeld, D. A, Hosler, B. A, Horvitz, H. R, & Brown, R. H. Jr. ((1997). Epidemiology of mutations in superoxide dismutase in amyotrophic lateral sclerosis. *Ann Neurol.* , 41, 210-221.

[21] Daube, J. R. (1995). Estimating the number of motor units in a muscle. *J Clin Neurophysiol.* , 12(6), 585-594.

[22] De Belleroche, J, Orrell, R, & King, A. J. (1995). Medical Genetics. Familial amyotrophic lateral sclerosis/motor neurone disease (FALS): a review of current developments. *J Med Genet.* , 32, 841-847.

[23] Doble, A. (1996). The pharmacology and mechanism of action of riluzole. *Neurology*. 47: S, 233-241.

[24] Eisen, A. (1995). Amyotrophic lateral sclerosis is a multifactorial disease. *Muscle Nerve.*, 18, 741-752.

[25] Felice, K. J. (1997). A longitudinal study comparing thenar motor unit number estimation to other quantitative tests in patients with amyotrophic lateral sclerosis. *Muscle Nerve.*, 20, 179-185.

[26] Figlewicz, D. A, Krizus, A, Martinoli, M. G, Meininger, V, Dib, M, Rouleau, G. A, & Julein, J. P. (1994). Variants of the heavy neurofilament subunit are associated with the development of amyotrophic lateral sclerosis. *Hum Mol Genet*, 3, 1757-1761.

[27] Gurney, M. E, Pu, H, & Chiu, A. Y. Dal Canto, M.C., Polchow, C.Y., Alexander, D.D., Caliendo, J., Hentati, A., Kwon, Y.W., Deng, H.X., Chen, W., Zhai, P., Sufit, R.L. & Siddique, T. ((1994). Motor neuro degeneration in mice that express a human Cu/Zn superoxide dismutase mutation. *Science.*, 264, 1772-1775.

[28] Gurney, M. E, Tomasselli, A. G, & Heinrikson, R. L. (1994). Stay the Executioner's hand. *Science* 2000;, 288, 283-284.

[29] bojan Hamilton, A, Balnave, R, & Adam, R. Grip strength reliability. *J Hand Therapy.*, 7(3), 163-170.

[30] Hand, C. K, & Rouleau, G. A. (2002). Familial Amyotrophic Lateral Sclerosis. *Muscle Nerve.*, 25, 135-159.

[31] Hanten, W. P, Chen, W. Y, Austin, A. A, Brooks, R. E, Carter, H. C, Law, C. A, Morgan, M. K, Sanders, D. J, Swan, C. A, & Vanderslice, A. L. (1993). Maximum grip strength in normal subjects from 20 to 64 years of age. *J. Hand Therapy.*, 12(3), 193-200.

[32] Haverkamp, L. J, Appel, V, & Appel, S. H. (1995). Natural history of amyotrophic lateral sclerosis in a database population. Validation of a scoring system and a model for survival prediction. *Brain.*, 118, 707-719.

[33] Hentati, A, Pericak-vance, M. A, Nijhawan, D, Ahmed, A, Yang, Y, Rimmler, J, Hung, W-Y, Schlotter, B, & Ahmed, A. Ben Hamida, M., Hentati, F., Siddique, T. ((1998). Linkage of a commoner form of recessive amyotrophic lateral sclerosis to chromosome 15q15-q22 markers. *Neurogenetics.*, 2, 55-60.

[34] Hoagland, R. J, Mendoza, M, Armon, C, Barohn, R. J, Byran, W. W, Goodpasture, J. C, Miller, R. G, Parry, G. J, Petjan, J. H, & Ross, M. A. the Syntex / Synergen Neuroscience Joint Venture rhCNTF ALS Study Group. ((1997). Reliability of maximal isometric contraction testing in multicenter study of patients with amyotrophic lateral sclerosis. *Muscle Nerve.*, 20, 691-695.

[35] Kong, J, & Xu, Z. (1998). Massive mitochondria degeneration in motor neurons triggers the onset of amyotrophic lateral sclerosis in mice expressing a mutant SOD1. *J Neurosci.*, 18, 3241-3250.

[36] Kosti, V, Jackson-lewis, V, & Bilbao, F. D. (1997). Bcl-2: prolonging life in a transgenic mouse model of familial amyotrophic lateral sclerosis. *Science*. 227: 577.

[37] Leigh, P. N. Amyotrophic lateral sclerosis and other motor neurone diseases. ((1997). *Current Opinion Neuro Neurosurg*. 3: 567.

[38] Li, M, Ona, V. O, Gueng, C, Chen, M, Jackson-lewis, V, Andrews, L. J, Olszewski, A. J, Steig, P. E, Przedborski, S, & Friendlander, R. M. (2000). Functional role of caspase-1 and caspase-3 in an ALS transgenic mouse model. *Science.*, 288, 335-339.

[39] Lomen-hoerth, C, & Slawnych, M. P. (2003). Statistical motor unit number estimation: From theory to practice. *Muscle Nerve.*, 28, 263-272.

[40] Lomen-hoerth, C, & Olney, R. K. Comparison of multiple point and statistical motor unit number estimation. Muscle Nerve. (2000). Oct;, 23(10), 1525-33.

[41] Mccomas, A. J. (1971). Functional compensation in partially denervated muscles. *J Neurol Neurosurg Psychiatry*, 34, 453-460.

[42] Mccomas, A. J. (1991). Motor unit estimation: Methods, results and present status. *Muscle Nerve.*, 14, 585-597.

[43] Mccomas, A. J, Fawcett, P. R. W, Campbell, M. J, & Sica, R. E. P. (1971). Electrophysiological estimation of the number of motor units within a human muscle. *J. Neurology, Neurosurgery and Psychiatry.*, 34, 121-131.

[44] Mcneil, D. (1996). Statistical Methods.1st Edition. New York. *Wiley & Sons*; 184.

[45] Mena, I, Marin, O, Fuenzalida, S, & Cotzias, G. C. (1967). Chronic manganese poisoning. Clinical picture and manganese turnover. *Neurology.*, 17, 128-136.

[46] Miller, R. G, Mitchell, J. D, Lyon, M, & Moore, D. H. (2007). Riluzole for amyotrophic lateral sclerosis (ALS / motor neuron disease (MND). *Cochrane Database Syst Rev.* 1: CD001447.

[47] Mu, X, He, J, & Anderson, M. (1996). Altered expression of bcl-2 and bax mRNA in amyotrophic lateral sclerosis spinal cord motor neurones. *Ann Neurol.* 40: 379.

[48] Mulder, D. W, & Howard, F. M. Jr. ((1976). Patient resistance and prognosis in amyotrophic lateral sclerosis. *Mayo Clin Proc.*, 51, 537-541.

[49] Mulder, D. W, Kurland, L. T, Offord, K. P, & Beard, C. M. (1986). Familial adult motor neurone disease: amyotrophic lateral sclerosis. *Neurology.*, 38, 511-517.

[50] Needleman, H. L. (1997). Exposure to lead: Sources and effects. *N Engl J Med.*, 297, 943-945.

[51] Noor, R, Mittal, S, & Iqbal, E. (2003). Superoxide dismutase- applications and relevance to human diseases. *Med Sci Monit.* , 8(9), 210-215.

[52] Olney, R. K, Yuen, E. C, & Engstrom, J. W. (2000). Statistical motor unit number estimation: Reproducibility and sources of error in patients with amyotrophic lateral sclerosis. *Muscle Nerve.* , 23, 193-197.

[53] Radunovic, A, & Leigh, P. N. (1996). Cu/Zn superoxide dismutase gene mutations in amyotrophic lateral sclerosis: correlation between genotype and clinical features. *J. Neurology, Neurosurgery and Psychiatry.* , 61, 565-572.

[54] Ringel, S. P, Murphy, J. R, Alderson, M. K, Byran, W, England, J. D, Miller, R. G, Petajan, J. H, Smith, S. A, Roelofs, R. I, Ziter, F, Lee, M. Y, Brinkmann, J. R, Almada, A, Gappmaier, E, Graves, J, Herbelin, L, Mendoza, M, Mylar, D, Smith, P, & Yu, P. (1993). The natural history of amyotrophic lateral sclerosis. *Neurology.* , 43, 1316-1322.

[55] Robberecht, W. (2000). Oxidative stress in amyotrophic lateral sclerosis. *J. Neuro.* 247 (Suppl. 1): 111-116.

[56] Rosen, D. R, Siddique, T, Patterson, D, Figlewicz, D. A, Sapp, P, Hentati, D, Donaldson, D, Goto, J, Regan, O, Deng, J. P, Rahmani, H. X, Krizus, Z, Mckenna-yasek, A, Cayabyab, D, Gaston, A, Berger, S, Tanzi, M, Halperin, R. E, Herzfeldt, J. J, Van Den, B, Bergh, R, Hung, W. Y, Bird, T, Deng, G, Mulder, D. W, Smyth, C, Laing, N. G, Soriano, E, Pericak-vance, M. A, Haines, J, Rouleau, G. A, Gusella, J. S, & Horvitz, H. R. Brown R.H., Jr. ((1993). Mutations in Cu, Zn superoxide dismutase gene are associated with familial amyotrophic lateral sclerosis. *Nature.*, 362, 59-62.

[57] Shaw, C. E, Enayat, Z. E, Powell, J. F, Anderson, V. E, Radunovic, A, Powell, J. F, & Leigh, P. N. (1998). Mutations in all five exons of SOD1 may cause ALS. *Ann Neurol.* , 43, 390-394.

[58] Shefner, J. M. (2001). Motor unit number estimation in human neurological diseases and animal models. *Clin Neurophysiolo.* , 112, 955-964.

[59] Shefner, J. M, Cudkowicz, M. E, Zhang, H, Schoenfiekd, D, & Jillapalli, D. (2004). Northeast ALS Consortium. The use of statistical MUNE in multicentre clinical trials. *Muscle Nerve.* , 30, 463-9.

[60] Shefner, J. M. (2009). Statistical motor unit number estimation and ALS trials: the effect of motor unit instability. *Suppl Clin Neurophysiol.*, 60, 135-41.

[61] Shefner, J. M, Watson, M. L, Simionescu, L, Caress, J. B, Burns, T. M, Maragakis, N. J, Benatar, M, David, W. S, Sharma, K. R, & Rutkove, S. B. Multipoint incremental motor unit number estimation as an outcome measure in ALS. *Neurology.* (2011). Jul 19; , 77(3), 235-41.

[62] Sica, R. E. P, Mccomas, A. J, Upton, A. R. M, & Longmire, D. (1974). Motor unit estimations in small muscles of the hand. *J Neurol Neurosurg Psychiatry.*, 37, 55-67.

[63] Siddique, T, & Deng, H. X. (1996). Genetics of amyotrophic lateral sclerosis. *Human Mol Gen.* , 5, 1465-1470.

[64] Siddique, T, Pericak-vance, M. A, & Brooks, B. R. (1989). Linkage analysis in familial amyotrophic lateral sclerosis. *Neurology.* , 39, 919-925.

[65] Siddique, T, Figlewicz, D. A, Pericak-vance, M. A, Haines, J. L, Rouleau, G. A, Jeffers, A. J, Sapp, P, Hung, W. Y, Bebout, J, Mckenna-yasek, D, Deng, G, Horvitz, H. R, Gusella, J. S, & Brown, R. H. Jr., Roses, A.D. and Collaborators. ((1991). Linage of a gene causing familial amyotrophic lateral sclerosis to chromosome 21 and evidence of genetic locus heterogenicity. *N Engl J Med.* , 324, 1381-1384.

[66] Sjalander, A, Beckman, G, & Deng, H. Z. A mutation results in a polymorphism of Cu/Zn superoxide dismutase that is prevalent in northern Sweden and Finland. Hum Mol Genet 1995; , 4, 1105-1108.

[67] Stein, R. B, & Yang, J. F. (1990). Methods of estimating the number of motor units in human muscles. *Ann Neurol.* , 28, 487 495.

[68] Talbot, K. (2002). Motor neurone disease. *Muscle Nerve.* , 25, 513-519.

[69] Trotti, D, Rolfs, A, Danbolt, N. C, & Brown, R. H. Jr, Hediger, M.A. ((1999). SOD1 mutations linked to amyotrophic lateral sclerosis selectively activates a glial glutamate transporter. *Na Neurosci.* , 19, 427-433.

[70] Vechio, J. D, Bruijn, L. I, Xu, Z, & Brown, R. H. Jr, ((1996). Cleveland,D.W. Sequence variants in the human neurofilament proteins: absence of linkage to familial amyotrophic lateral sclerosis. Ann Neurol 1996; , 40, 603-610.

[71] Yim, M. B, Chock, P. B, & Stadtman, E. R. (1990). Copper, zinc superoxide dismutase catalyses hydroxyl radial production from hydrogen peroxide. *Proc Natl Acad Sci.* , 87, 5006-5010.

Chapter 8

Changes in Motor Unit Loss and Axonal Regeneration Rate in Sporadic and Familiar Amyotrophic Lateral Sclerosis (ALS) — Possible Different Pathogenetic Mechanisms?

Tommaso Bocci, Elisa Giorli, Lucia Briscese,
Silvia Tognazzi, Fabio Giannini and
Ferdinando Sartucci

Additional information is available at the end of the chapter

http://dx.doi.org/10.5772/56561

1. Introduction

Amyotrophic Lateral Sclerosis (ALS) is a fatal, neurodegenerative disorder affecting upper and lower motor neurons; it's the commonest of the motor unit (MU) diseases in Europe and North America, characterized by a broad spectrum of clinical presentations [1, 2]. Striking asymmetry and selective involvement of individual groups of muscles, especially of hand and forearm, are typical early features of the disease. On average, delay from onset of symptoms to diagnosis is about 14 months and expected survival commonly ranges from months to a few years [3].

Five to ten percent of cases are familial and about 20% of these families have point mutations in the Cu/Zn superoxide dismutase-1 (SOD-1) gene. In mammalians, there are three SOD isoenzymes [4]: the cytosolic SOD1 (Cu/Zn-SOD), whose mutations are associated with familiar ALS, the mitochondrial Mn-SOD (SOD-2) and the secreted extracellular SOD (SOD-3). Most mutations in SOD-1 gene are autosomal dominant in inheritance, but there is one confirmed autosomal recessive mutation, predominant in Scandinavian ancestry, the D90A mutation in exon 4 [5].

More than 130 mutations in SOD-1 have been identified so far [6, 7]. Superoxide dismutase (SOD-1) is a well characterized enzyme, which exists as a homodimer whose sequence of 153 amino acids is remarkably well conserved across species. Sporadic and familial forms of the disease are clinically indistinguishable, suggesting they may share common mechanisms, but the pathogenic mechanisms underlying disease's induction in familiar cases are still largely controversial. The prevailing hypothesis is that familiar ALS, SOD-1 positive, could be caused by a neuronal damage due to a gradual accumulation of a toxic product SOD-1 derived; this cumulative damage leads to a disruption of the cytoskeleton and organelle trafficking within motor neuron dendrites. As the amount increases, a critical threshold may be reached, which overwhelms cellular homeostasis resulting in fast cell death [8, 9]. Aggregates do not exclusively occur in neurons, but also in glial cells, raising the question whether mutant SOD-1 expression in neurons is sufficient *per se* to induce pyramidal degeneration and sustain disease evolution over time [10-12]. Little is known about the differences both in motor unit loss and axonal regeneration rate between sporadic and familiar ALS and whether these changes underlie different pathogenetic mechanisms could represent a fascinating topic of debate.

2. Motor unit changes in familial ALS: What did we learn from animal studies?

To date, the more exhaustive study on the morphological differences between wild-type (WT) and transgenic SOD-1 motorneurons was made by Amendola and Durant [13]. By analyzing the arborizations of motorneurons in SOD-1^{G85R} mutant mice, they showed:

i. a dramatic increase in the total dendritic length;

ii. a significant proliferation of dendritic branches;

iii. a greater dendritic membrane area, as confirmed by intracellular recordings revealing a lower input resistance when compared with WT cells.

However, it's unclear whether these changes represent early compensatory modifications or a disease mechanism. Previous evidence emphasized an increased ratio of inhibitory to excitatory synapses in organotypic slice cultures derived from embryonic spinal cords of $SOD1^{G93A}$ mice [14] and a dampening in cholinergic transmission was also described in the lumbar spinal cord from adult $SOD1^{G93A}$ mice [15]. Conversely, an intrinsic hyperexcitability of mutant $SOD1^{G93A}$ spinal motorneurons was found in culture and in organotypic slice cultures [16, 17]. However, as the cells were not recorded from until they had been cultured for several weeks, the exact time course and progression rate of these changes are still largely obscure. Recently, Bories and colleagues showed motorneuron dysfunction appears centrally long before axonal degeneration [18], suggesting a pivotal role of these morphological changes in the core of disease mechanism.

Schwindt and Crill [19-21] proved that motorneurons have persistent inward currents (PICs) able both to potentiate and prolong synaptic firing rate after supraspinal input stopped: these currents are mainly generated in the dendritic regions, suggesting that motorneurons dendrites are not passive but active integrators of motor control. These conclusions fit with data in animals showing an increase in dendritic arborization in SOD-1 mutant mice compared with WT cells. High energy demands, due either to altered motorneuron

http://dx.doi.org/10.5772/56561

excitability or dendritic overbranching, destabilize calcium homeostasis [22-24]. These all changes make motor cells more susceptible to the axon transport, mitochondria and metabolic dysfunctions prominent in ALS, as motorneurons become heavily dependent on mitochondria for Ca^{++} buffering [25, 26].

In humans, these data were only in part reproduced by the pioneering study of Aggarwal [7, 27]. By evaluating MU changes in 87 subjects carrying mutations in SOD-1 gene, he showed that asymptomatic carriers of the SOD1 mutations, different from patients with sALS, have no significant difference in the number of motor neurons when compared with age and sex matched controls; as symptoms develop, a sudden and catastrophic loss of MU occurs. However, the significance of these differences is still largely misunderstood.

3. Use of Motor Unit Number Estimation (MUNE) and Macro-electromyography (Macro-EMG) in the diagnosis and management of ALS: A brief historical overview

Clinical neurophysiology in ALS plays a fundamental role both in the diagnosis of suspected disease and in the assessment of its severity and progression, offering a promising tool to quantify muscle involvement and evaluate response to therapy [28-30]. Electromyography (EMG) investigation, usually performed with concentric needle electrodes [31], plays an essential role in the diagnosis and monitoring of ALS [32-34]. Amplitude, duration, area, shape, stability on repeated discharges of MU and activity at full effort are parameters conventionally used to evaluate disease's stage. EMG may also assess the presence of activity of the denervation-reinnervation process and number of functioning motor units by evaluating recruitment-activation pattern [28, 35]. In Motor Neuron Diseases (MND), standard needle electromyography often reveals evidence of chronic reinnervation (increased motor unit action potential amplitudes and duration, with reduced recruitment), eventually associated with fasciculations and signs of denervation activity in progress, but provides little information about the extent of both motor neuron loss and axonal regeneration. The supramaximal CMAP amplitude also provides little evidence of the extent of motor neuron loss and normal CMAP amplitudes might mistakenly suggest that motor neuron loss has not occurred yet [36, 37].

A particular method to evaluate the full MU is the so-called macro-EMG [38-41]. This technique provides information from a larger area of the muscle than traditional needle EMG methods. The signal is recorded by most of the fibers inside the entire MU and is often employed to follow the degree of reinnervation. That represents a quantitative technique and can be applied to follow progression and study of putative therapies [33, 42] by evaluating size of individual MU [39, 43].

Among quantitative electrodiagnostic (EDX) techniques, the methodology of Motor Unit Number Estimation (MUNE) has been previously and widely employed in measuring loss of functioning MU in ALS patients [36, 44-49].

MUNE is very sensitive in documenting disease progression in ALS. Some studies combining MUNE and standard electromyography showed a highly significant correlation between motor unit loss, clinical quantitative features and changes in compound motor action potential (CMAP) amplitude over time [50]. That is not surprising considering their different targets; while MUNE assesses motor unit loss, changes in CMAP amplitude and duration also account for collateral reinnervation. A few longitudinal studies using MUNE in some ALS patients have been reported that MUNE decreases as the disease progresses and that MUNE is a very reliable and reproducible method in patients with ALS [36, 51-55]. Its inter-individual and intra-individual reproducibility linearly increases as disease progresses, making this technique particularly useful in the symptomatic stage of the disease [36, 55-57].

We routinely use the standard incremental technique, known as the McComas technique. Despite some limitations in comparison with statistical MUNE (alternation of motor unit, inability to recognize small motor units, small sample size), it is more reliable and less complex; in addiction, statistical MUNE cannot identify instable MUPs since it is based on the assumption that variability is due solely to the number of motor units responding in an intermittent manner [58]. More recently, Shefner and colleagues proposed a new method to follow over time motor unit loss in patients with ALS [59]: nerves were stimulated at 3 specified locations and 3 increments were obtained at each location. Average single motor unit action potential (SMUP) amplitude was calculated by adding the amplitude of the third increment at each location and dividing by 9; SMUP was divided into maximum CMAP amplitude to determine the MUNE. This approach needs further validation, but has some unquestionable advantages: it's easy to perform, well tolerated by patients and specialized equipment is not necessary. Most important, by applying the multipoint method MUNE values decline rapidly in patients with ALS, although the rate of decline is similar to that obtained with the standard incremental technique.

Use of Macro-EMG is limited to muscles from which electrical activity can be elicited without any interference from other muscles [60]; moreover, it's difficult to perform it in the hands during the course of the disease due to the strong wasting of the intrinsic hand muscles. Because of these limitations, our twenty-years experience led us to combine the two techniques in order to improve diagnostic sensitivity each other.

4. Different motor neuron impairment and axonal regeneration rate in patients with sporadic or familial Amyotrophic Lateral Sclerosis with SOD-1 mutations

4.1. Background and methodological considerations

In a previous study [61] we found that ALS patients with SOD-1 mutations have a higher number of MU at moment of diagnosis when compared with sporadic cases, as previously emerged from the work of Aggarwal in pre-symptomatic SOD-1 mutations carriers [27, 62]. Compared with previous studies, our innovatory ideas were:

i. taking into consideration simultaneously Macro-EMG and MUNE changes in proximal and distal muscles in the same sample of patients;

ii. following all our patients with a one-year follow-up;

iii. evaluating Macro-EMG and MUNE changes both in sporadic and familiar cases (sALs and fALS).

In the group of 15 symptomatic SOD-1 mutation carriers, two were found to have a point mutation in exon 4, codon 100, GAA to GGA-Glu100Gly; two were found to have a point mutation in exon 4, codon 113, ATT to ACT-Ile113Thr; five were found to have a point mutation in exon 5, codon 148, GTA to GGA-Val148Gly, and six with homozygous for aspartate to alanine mutations in codon 90 (homD90A), representing the most common SOD-1 mutation with a typical recessive fashion inheritance. Sixty ALS patients (34 males: mean age ± SD 60.0 ± 15.5 years; 26 females: mean age ± SD 62.0 ± 9.2 years) were enrolled in the study and examined basally (T0) and every 4 months (T1, T2, and T3). Fifteen of these patients are familial (SOD-1 mutation carriers, 9 males: mean age ± 1SD 46.3 ± 14.8 years; 6 females: mean age ± 1SD 49.0 ± 8.5 years). Macro Motor Unit Potentials (macro-MUPs) were derived from Biceps Brachialis (BB) muscle; MUNE was performed both in BB and Abductor Digiti Minimi (ADM) muscles of the same side. Thirty-three healthy volunteers (13 females and 20 males, mean age: 57.7 ± 13.8 years) served as controls. All patients had probable or definite ALS, according to the well known criteria of the World Federation of Neurology [18]. The sample group of patients included cases with a disease duration from clinical onset of symptoms to the time of the first examination less than 48 months (mean ± SD: 12.2 ± 11.0 months). Twenty-two patients presented a bulbar onset and the remaining a spinal one. As concerns symptoms and signs, among SOD-1 mutation carriers 10 have the spinal type, while only 5 patients have the bulbar type. Forty patients were in treatment with riluzole (Rilutek®, 50 mg) at a mean daily dosage of 100 mg throughout the period of EDX follow-up.

Standard macro-EMG method was applied [39]. The SFEMG recording surface was exposed 7.5 mm from the tip and the recording was made using two channels: the first one in whom the SFEMG activity was displayed (using the cannula as reference) and used to identify the MU and trigger the averaging procedure (band-pass filter for this channel: 500-10KHz); fiber density (FD) of the triggering single fibre electrode was recorded. The second channel averaged the activity from the cannula until a smooth baseline and a constant macro MUP was obtained (Filter pass-band: 5-10KHz). We measured from the averaged signal the total area between the curve and the baseline, the maximal peak-to-peak amplitude (macro-MUP) during the total sweep time of 70ms [63]. Results were expressed as individual area values from at least 20 trials. The relative macro amplitude was expressed as the obtained mean value [39]. Fibre density was expressed as number of time locked spikes obtained on the SFEMG channel [64]. In twenty-nine patients (subgroup 1: 19 males and 10 females; mean age ± 1SD: 60,0 ± 11,8 years; spinal/bulbar onset: 22/7; mean disease duration 29,7 months) macro-EMG was repeated after 4 months (T1). Among the second subgroup, eleven patients (subgroup 2: 8 males and 3 females; mean age ± SD: 57,0 ± 12,8 years; range 30–72 years; spinal/bulbar onset: 10/1; mean disease duration 31 months) were re-tested after 8 months (T2) and in 8 (subgroup 3; 7 males and 1 female; mean age ± SD: 58,0 ± 13,6 years; spinal/bulbar onset: 7/1; mean disease duration 37 months) after 12 months from the first examination.

MUNE technique was performed on the same Keypoint® EMG equipment (Medtronic Dantec, Copenhagen) provided with specific software for data acquisition and processing at same time and immediately after macro EMG on the same test session. The used technique relayed on manual incremental stimulation of the motor nerve, known as the McComas technique [46]. The use of specific software for MUNE detects "alternation", eliminates subjectivity and the sampling of artifactually small motor units in ALS patients [36, 46, 54]. Percutaneous stimuli were delivered over musculocutaneous nerve immediately below axilla, recording from BB muscles, and ulnar nerve at the wrist by recording from the ADM muscle of the same upper limb [36]. Signals were detected with common surface electrodes, Ag/AgCl type, tapered on the cutis over target muscles with a common muscle-belly tendon montage.

4.2. Main findings and possible explanations

MUNE values in ALS patients were behind normal limits in 55 (91.7%) and within normal limits in 5 (8.3%) in biceps brachialis (BB) muscle; in 58 (96.7%) and in 2 (3.3%) in ADM muscle, respectively [36]. In brief, we can summarize our findings in two main points:

- **i.** MUNE revealed a normal amount of motor units in fALS at the moment of diagnosis, followed by a dramatic loss of motor units, more pronounced than in patients with sALS (see Figure 1, top panels);
- **ii.** Macro-EMG in SOD-1 fALS showed increased fiber density and area values when compared with patients with sALS, likely suggesting a paradoxical more effective axonal sprouting in fALS (Figure 1, bottom panels).

Functioning MUs number progressively decreased in both muscles throughout the entire follow-up period. In ALS MUNE exhibited a parallel trends in proximal and distal muscles (BB and ADM), independently of disease duration; mean step area, instead, increased more in BB, especially in patients with longer disease duration. The MUNE's results as concerns patients with fALS, SOD-1 positive, were 80.2 ± 7.8 (T0), 21.8 ± 2.2 (T1), 16.8 ± 1.0 (T2) and 16.5 ± 2.2 (T3) for BB and 42.8 ± 6.6 (T0), 18.4 ± 3.1 (T1), 15.3 ± 2.1 (T2) and 9.0 ± 2.1 (T3) for ADM. Curiously, SOD-1 fALS patients showed a higher number of functioning motor units in the early stage of disease ($p<0.001$) and a more dramatic drop in later phases (Figure 1). These results suggest a normal pool of motor units in asymptomatic familiar ALS carriers [27]. No electrodiagnostic difference was found between patients with different SOD-1 point mutations. Moreover, we did not found any significant difference between spinal and bulbar-onset fALS in terms of surviving MU, for both BB and ADM muscles ($p>0.05$, Figure 2), as well as between males and females ($p>0.05$, Figure 3).

In sALS patients at T0, both Macro-motor Unit Potentials (Macro-MUPs) area and fiber density (FD) were above upper normal limits (for a global overview of Macro-EMG in healthy subjects, see Sartucci et al., 2007 and 2011): macro-MUP area was 4397.6 ± 255.9 μVms, mean FD 2.0 ± 0.2 (a summary of results is given in Figure 2). The macro-MUP area was abnormal in 57 (95.0%) and normal in 3 (5.0%) patients; in SOD-1 carriers baseline values of MUP area and FD matched

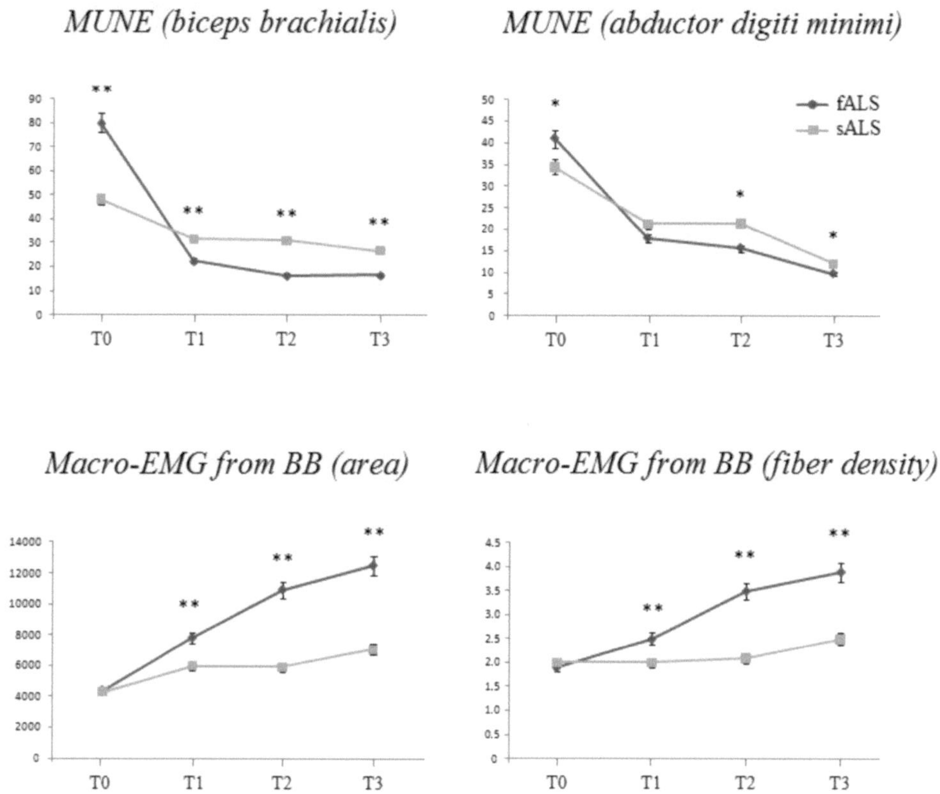

Figure 1. The top row shows MUNE values both for biceps brachialis, on the left, and abductor digiti minimi muscles, on the right, at different time points (at the moment of diagnosis and after 4, 8 and 12 months: T0, T1, T2 and T3). At the moment of diagnosis, motor units number is higher for familiar cases (black lines, fALS) compared with sporadic ones (gray lines, sALS). Bottom row shows time-trend of Macro-EMG parameters (fiber density, area) over time. All the values increase more steeply in familiar than in sporadic forms (black and gray lines, respectively), strengthening the idea that in the first group there is a paradoxical more effective axonal sprouting (modified from Bocci et al., *Int J Mol Sci* 2011; *p < 0.05; **p < 0.01).

with those of sALS patients (4378.9 ± 319.6 µVms and 1.9 ± 0.3, for Macro-MUPs area and FD respectively; p = 0.815 and p = 0.147). In sALS, Macro-MUPs area resulted progressively increased at every time, especially at T3, compared with T0 (Figure 1, bottom panels): Area: + 45.3% (T1); + 49.0% (T2); + 83.6% (T3); FD showed a trend to increase up to T3: +3.5% (T1); +15.4% (T2); +22.4% (T3). Interestingly, in SOD-1 carriers there was a much steeper increase at T1, T2 and T3 in respect to sporadic forms, as concerns both Macro-MUPs area and FD values. Macro-MUPs area was 7791.0 ± 953.4, 10922.8 ± 1123.7 and 12499.3 ± 1874.4 (p<0.01) µVms and mean FD 2.5 ± 0.3, 3.5 ± 0.6 and 3.9 ± 0.5 (p>0.01). As a whole, these results account both for a more severe involvement of alfa-motorneurons pool and a paradoxical more effective axonal sprouting in fALS compared with sALS.

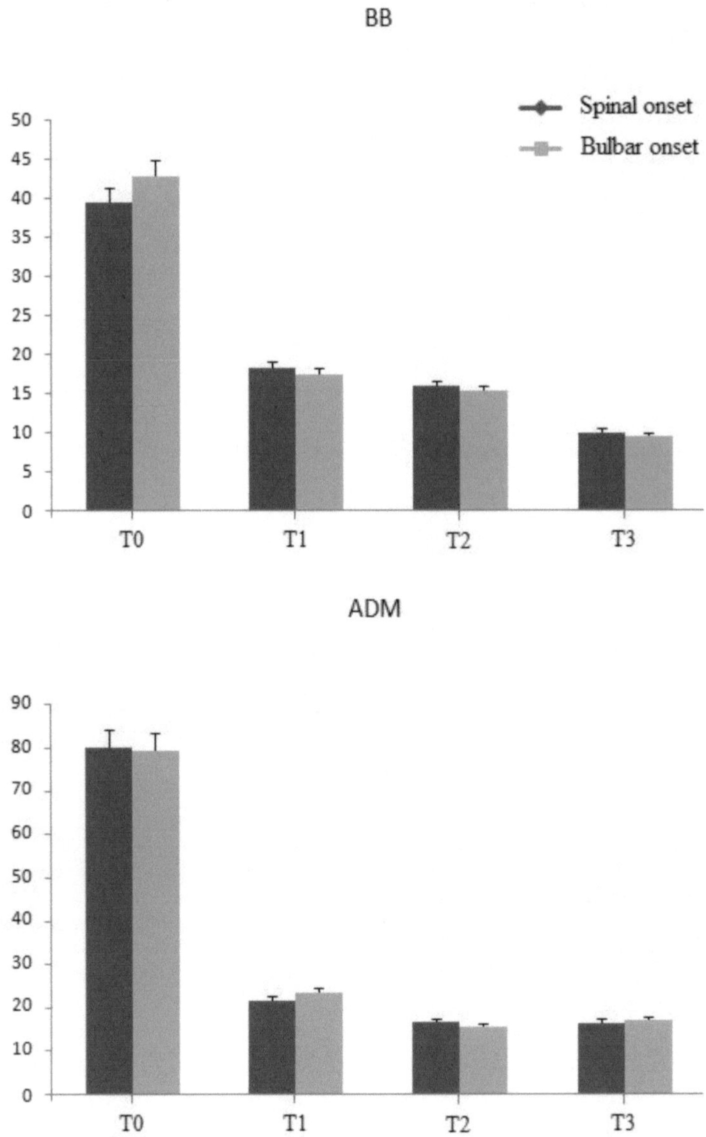

Figure 2. Histogram highlighting MUNE values in both BB (at the top) and ADM (bottom histogram) muscles at every time of follow-up, in males (gray columns) and females (black columns); the top row shows the evolution of motor unit loss in the familiar form, whereas the bottom one the trend in sporadic cases (modified from Bocci et al., *Int J Mol Sci* 2011).

Macro-MUP area and FD were beyond upper normal limits, as expected, in ALS [63, 65]. Our results indicate that carriers of SOD-1 mutations have a higher number of motor units at moment of diagnosis when compared with sporadic cases. On the other hand, in sALS the macro-EMG parameters progressively increased, displaying a gradual increment of correlation up to 8 months, suggesting that the process of MU rearrangement begins to fall after 8 months of disease course. In familiar SOD-1 form there isn't a specific time interval in which the axonal regeneration and the collateral sprouting can balance the neuronal damage. Paradoxically, despite faster loss of motor units, in fALS we have undisclosed a more effective axonal sprouting in the few surviving motor fibers. Compared with sporadic forms, in SOD-1 fALS the substantial lack of a fleeting stabilization of motor unit number within eight months from clinical onset, as emerged from MUNE, could indicate that damage of cell types different from motor neurons is a critical factor for the progression of corticospinal degeneration [66, 67]. Our results strengthen the idea that accelerated disease progression does not alter the timing of disease onset. These data are consistent with those reported by Yamanaka and colleagues [67]: using chimeras derived from embryonic cells of SOD-1^{G37R} mice, they postulated that multiple cell types drive non-cell-autonomous onset of motor degeneration. That could also explain the wide variability in terms of age of onset, clinical presentation and rate of progression in familiar forms of ALS. This is in line with previous papers showing a differential pyramidal tract degeneration in homozygous SOD-1^{D90A} ALS and sALS [68-70]; e.g., Blain and colleagues have recently reported a marked reduction in fractional anisotropy in the corticospinal tract in patients with sALS and fALS, despite similar levels of upper motor neurons dysfunction and overall clinical disability [68]. ALS is featured by repetitive cycles of denervation/reinnervation and the mechanism lead to a variation in FD within a given motor unit [33, 42]. SOD-1 carriers had a full complement of motor neurons during the asymptomatic phase, indicating that SOD-1 mutation carriers have normal survival of motor neurons until sudden catastrophic cell death occurs. This significant gradual preclinical loss does not occur in SOD-1 mutation carriers. Despite the small sample of fALS patients, we also tried to detect significant differences in motor unit pool between spinal and bulbar forms, for both BB and ADM muscles (Figure 2). Interestingly, we did not found any difference suggesting the rate and amount of motor units decrease are approximately similar in proximal and distal muscles. That confirms the non length-dependent and all-or-none nature of pathological processes underlying progression of fALS. A possible explanation could be based on an epigenetics approach: it has been proposed that epigenetic silencing of genes vital for motor neuron function could underlie ALS [44,45]. The promoters of genes thought to be implicated in sALS, SOD-1 and VEGF, or that of MT-Ia and MT-II (the most common human isoforms of the metallothionein (MT) family of proteins), have been found with inappropriate methylation levels [46]. There's an increasing interest in this field, despite no conclusive remark has been collected in human models so far. That's likely due to the discrepancy between humans patients and animal models, in terms of disease and pre-symptomatic phase duration, absence of sensitive biological markers and different pathogenesis. Our findings agree with those described by Aggarwal both in symptomatic and asymptomatic SOD-1 mutation carriers [27]: symptomatic fALS could represent an all-or none process and it is not the final result of a slow attrition of motor neurons.

Another interesting finding is about the lack of significant differences in motor unit depletion over time between females and males in SOD-1 type, both in fALS and sALS form (see Figure 3): the antioxidant effects of estrogens and their proved role in preventing glutamate related

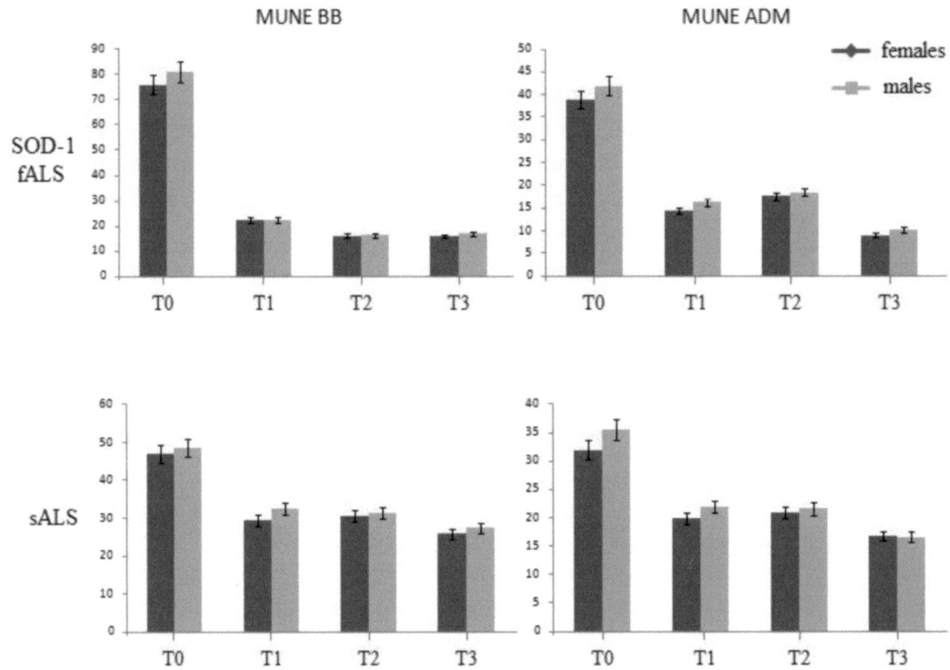

Figure 3. Histogram highlighting MUNE values in both BB (left) and ADM (right) muscles at every time of follow-up, in males (gray columns) and females (black columns); the top row shows the evolution of motor unit loss in the familiar form, whereas the bottom one the trend in sporadic cases. The lack of significant differences between males and females, in sporadic as well as in familiar forms, is consistent with results recently reported in recent literature [71, 72]. (modified from Bocci et al., *Int J Mol Sci* 2011: *p<0.05; **p<0.01).

toxicity in vitro [71, 72] could not delay both the early retraction of nerve terminals from neuromuscular end-plates and the dying-back of axons during asymptomatic phase in vivo.

5. Conclusions and future directions

Although our preliminary results cannot be directly compared with those found in animals, these data could expand current knowledges about morphological and functional differences between mutant and wild type motorneurons in ALS.

We speculate that overbranching occurs not only in dendrites but also in the few surviving axons. This increased complexity of axonal arborization, compared both with healthy and sALS subjects, is still largely undervalued and whether that represents a pointless neuroprotective response of nervous system or a disease mechanism is an intriguing matter of debate. However, as suggested in animal models [73], our Macro-EMG data seem to suggest that overbranching might be one way to mitigate loss of function along corticospinal pathways. These evidences highlight a novel hypothesis for the adult onset of fALS symptoms, namely that they result from age-related factors (e.g., neuron loss or other traumatic insults) that cause a breakdown of homeostatic compensatory processes for neuronal hyperactivity.

Further studies are needed to solve these dilemmas, especially in familiar forms different from those related to mutations pertaining to Cu/Zn superoxide dismutase gene. Particularly, it could be very interesting if a combined MUNE/Macro-EMG protocol was applied to subjects carrying mutations in C9ORF72 gene; these patients, although very rare in the Mediterranean area, typically have upper motor neuron-predominant variants, show memory and executive dysfunctions and account for about 30% of the cases of fALS [74-77]. Most important, the increasing interest in C9ORF72 mutations are due to the frequent association with extra-pyramidal features and Frontotemporal Dementia spectrum.

Author details

Tommaso Bocci[1,2], Elisa Giorli[1,2], Lucia Briscese[1], Silvia Tognazzi[3], Fabio Giannini[2] and Ferdinando Sartucci[1,3,4*]

*Address all correspondence to: f.sartucci@neuro.med.unipi.it

1 Department of Neuroscience, Unit of Neurology, Pisa University Medical School, Pisa, Italy

2 Department of Neuroscience, Neurology and Clinical Neurophysiology Section, Siena University Medical School, Siena, Italy

3 Department of Neuroscience, Cisanello Neurology Unit, Azienda Ospedaliera Universitaria Pisana, Pisa, Italy

4 CNR Neuroscience Institute, Pisa, Italy

References

[1] Juergens, S.M., et al., *ALS in Rochester, Minnesota, 1925-1977.* Neurology, 1980. 30(5): p. 463-70.

[2] Swash, M., *ALS and motor neuron disorders today and tomorrow.* Amyotroph Lateral Scler Other Motor Neuron Disord, 2001. 2(4): p. 171-2.

[3] Andersen, P.M., et al., *Good practice in the management of amyotrophic lateral sclerosis: clinical guidelines. An evidence-based review with good practice points. EALSC Working Group.* Amyotroph Lateral Scler, 2007. 8(4): p. 195-213.

[4] Rosen, D.R., et al., *Mutations in Cu/Zn superoxide dismutase gene are associated with familial amyotrophic lateral sclerosis.* Nature, 1993. 362(6415): p. 59-62.

[5] Andersen, P.M., et al., *Phenotypic heterogeneity in motor neuron disease patients with CuZn-superoxide dismutase mutations in Scandinavia.* Brain, 1997. 120 (Pt 10): p. 1723-37.

[6] de Belleroche, J., R. Orrell, and A. King, *Familial amyotrophic lateral sclerosis/motor neurone disease (FALS): a review of current developments.* J Med Genet, 1995. 32(11): p. 841-7.

[7] Aggarwal, A. and G. Nicholson, *Detection of preclinical motor neurone loss in SOD1 mutation carriers using motor unit number estimation.* J Neurol Neurosurg Psychiatry, 2002. 73(2): p. 199-201.

[8] Clarke, G., C.J. Lumsden, and R.R. McInnes, *Inherited neurodegenerative diseases: the one-hit model of neurodegeneration.* Hum Mol Genet, 2001. 10(20): p. 2269-75.

[9] Johnston, J.A., et al., *Formation of high molecular weight complexes of mutant Cu, Zn-superoxide dismutase in a mouse model for familial amyotrophic lateral sclerosis.* Proc Natl Acad Sci U S A, 2000. 97(23): p. 12571-6.

[10] Bruijn, L.I., et al., *ALS-linked SOD1 mutant G85R mediates damage to astrocytes and promotes rapidly progressive disease with SOD1-containing inclusions.* Neuron, 1997. 18(2): p. 327-38.

[11] Deng, H.X., et al., *Conversion to the amyotrophic lateral sclerosis phenotype is associated with intermolecular linked insoluble aggregates of SOD1 in mitochondria.* Proc Natl Acad Sci U S A, 2006. 103(18): p. 7142-7.

[12] Kong, J. and Z. Xu, *Massive mitochondrial degeneration in motor neurons triggers the onset of amyotrophic lateral sclerosis in mice expressing a mutant SOD1.* J Neurosci, 1998. 18(9): p. 3241-50.

[13] Amendola, J. and J. Durand, *Morphological differences between wild-type and transgenic superoxide dismutase 1 lumbar motoneurons in postnatal mice.* J Comp Neurol, 2008. 511(3): p. 329-41.

[14] Avossa, D., et al., *Early signs of motoneuron vulnerability in a disease model system: Characterization of transverse slice cultures of spinal cord isolated from embryonic ALS mice.* Neuroscience, 2006. 138(4): p. 1179-94.

[15] Schutz, B., *Imbalanced excitatory to inhibitory synaptic input precedes motor neuron degeneration in an animal model of amyotrophic lateral sclerosis.* Neurobiol Dis, 2005. 20(1): p. 131-40.

[16] Pieri, M., et al., *Altered excitability of motor neurons in a transgenic mouse model of familial amyotrophic lateral sclerosis.* Neurosci Lett, 2003. 351(3): p. 153-6.

[17] Kuo, J.J., et al., *Hyperexcitability of cultured spinal motoneurons from presymptomatic ALS mice.* J Neurophysiol, 2004. 91(1): p. 571-5.

[18] Bories, C., et al., *Early electrophysiological abnormalities in lumbar motoneurons in a transgenic mouse model of amyotrophic lateral sclerosis.* Eur J Neurosci, 2007. 25(2): p. 451-9.

[19] Schwindt, P. and W.E. Crill, *A persistent negative resistance in cat lumbar motoneurons.* Brain Res, 1977. 120(1): p. 173-8.

[20] Schwindt, P.C. and W.E. Crill, *Properties of a persistent inward current in normal and TEA-injected motoneurons.* J Neurophysiol, 1980. 43(6): p. 1700-24.

[21] Schwindt, P.C. and W.E. Crill, *Factors influencing motoneuron rhythmic firing: results from a voltage-clamp study.* J Neurophysiol, 1982. 48(4): p. 875-90.

[22] ElBasiouny, S.M., J.E. Schuster, and C.J. Heckman, *Persistent inward currents in spinal motoneurons: important for normal function but potentially harmful after spinal cord injury and in amyotrophic lateral sclerosis.* Clin Neurophysiol, 2010. 121(10): p. 1669-79.

[23] Carriedo, S.G., H.Z. Yin, and J.H. Weiss, *Motor neurons are selectively vulnerable to AMPA/kainate receptor-mediated injury in vitro.* J Neurosci, 1996. 16(13): p. 4069-79.

[24] Carriedo, S.G., et al., *AMPA exposures induce mitochondrial Ca(2+) overload and ROS generation in spinal motor neurons in vitro.* J Neurosci, 2000. 20(1): p. 240-50.

[25] Magrane, J., et al., *Mutant SOD1 in neuronal mitochondria causes toxicity and mitochondrial dynamics abnormalities.* Hum Mol Genet, 2009. 18(23): p. 4552-64.

[26] Magrane, J. and G. Manfredi, *Mitochondrial function, morphology, and axonal transport in amyotrophic lateral sclerosis.* Antioxid Redox Signal, 2009. 11(7): p. 1615-26.

[27] Aggarwal, A. and G. Nicholson, *Normal complement of motor units in asymptomatic familial (SOD1 mutation) amyotrophic lateral sclerosis carriers.* J Neurol Neurosurg Psychiatry, 2001. 71(4): p. 478-81.

[28] Brooks, B.R., et al., *El Escorial revisited: revised criteria for the diagnosis of amyotrophic lateral sclerosis.* Amyotroph Lateral Scler Other Motor Neuron Disord, 2000. 1(5): p. 293-9.

[29] Beghi, E., et al., *Reliability of the El Escorial diagnostic criteria for amyotrophic lateral sclerosis.* Neuroepidemiology, 2002. 21(6): p. 265-70.

[30] Olney, R.K. and C. Lomen-Hoerth, *Motor unit number estimation (MUNE): how may it contribute to the diagnosis of ALS?* Amyotroph Lateral Scler Other Motor Neuron Disord, 2000. 1 Suppl 2: p. S41-4.

[31] Daube, J.R., et al., *Motor unit number estimation (MUNE) with nerve conduction studies.* Suppl Clin Neurophysiol, 2000. 53: p. 112-5.

[32] Bromberg, M.B., et al., *Motor unit number estimation, isometric strength, and electromyographic measures in amyotrophic lateral sclerosis.* Muscle Nerve, 1993. 16(11): p. 1213-9.

[33] de Carvalho, M., J. Costa, and M. Swash, *Clinical trials in ALS: a review of the role of clinical and neurophysiological measurements.* Amyotroph Lateral Scler Other Motor Neuron Disord, 2005. 6(4): p. 202-12.

[34] Eisen, A., *Clinical electrophysiology of the upper and lower motor neuron in amyotrophic lateral sclerosis.* Semin Neurol, 2001. 21(2): p. 141-54.

[35] Finsterer, J. and A. Fuglsang-Frederiksen, *Concentric-needle versus macro EMG. II. Detection of neuromuscular disorders.* Clin Neurophysiol, 2001. 112(5): p. 853-60.

[36] Sartucci, F., et al., *Motor unit number estimation (mune) as a quantitative measure of disease progression and motor unit reorganization in amyotrophic lateral sclerosis.* Int J Neurosci, 2007. 117(9): p. 1229-36.

[37] Sartucci, F., et al., *Macro-EMG and MUNE changes in patients with amyotrophic lateral sclerosis: one-year follow up.* Int J Neurosci, 2011. 121(5): p. 257-66.

[38] Stålberg, E., *Macro EMG, a new recording technique.* J Neurol Neurosurg Psychiatry, 1980. 43(6): p. 475-82.

[39] Stålberg, E., *Macro EMG.* Muscle Nerve, 1983. 6(9): p. 619-30.

[40] Stalberg, E. and P.R. Fawcett, *Macro EMG in healthy subjects of different ages.* J Neurol Neurosurg Psychiatry, 1982. 45(10): p. 870-8.

[41] Dengler, R., et al., *Amyotrophic lateral sclerosis: macro-EMG and twitch forces of single motor units.* Muscle Nerve, 1990. 13(6): p. 545-50.

[42] de Carvalho, M., et al., *Neurophysiological measures in amyotrophic lateral sclerosis: markers of progression in clinical trials.* Amyotroph Lateral Scler Other Motor Neuron Disord, 2005. 6(1): p. 17-28.

[43] Guiloff, R.J., et al., *Short-term stability of single motor unit recordings in motor neuron disease: a macro EMG study.* J Neurol Neurosurg Psychiatry, 1988. 51(5): p. 671-6.

[44] Daube, J.R., *Estimating the number of motor units in a muscle.* J Clin Neurophysiol, 1995. 12(6): p. 585-94.

[45] Daube, J.R., *Motor unit number estimates--from A to Z.* J Neurol Sci, 2006. 242(1-2): p. 23-35.

[46] McComas, A.J., *Motor unit estimation: anxieties and achievements.* Muscle Nerve, 1995. 18(4): p. 369-79.

[47] Wang, F.C. and P.J. Delwaide, *Number and relative size of thenar motor units in ALS patients: application of the adapted multiple point stimulation method.* Electroencephalogr Clin Neurophysiol, 1998. 109(1): p. 36-43.

[48] Gooch, C.L. and J.M. Shefner, *ALS surrogate markers. MUNE.* Amyotroph Lateral Scler Other Motor Neuron Disord, 2004. 5 Suppl 1: p. 104-7.

[49] McComas, A.J., et al., *Electrophysiological estimation of the number of motor units within a human muscle.* J Neurol Neurosurg Psychiatry, 1971. 34(2): p. 121-31.

[50] Liu, X.X., et al., *Stratifying disease stages with different progression rates determined by electrophysiological tests in patients with amyotrophic lateral sclerosis.* Muscle Nerve, 2009. 39(3): p. 304-9.

[51] Boe, S.G., D.W. Stashuk, and T.J. Doherty, *Motor unit number estimates and quantitative motor unit analysis in healthy subjects and patients with amyotrophic lateral sclerosis.* Muscle Nerve, 2007. 36(1): p. 62-70.

[52] Kwon, O. and K.W. Lee, *Reproducibility of statistical motor unit number estimates in amyotrophic lateral sclerosis: comparisons between size- and number-weighted modifications.* Muscle Nerve, 2004. 29(2): p. 211-7.

[53] Olney, R.K., E.C. Yuen, and J.W. Engstrom, *Statistical motor unit number estimation: reproducibility and sources of error in patients with amyotrophic lateral sclerosis.* Muscle Nerve, 2000. 23(2): p. 193-7.

[54] Hong, Y.H., et al., *Statistical MUNE: a comparison of two methods of setting recording windows in healthy subjects and ALS patients.* Clin Neurophysiol, 2007. 118(12): p. 2605-11.

[55] Sartucci, F., et al., *Macro-EMG and MUNE Changes in Patients with Amyotrophic Lateral Sclerosis: One-Year Follow Up.* Int J Neurosci, 2011.

[56] Shefner, J.M., M.E. Cudkowicz, and R.H. Brown, Jr., *Comparison of incremental with multipoint MUNE methods in transgenic ALS mice.* Muscle Nerve, 2002. 25(1): p. 39-42.

[57] Zhou, C., et al., *A method comparison in monitoring disease progression of G93A mouse model of ALS.* Amyotroph Lateral Scler, 2007. 8(6): p. 366-72.

[58] Shefner, J.M., et al., *Revised statistical motor unit number estimation in the Celecoxib/ALS trial.* Muscle Nerve, 2007. 35(2): p. 228-34.

[59] Shefner, J.M., et al., *Multipoint incremental motor unit number estimation as an outcome measure in ALS.* Neurology, 2011. 77(3): p. 235-241.

[60] de Koning, P., et al., *Estimation of the number of motor units based on macro-EMG.* J Neurol Neurosurg Psychiatry, 1988. 51(3): p. 403-11.

[61] Bocci, T., et al., *Differential Motor Neuron Impairment and Axonal Regeneration in Sporadic and Familiar Amyotrophic Lateral Sclerosis with SOD-1 Mutations: Lessons from Neurophysiology.* Int J Mol Sci, 2011. 12(12): p. 9203-15.

[62] Aggarwal, A., *Motor unit number estimation in asymptomatic familial amyotrophic lateral sclerosis.* Suppl Clin Neurophysiol, 2009. 60: p. 163-9.

[63] Bauermeister, W. and J.F. Jabre, *The spectrum of concentric macro EMG correlations. Part I. Normal subjects.* Muscle Nerve, 1992. 15(10): p. 1081-4.

[64] Sanders, D.B. and E.V. Stalberg, *AAEM minimonograph #25: single-fiber electromyography.* Muscle Nerve, 1996. 19(9): p. 1069-83.

[65] Gan, R. and J.F. Jabre, *The spectrum of concentric macro EMG correlations. Part II. Patients with diseases of muscle and nerve.* Muscle Nerve, 1992. 15(10): p. 1085-8.

[66] Ilieva, H.S., et al., *Mutant dynein (Loa) triggers proprioceptive axon loss that extends survival only in the SOD1 ALS model with highest motor neuron death.* Proc Natl Acad Sci U S A, 2008. 105(34): p. 12599-604.

[67] Yamanaka, K., et al., *Mutant SOD1 in cell types other than motor neurons and oligodendrocytes accelerates onset of disease in ALS mice.* Proc Natl Acad Sci U S A, 2008. 105(21): p. 7594-9.

[68] Blain, C.R., et al., *Differential corticospinal tract degeneration in homozygous 'D90A' SOD-1 ALS and sporadic ALS.* J Neurol Neurosurg Psychiatry. 82(8): p. 843-9.

[69] Agosta, F., et al., *Assessment of white matter tract damage in patients with amyotrophic lateral sclerosis: a diffusion tensor MR imaging tractography study.* AJNR Am J Neuroradiol. 31(8): p. 1457-61.

[70] Agosta, F., et al., *The present and the future of neuroimaging in amyotrophic lateral sclerosis.* AJNR Am J Neuroradiol. 31(10): p. 1769-77.

[71] Hegedus, J., C.T. Putman, and T. Gordon, *Progressive motor unit loss in the G93A mouse model of amyotrophic lateral sclerosis is unaffected by gender.* Muscle Nerve, 2009. 39(3): p. 318-27.

[72] Nakamizo, T., et al., *Protection of cultured spinal motor neurons by estradiol.* Neuroreport, 2000. 11(16): p. 3493-7.

[73] van Zundert, B., et al., *Neonatal neuronal circuitry shows hyperexcitable disturbance in a mouse model of the adult-onset neurodegenerative disease amyotrophic lateral sclerosis.* J Neurosci, 2008. 28(43): p. 10864-74.

[74] Ratti, A., et al., *C9ORF72 repeat expansion in a large Italian ALS cohort: evidence of a founder effect.* Neurobiol Aging, 2012. 33(10): p. 2528 e7-2528 e14.

[75] Chio, A., et al., *ALS/FTD phenotype in two Sardinian families carrying both C9ORF72 and TARDBP mutations.* J Neurol Neurosurg Psychiatry, 2012. 83(7): p. 730-3.

[76] Renton, A.E., et al., *A hexanucleotide repeat expansion in C9ORF72 is the cause of chromosome 9p21-linked ALS-FTD.* Neuron, 2011. 72(2): p. 257-68.

[77] Sabatelli, M., et al., *C9ORF72 hexanucleotide repeat expansions in the Italian sporadic ALS population.* Neurobiol Aging, 2012. 33(8): p. 1848 e15-20.

Chapter 9

Eye-Gaze Input System Suitable for Use under Natural Light and Its Applications Toward a Support for ALS Patients

Abe Kiyohiko, Ohi Shoichi and
Ohyama Minoru

Additional information is available at the end of the chapter

http://dx.doi.org/10.5772/56560

1. Introduction

Recently, eye-gaze input systems have been developed as novel human–machine interfaces [1-10]. Their operation requires only eye movements by the user. Based upon such systems, many communication aids have been developed for people with severe physical disabilities, such as amyotrophic lateral sclerosis (ALS). Eye-gaze input systems commonly employ non-contact eye-gaze detection for which an incandescent, fluorescent, or LED lamp can be used as the source of infrared or natural light. Detection based on infrared light can detect eye gaze with a high degree of accuracy [1-3] but requires an expensive device. Detection based on natural light uses ordinary devices and is therefore cost-effective [4,5]. However, an eye-gaze input system for natural light has a low degree of accuracy.

We have previously developed an eye-gaze input system for people with severe physical disabilities [8-10]. This system uses a personal computer (PC) and a home video camera to detect eye gaze under natural light. The camera (e.g., a DV camera) can easily be connected to a PC through an IEEE 1394 interface. The frames taken by the camera can be analyzed in real time using the DirectShow library by Microsoft. We developed image analysis software to detect eye gaze. Our eye-gaze input system runs the software on Windows. This system does not require any special devices and is easily customizable. Therefore, this system is not only cost-effective but also versatile. Moreover, it can be operated under natural light and thus is suitable for personal use.

2. Current eye-gaze input systems

Many systems or devices have been developed as communication aids for ALS patients. For example, the E-tran (eye transfer) frame is used for communication between ALS patients and others. The E-tran frame is a conventional device and its structure is very simple. It is a transparent plastic board with characters, such as the alphabet, printed on it. When using the E-tran frame, a communication partner (helper) holds it over the user's face. Specifically, the user gazes at the place where the character that the user wishes to communicate is positioned. The helper moves the E-tran frame until the eye gaze of the user corresponds with that of the helper. Therefore, the helper can determine the character from the user's eye gaze. A user who can gaze at the characters on the E-tran frame can also communicate with others. In addition, the E-tran frame does not require power supply and is therefore highly portable. However, considerable skill is required to use the E-tran frame.

The row–column scanning system is also used to aid the communication of ALS patients. This system can be operated with one switch. In other words, the user can input characters or operate a PC by using their physical residual function. The row–column scanning system is configured to exploit simple hardware. For example, if the user employs the screen keyboard that is installed on Windows, the user can operate many of the Windows software applications. It takes considerable time to input using the row–column scanning system, because this system operates by scanning the rows and columns of keyboards using only one switch. To improve upon this situation, a new method for row–column scanning has been reported [11]. This method optimizes the speed of row-column scanning by using a Bayesian network for machine learning. However, a patient with severe ALS cannot use the row–column scanning system, despite its single switch.

Our eye-gaze input system mitigates these weaknesses. In a general eye-gaze input system, the icons displayed on the PC monitor are selected by the user gazing at them, as shown in Figure 1. These icons are called indicators and are assigned to characters or functions of the application program. The eye-gaze input has to detect the user's gaze in order to ascertain the selected indicator. Many eye-gaze detection methods have been developed in the past. Several systems use the EOG(electro-oculogram) method for eye-gaze detection [7], which detects eye gaze by the difference in the electrical potential between the cornea and the retina. It is a contact method that uses electrodes placed around the eye. Although cost-effective, some users find that long-term use of the electrodes is uncomfortable. Therefore, many systems detect eye gaze using non-contact methods [1-10]. Specifically, the user's gaze is detected by analyzing images of the eye (and its surrounding skin) captured by a video camera. To classify the many indicators, most conventional systems use special devices such as infrared light [1-3] or multiple cameras [6]. Nevertheless, in order to be suitable for personal use, the system should be inexpensive and user-friendly. Therefore, a simple system using a single camera in natural light is desirable [4-6]. However, natural-light systems often have low accuracy and are capable of classifying only a few indicators [4]. This makes it difficult for users to perform a task that requires many functions, such as text input. To solve these problems, a simple eye-gaze input system that can classify many indicators is needed.

http://dx.doi.org/10.5772/56560

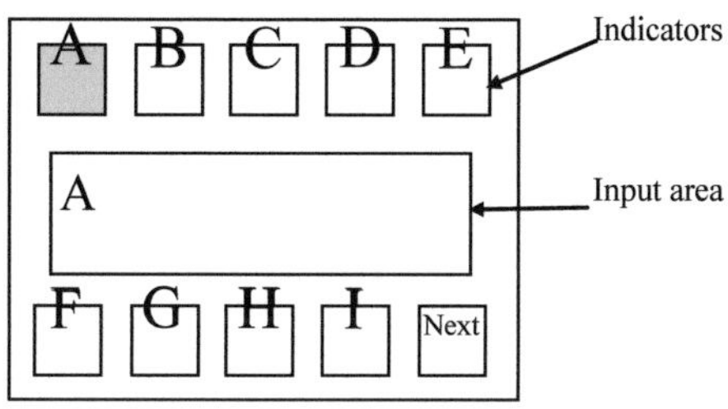

Figure 1. Overview of eye-gaze input

3. Eye-gaze detection by image analysis

Eye gaze is defined as a unit vector in a three-dimensional coordinate space. The origin of this unit vector is the center of the eyeball. Generally, the user's gaze is detected on a two-dimensional plane. It has horizontal and vertical components. The method of tracking the iris (the colored part of the eye) is the most popular method for eye-gaze detection using image analysis in natural light [4-6]. For example, if the edge between the iris and the sclera (the white part of the eye) is estimated by image processing, the appropriately approximated ellipse of the edge shows the location of the iris. However, it is difficult to distinguish the iris and the sclera by image analysis, because the edge between the iris and the sclera is not sharp. In addition, if a large part of the iris is hidden by the upper and lower eyelids, the measurement errors increase, because the obscuring of the iris by the eyelids causes estimation errors in the delineation of the iris. To resolve these issues, we propose a new image analysis method for detecting eye gaze using both the horizontal and vertical directions. This detection method is based on the limbus tracking method. Our eye-gaze detection method can obtain the coordinates of the user's gaze point.

In our eye-gaze detection method, the video camera records images of the user's eye from a distant location (the distance between the user and camera is approximately 70 cm), and then this image is enlarged. The head movements of the user induce a large error in the detected gaze. We compensated for the head movements by tracing the location of a corner within the eye.

3.1. Horizontal gaze detection

The limbus tracking method is an eye-gaze detection method using the difference in reflectance between the iris and the sclera. By this method, eye gaze can be estimated with relative ease, and therefore it has been used since the 1960s [12]. The general eye-gaze detection system using the limbus tracking method irradiates an eyeball of a subject with infrared light. The eye gaze of the subject is detected by measuring the reflected light using optical sensors such as photodiodes.

We have developed a new eye-gaze detection method that is used under natural light [8,9]. An overview of the proposed horizontal gaze detection method is shown in Figure 2. The difference in reflectance between the iris and the sclera is used as follows: the gaze is estimated from the difference between the integral values of the light intensities in Areas A and B, as shown in Figure 2. We designate this differential value as the horizontal eye-gaze value, which gives a value for the horizontal gaze component. The relation between the horizontal eye-gaze value and the angle of sight is nearly proportional. Therefore, the system can be calibrated using this relation.

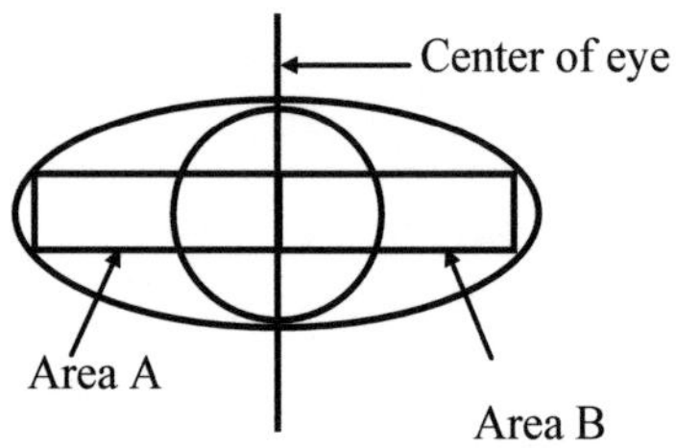

Figure 2. Detection of horizontal gaze

3.2. Vertical gaze detection

An overview of the proposed vertical gaze detection method is shown in Figure 3. The vertical eye-gaze is also detected by the limbus tracking method. In other words, the light intensity of the eye image is used to detect the vertical eye gaze. Specifically, the vertical eye gaze is estimated from the integral value of the light intensity in Area C that is not hidden by the eyelids [10]. We designate this integral value as the vertical eye-gaze value, which gives a value for the vertical gaze component. The relation between the vertical eye-gaze value and the angle of sight is a characteristic function. Therefore, the system can be calibrated using this relation. Many application programs for eye-gaze input need low-accuracy measurements that involve only three directions of vertical eye gaze (top, center, and bottom). Therefore, our practical eye-gaze input system detects only three general directions of vertical eye gaze.

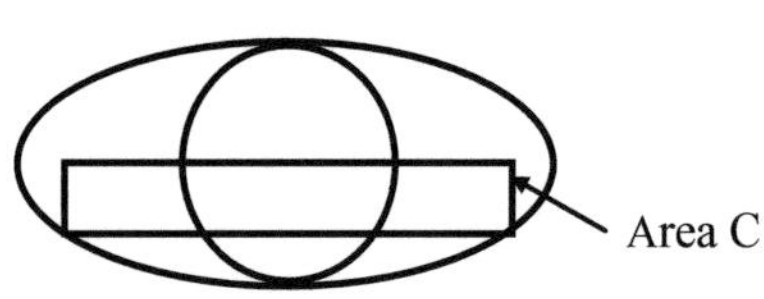

Figure 3. Detection of Vertical gaze (Method 1)

In reality, the light-intensity distribution of the eye image changes with iris movement, and vertical gaze can be detected using this change [9]. The system stores vertically aligned images of the eye gazing at the indicators. The light-intensity distributions (the results of a one-dimensional projection) are calculated from these eye images as reference data. The user's vertical gaze can be detected by pattern matching based on these reference data. An overview of the method is shown in Figure 4, which illustrates the detection of each of the three gaze directions: top, center, and bottom. The wave patterns at the right of the eye illustrations show the light-intensity distributions. We confirmed that with increasing reference data the method can distinguish five to seven vertical gaze directions.

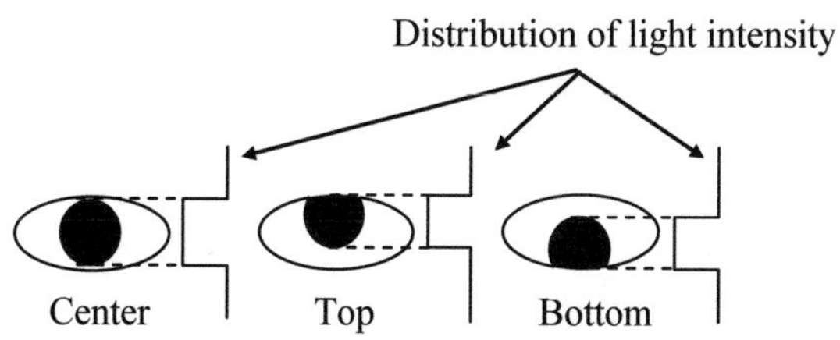

Figure 4. Detection of Vertical gaze (Method 2)

4. Input interfaces based on eye gaze

We developed a new eye-gaze input system using the methods discussed in Section 3. This system detects the eye gaze of a user under natural light and operates the application programs for communication aids such as text input. Two interfaces to operate the application programs have been developed. One of the interfaces has indicators displayed on the PC monitor. The functions of application programs are executed by gazing at these indicators. The other interface allows eye gaze to control the mouse cursor. By means of this interface, a user can operate the general Windows software. We describe our eye-gaze input system and its input interface below.

4.1. Eye-gaze input system

Our eye-gaze input system comprises a PC, a home video camera, and an IEEE 1394 interface for image capture from the camera. For eye-gaze detection, the computer runs image analysis software on Windows (XP, Vista, or 7). This system (illustrated in Figure 5) does not require a device exclusively for image processing. The characteristics of eye gaze vary from one individual to another. Therefore, the eye-gaze input system requires calibration. The indicators for calibration are shown in Figure 6. Users must calibrate the system before using it for tasks. After the camera location is adjusted, the calibration begins. While the calibration is being performed, users gaze at each indicator when its color switches to red. Our eye-gaze input system has two types of indicators, which are specific to each application. In particular, the five calibration indicators shown in Figure 6(a) are used for the input interface with a workspace displayed at the center of the PC monitor. The workspace is used for displaying an application software window. In addition, the nine calibration indicators shown in Figure

6(b) are used for the interface to operate the mouse cursor, because this interface requires a higher accuracy of measurement.

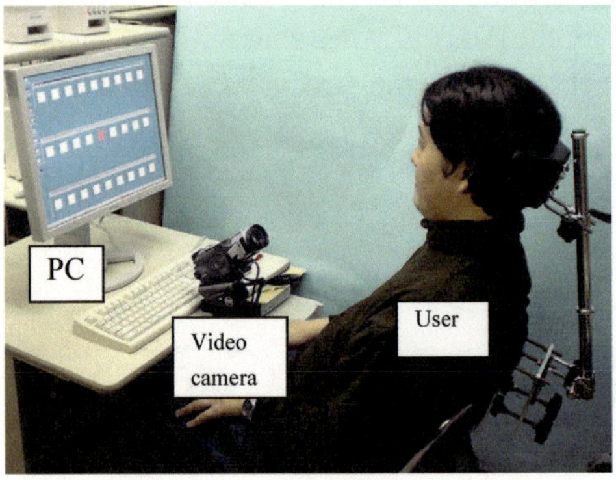

Figure 5. Appearance of proposed system

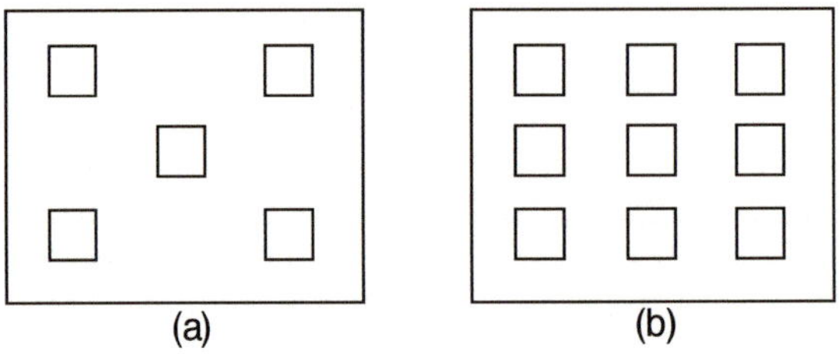

Figure 6. Indicators for calibration

4.2. Interface using indicators displayed on PC monitor

An interface suitable for eye-gaze input can be designed when developing application programs for an eye-gaze input system. For example, an interface using indicators is most commonly used. The indicators are displayed on the windows of the application program and are selected by the gaze of the user. The arrangement of indicators depends on the measurement accuracy of the eye-gaze input system. Our system treats each indicator as one of 27 indicators (3 rows and 9 columns), which permits high accuracy. However, in the interest of usefulness, our practical eye-gaze input system utilizes an interface with 5 to 12 indicators. The arrangement patterns of the indicators are shown in Figure 7.

The arrangement pattern in Figure 7(a) is used when the eye-gaze input system needs fewer than five indicators. This arrangement pattern can be used when the application program requires a small number of indicators. However, it can demand a wide display area for the application program. Therefore, this arrangement is best used by application programs such as a television program viewer. The arrangements in Figures 7(b) and (c) are used when the eye-gaze input system needs 6 to 12 indicators. In particular, some kinds of application programs require 6 to 10 indicators. These application programs utilize the arrangement in Figure 7(b). For example, fixed-phrase mailers or Web browsers use this arrangement pattern.

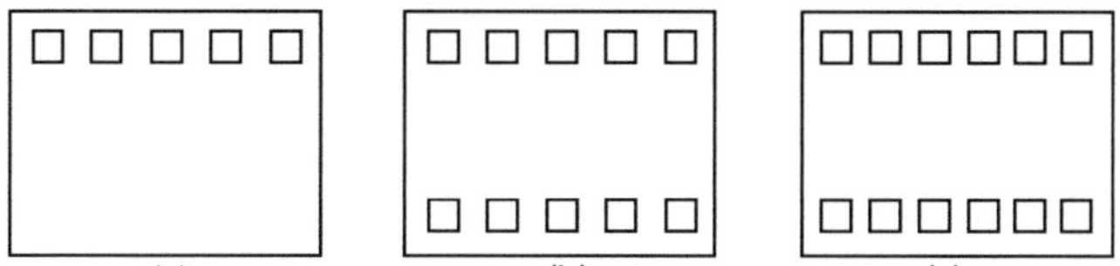

Figure 7. Arrangement patterns of indicators

In addition, text input is a popular application for eye-gaze input. Around 60 indicators are required to input Japanese text. In fact, English text input systems require a similar number of indicators, because the English language contains uppercase letters, lowercase letters, and punctuation marks. Moreover, control keys are required for text input. If around 60 indicators are displayed on a screen, the window for text input cannot be arranged on the same screen. In other words, its operability is greatly decreased. Therefore, we developed a text input system for Japanese and English using the indicators shown in Figure 7(c). Its interface requires two selections: one for character group selection and another for character input (the details are given in Section 5). For an eye-gaze input system with the indicators shown in Figure 7(a), (b), or (c), there is no necessity to detect eye gaze when the user gazes at the center of the PC monitor. Therefore, an eye-gaze input system using any of these arrangements is calibrated with the simple indicators shown in Figure 6(a).

Generally, the eye-gaze input decision with such an interface requires the detection of not only the user's gaze point but also the user's command for an indicator (assigned character) selection. An input decision can be made by using eye fixation, measuring the time for which the eye fixates on a target such as one of the indicators. The abovementioned interface using indicator selection requires special application programs. However, the operability of the system can be increased by using suitably designed indicators. The users need to sufficiently practice operating this system to operate the application programs at a faster pace.

4.3. Interface for mouse operation

When users operate a PC with the mouse, they gaze at the mouse cursor routinely. In other words, if the mouse cursor can be moved to the user's gaze point, the eye gaze of the user can be utilized for an input interface. Our eye-gaze input system can obtain the coordinates of the user's gaze point. In other words, when a user gazes at a point on the PC screen, the mouse cursor moves to that point.

If the mouse cursor is controlled by eye gaze, the user gazes over the entire area of screen. Hence, the eye gaze of the user must be detected with a high degree of accuracy. Therefore, a system with this interface is calibrated using the indicators shown in Figure 6(b). By using an interface for mouse operation, the general Windows software can be operated without any special application programs. In addition, Windows operations such as copying a file can be performed by eye gaze. The method for operating this interface is clear and simple; therefore, this interface is user-friendly.

We developed special application programs for eye-gaze input. However, users may want to run other Windows software. By selecting the abovementioned interface, users can fulfill this desire. However, the icons and menu items of the general Windows software are small for eye-gaze input. In other words, it is difficult to select the icons and menu items with mouse operations by eye gaze. When users gaze at one point on the object viewed, their eye fixation has micromotions (called involuntary eye movements). Therefore, it is difficult to keep the mouse cursor on the viewed object for the time required for eye-gaze input. In addition, the general Windows software and the eye-gaze detection software are executed on Windows separately. Hence, the general Windows software cannot recognize the icon or menu item that is gazed at by the user.

To resolve these issues, the interface for mouse operation requires a different method for input decisions. We think that an eye blink should provide the information used in this input decision method. The details of this method are given in Section 6.

5. Application programs for eye-gaze input

Our research group has developed application programs for eye-gaze input to assist ALS patients. The interface of the application programs employs indicators displayed on the PC monitor, as shown in Section 4-2. We present our application programs below.

5.1. Text input system

Text input is the most important function to aid communication by ALS patients. Inputting text by eye gaze increases the convenience of their communication. We designed indicators for text input by eye gaze, considering the success rate of gaze selection with our proposed system [9]. There are 12 indicators (2 rows and 6 columns). With this system, users can input Japanese or English text at a faster pace. However, around 60 indicators are required to input Japanese text. Similarly, 12 indicators are insufficient for English text input, because the English language contains uppercase letters, lowercase letters, and punctuation marks. To resolve this problem, we designed a new interface through which users can select any character (English or Japanese) by first choosing the indicator group. An overview of the interface is shown in Figure 8.

This interface requires two selections: one for character group selection (e.g., Group "A–E") and another for character input. Letters require two selections, and punctuation marks ("etc." in Figure 8) also require two. However, commonly used characters such as the space ("SPC" in Figure 8) require just one selection. To input the character "C," the user first selects the indicator for Group "A–E" and then the indicator for the uppercase letter "C." Japanese characters can be input in the same way.

http://dx.doi.org/10.5772/56560

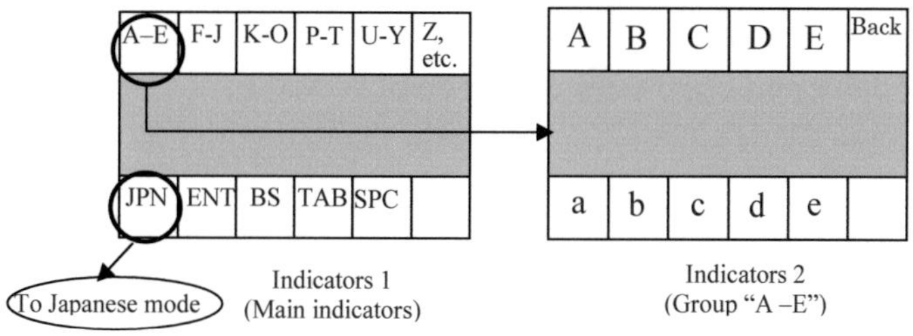

Figure 8. Text input system

5.2. Support system for personal computer operation

If users can operate general Windows functions by eye gaze, they can operate commonly used application programs such as mailers and Web browsers. Users can input text to these applications using the abovementioned interface for text input. Such applications are normally operated by keyboard or mouse, especially the latter. When an eye-gaze input system is used, the functions of the application programs must be assigned to indicators. We have extended our system to general Windows functions. Many guidelines have been proposed for the development of application programs for the disabled. To satisfy these guidelines, we assign the following Windows functions to indicators: cursor control; execution of application programs; use of shortcut keys to copy, cut, and paste; and selection of items from a menu bar. Hence, commercial applications can be used with our system [9]. The Windows functions are organized as shown in Figure 9, and the user can switch indicator group. The "main operation screen" has indicators for cursor operation, object selection, decision input (enter), etc. The "extended operation screen" has indicators for operating the mouse, activating the desktop, switching, or closing the window, etc. Using these indicators, all general Windows functions can be performed.

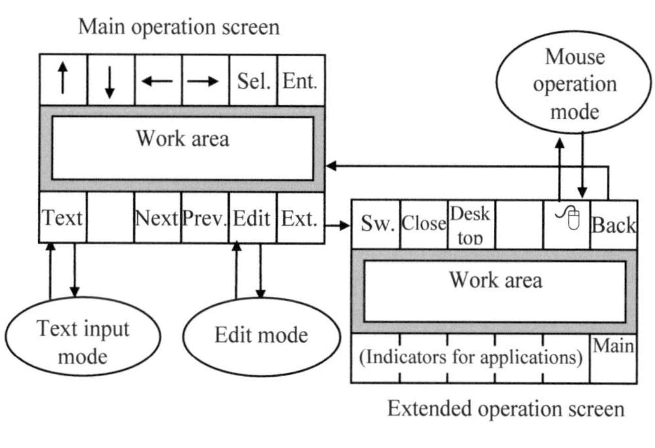

Figure 9. Support system for personal computer operation

As described in Section 4-3, general Windows functions can be extended by controlling the mouse cursor by eye gaze. However, indicators that include the commonly used functions actualize a comfortable and high-speed operation of Windows.

5.3. Mailer software for sending fixed phrases

By using the text input system described in Section 5-1, users can input English text by eye gaze at approximately 16 characters per minute [9]. This input rate is not adequate to send an emergency message. To resolve this concern, we developed mailer software for sending fixed phrases by eye gaze. This software requires only a few steps for sending a message. In addition, combinations of the fixed phrases can be sent, and each phrase is customizable. Users can send a message to a pager or a smart phone outside the room. Therefore, users can communicate their requests (such as "I would like a drink of water") to their helpers. A screenshot of this mailer software is shown in Figure 10.

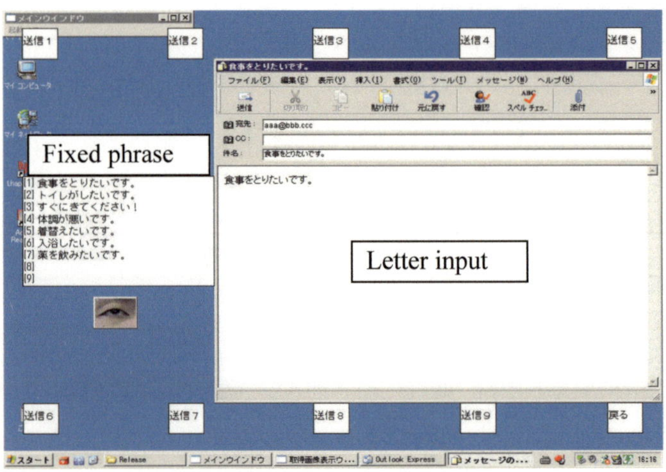

Figure 10. Mailer software for sending fixed messages

5.4. Web browser using eye gaze

With the popularization of the Internet, people now frequently browse Web pages to collect information. We paid great attention to this point; hence, we developed a Web browser for the eye-gaze input system. Generally, a Web page is related to others via hyperlinks. In addition, users often input text to a Web page when using a social networking service (SNS), online shopping, etc. When browsing these Web pages, the users make selections via hyperlinks, radio buttons, and text boxes that must be detected on the Web pages. Our system determines the locations of these selectable objects on a Web page. The system then stores the locations of these objects. Consequently, the mouse cursor jumps to the object of the candidate input. Therefore, our system enables Web browsing at a faster pace. An overview of the object selection method that uses information on the arrangement is shown in Figure 11.

http://dx.doi.org/10.5772/56560

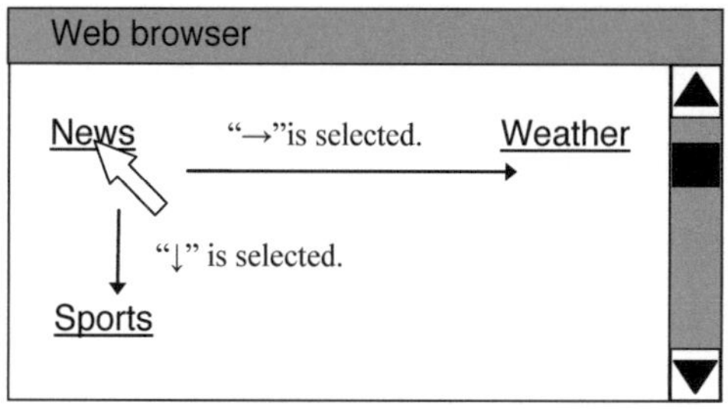

Figure 11. Object selection method using arrangement information

5.5. Television program viewing system

Studies have reported that the three principal functions of an environmental control system are for a television, reclining bed, and air conditioner. In other words, physically disabled people such as ALS patients would like to operate the functions of these devices. We focused our attention on a PC with a television tuner, and developed a television program viewing system for eye-gaze input. This system displays television programs on the PC screen along with the indicators for function control. The five indicators for the television program viewing system are displayed in the upper part of the screen as shown in Figure 12. The functions of a channel selector, volume control, and power switch are assigned to the five indicators. When users view television programs, the indicators are not required. Therefore, we set up two modes designated as viewer mode and control mode. In control mode, the five indicators are displayed on the screen. In viewer mode, the five indicators are not displayed, but an indicator for mode change is displayed. If the user gazes at the indicator for mode change, the other five indicators appear instead.

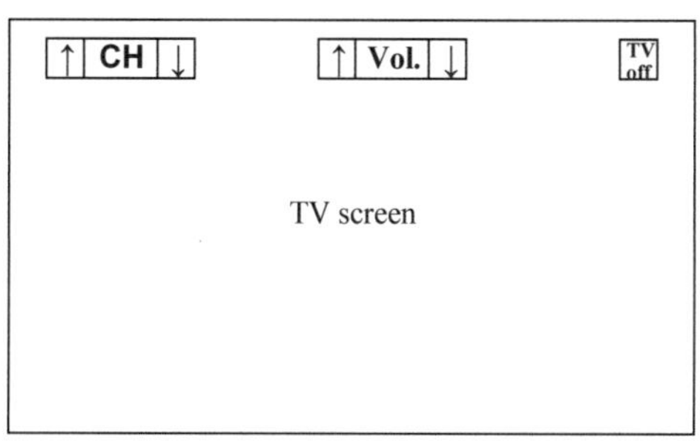

Figure 12. Television program viewing system

6. Next-generation eye-gaze input system

As described above, we have developed not only an eye-gaze input system for natural light but also an application system. When the application programs are used in combination, the quality of life (QoL) of ALS patients is improved. However, in order to provide additional improvements in QoL, a more versatile environment for eye-gaze input is required. For example, some users would like to explore the newer Web services, such as Facebook and Twitter. It is difficult to develop new software for these users individually. To resolve this problem, we need to improve our interface for mouse operation by eye gaze (presented in Section 4-3).

As shown in Section 4-2, if a user gazes at the indicator for a desired input, that input is easily decided upon, because the application program can recognize the indicator viewed. The interface for mouse operation can move the cursor to the gaze point of the user; however, it is difficult for this type of interface to recognize the icon viewed. To resolve this problem fundamentally, we are developing an interface that utilizes information on eye gaze and eye blinks. Many such interfaces have been proposed, but no truly practical system has been developed. When using this type of interface, unconscious eye blinks occur. In other words, the input errors are often attributable to unconscious blinks. This phenomenon is known as the "Midas touch problem."

We think that if involuntary (unconscious) blinks can be recognized, the input errors can be significantly decreased. In fact, we are presently developing an eye-gaze input system that can recognize voluntary blinks. Most conventional methods for measuring eye blinks analyze images of the eye (and its surrounding skin) captured by a video camera. Commonly used NTSC video cameras are capable of detecting eye blinks. However, it is difficult for these cameras to measure the detailed temporal changes that occur during the process of eye blinking, because an eye blink occurs relatively fast (within a few hundred milliseconds). The eye-gaze input system also uses an NTSC camera and therefore it is necessary to take account of this problem.

NTSC video cameras capture moving images at 60 fields/s, and these field images are mixed to produce field-interlaced images at a rate of 30 frames/s (fps). We have proposed a new method for using NTSC video cameras to measure eye blinks [13]. This method utilizes the non-interlaced eye images captured by an NTSC video camera. These images are odd- and even-field images in the NTSC format and are generated by splitting NTSC frames (interlaced images). The proposed method has a time resolution that is twice that of the NTSC format. Therefore, the detailed temporal changes that occur during the process of eye blinking can be measured. By using this new method for eye blink detection, we can develop a next-generation eye-gaze input system that is more user-friendly.

7. Conclusions

We have developed a new eye-gaze input system for people with severe physical disabilities. This system detects the horizontal and vertical eye-gaze components of users under natural light such as that from an incandescent, fluorescent, or LED lamp. By using this system, users can input text or commands to a PC. We have also developed application programs for the eye-gaze input system, including a text input system, PC operation support system, fixed-

http://dx.doi.org/10.5772/56560

phrase mailer, Web browser, and television program viewing system. When these programs are used in combination, the QoL of ALS patients is improved.

Our eye-gaze input system can obtain the coordinates of the user's gaze point. Accordingly, when a user gazes at a point on the PC screen, the mouse cursor moves to that point. By using this input interface, users can operate the general application software of Windows. In addition, our system is expected to contribute to the development of a next-generation eye-gaze input system. This new eye-gaze input system will be developed using our new method for eye-gaze and eye-blink detection. We believe that our new eye-gaze input system can ameliorate the QoL of ALS patients.

Author details

Abe Kiyohiko[1], Ohi Shoichi[2] and Ohyama Minoru[2]

*Address all correspondence to: abe@kanto-gakuin.ac.jp

1 College of Engineering, Kanto Gakuin University, Kanazawa-ku, Yokohama-shi, Kanagawa, Japan

2 School of Information Environment, Tokyo Denki University, Inzai-shi, Chiba, Japan

References

[1] Huchinson T.E., White K.P., Martin W.N. Jr., Reichert K.C., Frey, L.A. Human-computer Interaction using Eye-gaze Input. IEEE Transactions on Systems, Man, and Cybernetics, 1989;19(7) 1527-1534.

[2] Ward D.J., MacKay D.J.C. Fast Hands-free Writing by Gaze Direction. Nature, 2002 418; 838.

[3] Hansen J.P., Torning K., Johansen A.S., Itoh K., Aoki H. Gaze Typing Compared with Input by Head and Hand. Proceedings of Eye Tracking Research and Applications Symposium on Eye Tracking Research and Applications, 2004, 131-138

[4] Corno F., Farinetti L., Signorile I. A Cost-effective Solution for Eye-gaze Assistive Technology. Proceedings of IEEE International Conference on Multimedia and Expo, 2002;2.433-436.

[5] Kim K.N., Ramakrishna R.S. Vision-based Eye-gaze Tracking for Human Computer Interface. Proceedings of IEEE International Conference on Systems, Man and Cybernetics, 1999;2, 324-329.

[6] Wang J.G., Sung E. Study on Eye Gaze Estimation. IEEE Transactions on Systems, Man and Cybernetics, 2002;32(3) 332-350.

[7] Gips J., DiMattia P., Curran F.X., Olivieri P. Using EagleEyes - an Electrodes Based Device for Controlling the Computer with Your Eyes - to Help People with Special Needs. Proceedings of 5th International Conf. on Computers Helping People with Special Needs, 1996, 77-83

[8] Abe K., Ohi S., Ohyama M. An Eye-gaze Input System based on the Limbus Tracking Method by Image Analysis for Seriously Physically Handicapped People. Adjunct Proceedings of 7th ERCIM Workshop "User Interfaces for All," 2002, 185-186

[9] Abe K., Ohi S., Ohyama M. An Eye-Gaze Input System Using Information on Eye Movement History. Proceedings of 12th International Conference on Human-Computer Interaction, 2007;6, 721-729.

[10] Abe K., Ohi S., Ohyama M. Eye-gaze Detection by Image Analysis Under Natural Light. Proceedings of 14th International Conference on Human-Computer Interaction, 2011;2,19-26.

[11] Simpson RC, Koester HH. Adaptive one-switch row-column scanning. IEEE Transactions on Rehabilitation Engineering 1999;7(4) 464-73.

[12] Stark L., Vossius G., Young L.R. Predictive Control of Eye Tracking Movements. IRE Transactions on Human Factors in Electronics, 1962; 3, 52-57.

[13] Abe K., Ohi S., Ohyama M. Automatic Method for Measuring Eye Blinks Using Split-Interlaced Images. Proceedings of 13th International Conference on Human-Computer Interaction, 2009;1, 3-11.